Chemotherapy of gliomas

Chemotherapy of gliomas

Basic research, experiences and results

Edited by
D. Voth and P. Krauseneck

In collaboration with
C. Langmaid and P. Glees

Walter de Gruyter
Berlin · New York 1985

Prof. Dr. med. Dieter Voth
Klinikum der Johannes-Gutenberg-Universität
Neurochirurgische Klinik und Poliklinik
Langenbeckstr. 1
D-6500 Mainz

Prof. Dr. med. Peter Krauseneck
Neurologische Universität Würzburg
Maillingerstr. 13
D-8700 Würzburg

This book contains 163 illustrations and 92 tables

CIP-Kurztitelaufnahme der Deutschen Bibliothek

Chemotherapy of gliomas : basic research, experiences and results / ed. by D. Voth and P. Krauseneck. In collab. with C. Langmaid and P. Glees. – Berlin ; New York: de Gruyter, 1984.
ISBN 3-11-009990-X
NE: Voth, Dieter [Hrsg.]

Library of Congress Cataloging in Publication Data

Main entry under title:

Chemotherapy of gliomas.

Papers presented at the 4th Mainzer Herbsttagung, held Oct. 13–15, 1983.
Includes bibliographies and indexes.
1. Gliomas -- Chemotherapy -- Congresses. 2. Gliomas -- Treatment -- Congresses. I. Voth, D. (Dieter), 1935- II. Krauseneck, P. (Peter) III. Mainzer Herbsttagung (4th : 1983 Oct. 13–15) [DNLM: 1. Brain Neoplasms -- congresses. 2. Glioma -- congresses. WL 358 C517 1983]
RC280.B7C43 1984 616.99'481 84-22980

ISBN 3-11-009990-X

 Typesetting and Printing: Buch- und Offsetdruckerei Wagner GmbH, Nördlingen. – Binding: Lüderitz & Bauer, Buchgewerbe GmbH, Berlin. – Cover design: Rudolf Hübler. – Printed in Germany.

Dedicated in cordialityto
Prof. Dr. Dr. h. c. K. Schürmann
on the occasion of his 65th birthday.

Dieter Voth (editor),

the co-workers of the
Fourth Mainz Autumnal Congress

K. Dei-Anang,
M. Henn,
N. Hüwel,
W. Kahl,
G. Keßel,
E. Mahlmann,
M. Schwarz

and all the staff of the
Neurosurgical Department Mainz

Foreword

Chemotherapy has now become a standard treatment in the management of a whole range of tumours, with relatively well-recognised prospects of success, so that in many diseases there has been a striking improvement in the prognosis, particularly in paediatric oncology.

Unfortunately for a long time our results in the treatment of intrinsic brain tumours have been completely otherwise. If at least in the case of medulloblastomas the efficacy of chemotherapy can be proved, the results with the supratentorial gliomas are strikingly different and inconsistent. Such contradictory findings as regards our results give rise to justifiable doubts regarding chemotherapy for astrocytomas and also, unfortunately for glioblastomas.

In the interdisciplinary setting of the Fourth Mainz Autumnal Congress 1983 the participants endeavoured to define the problems of the gliomas by going back to pathological findings, against the background of basic research and in cooperation with modern clinical methods. They also sought to review the theoretical basis of chemotherapy and to examine and to interpret the fundamental principles and results which have so far been acquired.

In addition, after the deliberations of this meeting we hoped for a pronouncement as to which method of chemotherapy might promise the best results, if our current concept is capable of development or if we going up a blind alley. Finally with our treatment we must access what relationship the side-effects bear to the possible, or even the hoped-for effects, an if we – and this is indeed the most important maxim of all medical treatment – are doing good to our patients or harming them.

Mainz–Würzburg 1984 D. Voth and P. Krauseneck

Contents

I Special and comparative pathology of the gliomas – experimental findings

II General and specialised diagnosic methods for intrinsic brain tumours

III Principles of operative treatment and radiation therapy

I Special and comparative pathology of the gliomas – experimental findings

Classification of supratentorial gliomas

H. D. Mennel

Introduction

In the morphologist's language and thinking, the expression "supratentorial gliomas" stands in the very first line for the problems arising in intracranial and intraspinal newgrowth, due to the limited space of these cavities. For the neurosurgeon, this "group" rather represents a technical problem. The neuropathologist, however, would not consider this group as an entity in the strict sense. With these few remarks, the question of classification of intracranial tumors is already posed. There are different approaches to the classification. This interaction of different approaches has deeply influenced neuro-oncology since its beginnings. We will briefly trace these developments in order to explain the remaining open questions.

Historical aspects

The morphological investigation of the nervous system was an offspring of clinical neurology and psychiatry, as documented in the schools of the Salpetrière in Paris or of the Deutsche Forschungsanstalt für Psychiatrie, Munich, just to mention two outstanding historical places. In contrast, strong and lasting influences for neuro-oncology came from developing neurosurgery: It was the collaboration of Harvey Cushing and Percival Bailey, which led to the evolution of todays classification and grading. Bailey's tumours of the glioma group (1926) contained several groups, which were continously reduced in later editions, since some of them were ill-defined [1–5].

Attempts to correlate survival time with morphology especially reflected the needs of neurosurgery in tumour classification. Wilder Penfield [17] and H. Bergstrand [7, 8] have critically followed the evolution of the Bailey and Cushing classification; it somehow gained its final form in Zülch's classification proposed in 1956 [24], based on one of the largest tumour collections. This classification comprised some 25 entities.

Yet, the work of Bailey and Cushing as well as the further development of their classification started from the cytogenetic concept, as documented in the nomenclature. Various other schemes have been proposed and used, e. g. by Del Rio Hortega [10], Roussy-Oberling [20] and Russell-Rubinstein [21], just to enumerate some comprehensive contributions of maior influence. All of these classification-schemes mentioned were more or less cytogenetic i. e. based on the comparison of tumour cytology with the constituent cells of the nervous system and their precursor.

Kernohan et al. [11] rigourously cut down the number of entities, but introduced a system of grading, which would give an indication as to the inherent malignancy of the tumour and some kind of prognosis. There is no room in this contribution to describe the whole controversial history of the concept of malignancy within the nervous system. Only it should once more be stated, that the rules of malignant behaviour of general pathology are less suited for nervous system tumours and that differing grading schemes have been proposed [19, 25].

Thus, some confusion from equivocal nomenclature and grades of malignancy which are not comparable aroused and demanded unification and simplification. This has been attempted several times, most recently through the work of the World Health Organization [23]. Yet, even this largely accepted compromise did not meet common acceptance. This fact is sometimes not understood by the clinical worker, who thinks, that the remaining controversies are purely academic. To explain these controversies, one has to be aware, that there are different lines of thinking, which underly controversial statements.

Concepts

Three main influences may be distinguished:

1. The cytogenetic concept: This approach, which serves as background for the morphological analysis of tumours in general pathology [14], was introduced in the study of brain tumours by Pick and Bielschowsky [18]. There is no doubt, that the comparison of tumours with constituent cells of the nervous system and their precursors is important in defining entities and their neoplastic behaviour. On the other hand, the cytogenetic concept led to some misinterpretations. It favoured the Cohnheim-Ribbert dysontogenetic hypothesis for the aetiology of intracranial tumours, it wrongly paralleled malignancy with the stage of differentiation of the corresponding cell groups and led to very heterogeneous groups of tumours (fig. 1).

2. The pragmatic approach: In particular this last point, the heterogeneity of tumours, induced a "pragmatic" clearing of the system of tumours. It soon became clear, that some groups are frequent and important – especially the "supratentorial gliomas" – while others remained questionable and ill defined. The existence and significance of large groups was further corroborated by the fact, that many of them were biologically defined through age, sex and site predilection. In addition, most entities had defined malignancies: increasing collections showed, which diagnoses

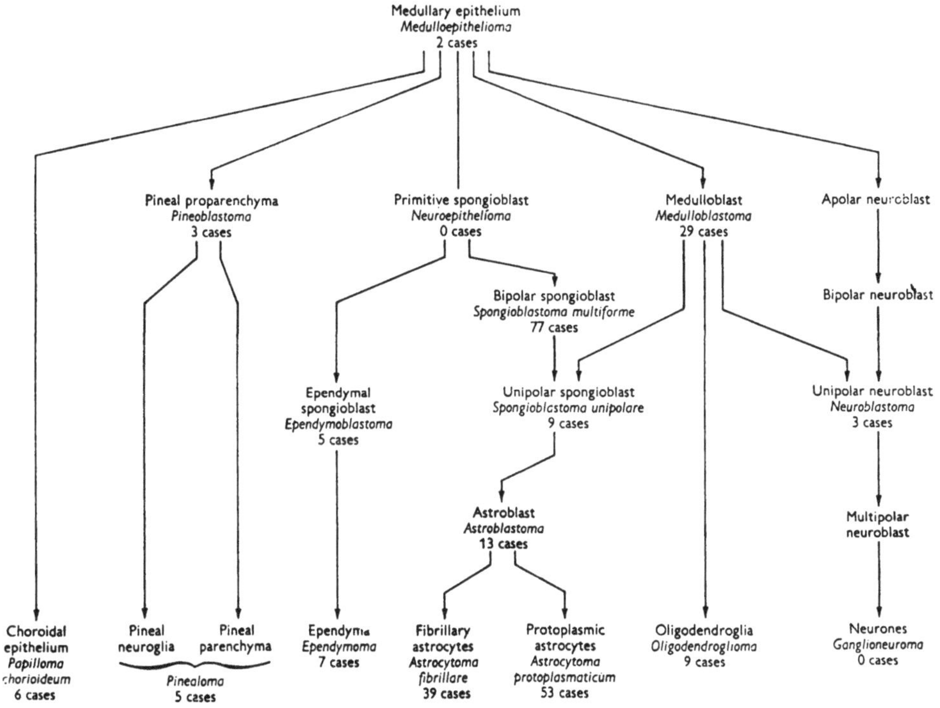

Fig. 1 Cytogenetic "tree" of nervous tumours, from by Bailey and Cushing "Tumors of the glioma group" [4]. The diagram shows clearly the unequal number falling into the different group. In the group neuroepithelioma, no cases have so far been found.

were important and how long patients could survive with them. This had been initiated by the work of Bailey and Cushing (tab. 1) and became the basis of Zülch's grading system (tab. 2).

This pragmatic approach preserved the essential and neglected the ill-defind, questionable and outstanding. It was one of the special merits of Zülch, to put this point in the centre of the neuropathologist's attentions. Zülch's group contained in Olivecrona's textbook comprised some twenty-five groups, all well defined and most with constant biological behaviour.

3. The surgical problem posed by intracranial tumours demanded further simplification and/or grading. This problem consists in the fact, that each growing lesion in the skull and spinal cord needs intervention; this holds especially true for the skull, where any growing space occupying lesion will have a fatal outcome, regardless of the inherent growth rate of the tumour. There are only few exceptions, e. g. slowly growing tumours in older patients. Intervention, especially surgical, in the nervous system however is dangerous for life and personality. The neurosurgeons interest therefore is to gain all possible information which may tell him the tumours prognosis.

Table 1 Average survival period of different histological tumour types

Type of tumour	Average survival period (mths)
Medulloepithelioma	8
Pineoblastoma	12
Spongioblastoma multiforme	12
Medulloblastoma	17
Pinealoma	18
Ependymoblastoma	19
Neuroblastoma	25
Astroblastoma	28
Ependymoma	32
Spongioblastoma unipolare	46
Oligodendroglioma	66
Astrocytoma protoplasmaticum	67
Astrocytoma fibrillare	86

Survival chart from Bailey and Cushing's book. This chart can with some minor alterations be considered equivalent to todays grading system.

Table 2 Classification of brain tumours and their different degrees of malignancy

Degree of malignancy	Prognosis after 'total' removal	Tumours extracerebral	intracerebral
Grade I *benign*	Cure or at least survival time of 5 and more years	Neurinomas Meningiomas Pituitary adenomas Craniopharyngiomas	Gangliocytomas (temporo-basal) Ependymomas, ventricular Plexus papillomas Spongioblastomas Pinealomas, isomorphous Angioblastomas (Lindau)
Grade II *semi-benign*	Postoperative survival time: 3–5 years	Pituarity adenomas, polymorphous	Gangliocytomas of other location Ependymomas, extraventricular Astrocytomas, isomorphous Oligodendrogliomas, isomorphous Pinealomas, anisomorphous
Grade III *semi-malignant*	Postoperative survival time: 2–3 years	Meningiomas, polymitotic, Neurinomas, polymitotic	Gangliocytomas, polymorphous Ependymomas, polymorphous Plexus papillomas, polymorphous Astrocytomas, polymorphous Oligodendrogliomas, polymorphous Pinealomas, polymorphous
Grade IV *malignant*	Postoperative survival time: 6–15 months	Sarcomas	Glioblastomas Medulloblastomas Primary sarcomas

Zülch's grading, which attributes to the tumour entities one or two, seldom three "grades of malignancy" which are considered to be well correlated with mean survival times after tumour removal.

This was the rationale of Kernohan's (tab. 3) and Ringertz (fig. 2) grading systems. Both of them however gained limited acceptance, since the simplification was going too far. Zülch and Wechsler [25] proposed an reasonable compromise (tab. 4).

These consideration should not be forgotten, when tumour diagnoses are made and prognoses are evaluated. Yet, their rigid application led to the different classification schemes, held by "schools", and to confusion of terminology, which urgently demanded common agreement; this was repeatedly attempted and regularly failed [22, 26]. The reason why lies in the fact, that these same lines of thinking (and working) naturally continue in other forms, corroborated by fieldings using modern methods of morphological investigation. There are many examples to underline this statement; we shall mention only few concerning the further development of morphological methods and neurosurgical techniques.

New development

The first few examples show, how cytogenetic concepts continously change with increasing knowledge in this field.

The first example concerns one of the most frequent intracranial tumours and its common variant: endotheliomatous meningioma. The nomenclature indicates, that

Table 3 Kernohan's grades; the number of diagnoses were cut down to five, each with four grades of malignancy. Old names were forced into the different grades, which again brought inconsistencies

New names	Old names (with new names in parentheses)
Astrocytoma grades I–IV	Astrocytoma (astrocytoma grade I)
	Astroblastoma (astrocytoma grade II)
	Spongioblastoma polare (left out)
	Glioblastoma multiforme (astrocytoma grades III and IV)
Ependymoma grades I–IV	Ependymoma (ependymoma grade I)
	Ependymoblastoma (ependymoma grades II–III)
	Neuroepithelioma (left out)
	Medulloepithelioma (ependymoma grade IV)
Oligodendroglioma grades I–IV	Oligodendroglioma (oligodendroglioma grade I)
	Oligodendroblastoma (oligodendroglioma grades II–IV)
Neuroastrocytoma	Neurocytoma
	Ganglioneuroma (neuroastrocytoma grade I)
	Gangliocytoma
	Ganglioglioma
	Neuroblastoma
	Spongioneuroblastoma (neuroastrocytoma grades II–IV)
	Glioneuroblastoma
Medulloblastoma	Medulloblastoma

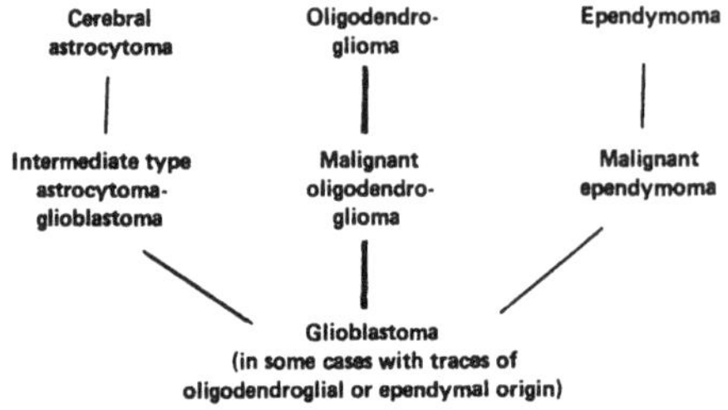

Fig. 2 Ringertz' three grade system can be considered as the appropriate grading for most (but not all) supratentorial gliomas.

these tumours originate from the meninges; the exact cytological derivation however is not entirely clear. The different subtypes of meningioma prompted the conclusion that the Pacchionian granulations might be the parent tissue.

Electron microscopic investigation however brought further elucidation of the relations of the tumour cells. In addition to the conspicuous onion bulb formations and psammoma bodies, which were known from light microscopical pictures, intense cell-to-cell contacts were found. The ultrastructural characteristics of these tumours are the numerous interdigitations of cellular processes giving the impression of interwaving foldings of cell membrane (fig. 3 a). Yet, cellular processes can remain unattached to each other within the tumours. Clefts between single tumour cells then arise (fig. 3 b, c). In the membranes, junctional complexes are regularly found. Such identical membrane foldings and intercellular clefts, as well as junctions, are found in the outermost layer of the arachnoid in several species [15]. Thus, both conventional and electron microscopy reveal the outstanding "enveloping" potentiality of these cells. Even the *in vitro* behaviour of meningioma cells illustrates the strong tendency to form concentric cellular sheets around a central structure, which in this case cannot be anything but another tumour cell (fig. 3 d). By these investigations, the outermost enveloping cells of the arachnoid could be identified as almost certain candidates for the cytological derivation of meningioma. There are no major difficulties in explaining other subgroups by similar findings of normal anatomy.

On the other hand, the second example concerns one of the rare and controversial tumours of nervous tissue, i. e. the neuroblastoma growing in the olfactory region and often extending into the frontal lobe, widely known as Berger's [6] ésthésio-neuroepithéliome olfactif. This tumour is difficult to diagnose by light microscopy, if characteristic formations, such as rosettes or demonstrable axons are absent. By electron microscopy the occurrence of dense core vesicles within the tumour cells and within the cellular processes, could be demonstrated (fig. 4 a). This linked these tumours with other neoplasms of the peripheral nervous system – the peripheral neuroblastomas and other tumours of the APUD system [16]. However it created new problems, since it seemed reasonable to assume that the olfactory mucosa, which does not belong to the APUD-system, is the tissue of origin of those tumours.

Table 4 The grades of Zülch and Wechsler [25] which avoid the forcing of established entities into rigid grades. This has been the precursor of the grade indication in the WHO classification

Tumours	Grade I benign	Grade II semi-benign	Grade III semi-malignant	Grade IV malignant
Gangliocytoma				
isomorphous	+	+		
polymorphous			+	
Ependymoma				
isomorphous	+	+		
polymorphous			+	
Plexus papilloma				
isomorphous	+			
polymorphous			+	
Astrocytoma				
isomorphous		+		
polymorphous			+	
Oligodendroglioma				
isomorphous		+		
polymorphous			+	
Glioblastoma				+
Spongioblastoma				
isomorphous	+			
polymorphous			+	
Medulloblastoma				+
Pinealoma				
isomorphous	+			
anisomorphous		+		
polymorphous			+	
Neurinoma				
amitotic	+			
polymitotic			+	
Meningioma				
amitotic				
oligomitotic	+			
polymitotic			+	
Angioblastoma				
(Lindau)	+			
Sarcoma				+
Pituitary adenoma				
isomorphous	+			
polymorphous		+		
Craniopharyngioma	+			

Other organelles however, found ultrastructurally in these neoplasms, were in good agreement with their true "neurosensorial" nature [9]. These include synaptic or synaptic-like formations (fig. 4 b) and bulbous expansions, considered to be axonal growth cones (fig. 4 c). Our own investigations have shown, that there is a wealth of

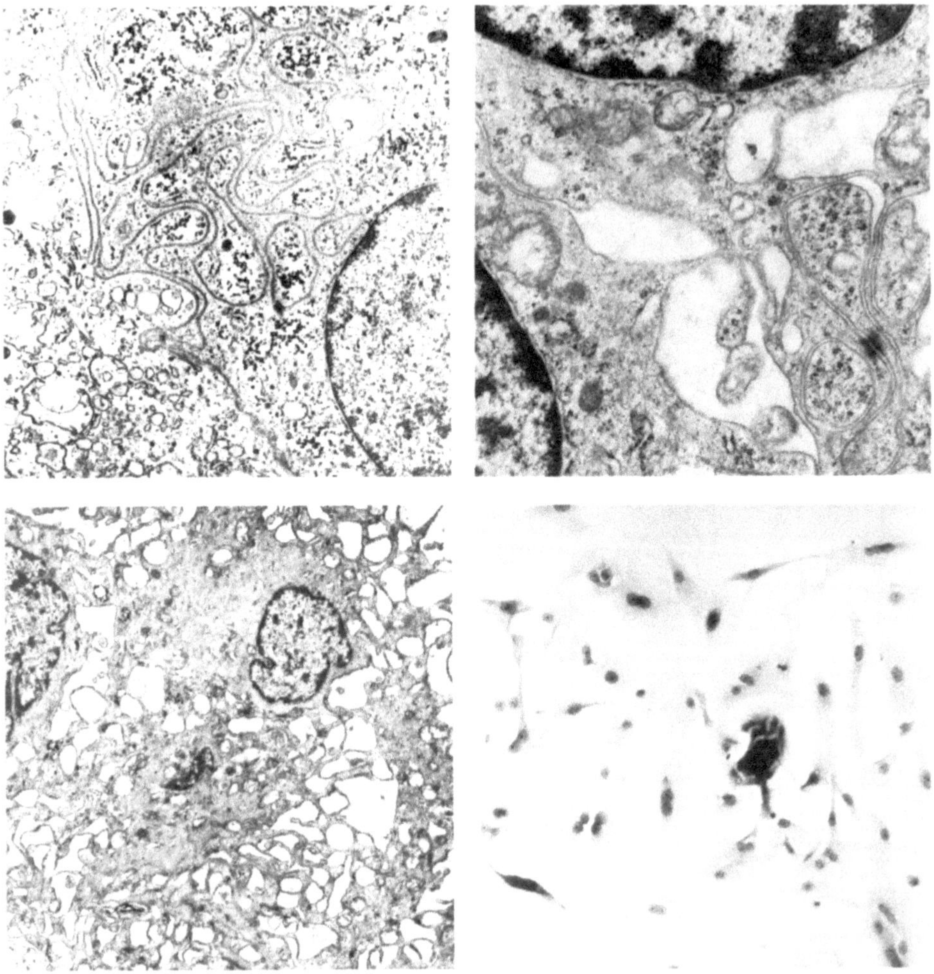

a) b) c) d)

Fig. 3 The meningioma has very typical features ultrastructurally:
a) Cell membranes with close contacts and membrane specifications form conspicuous interdigitations x 4900.
b) The adjacent membranes often form clefts. Note desmosome in right lower angle x 7500.
c) These clefts, if abundant, give a spongy picture x 1800.
d) Tissue culture picture of meningioma: Cells form envelopes around central whorls. H & E, x 360.

differently sized vesicles, albeit dense core or clear ones, which could well be interchangeable, since intermediate forms are found (fig. 4 d). Thus, olfactory neuroblastoma may well form some kind of link between central and neural-crest neuroblastoma. Our ultrastructural investigations of olfactory mucosa do not contradict this assumption.

The third example is taken from experimental neuro-oncology. Tumours induced in rodents are a very valuable model for neuro-oncological investigations in man, under

a) b)

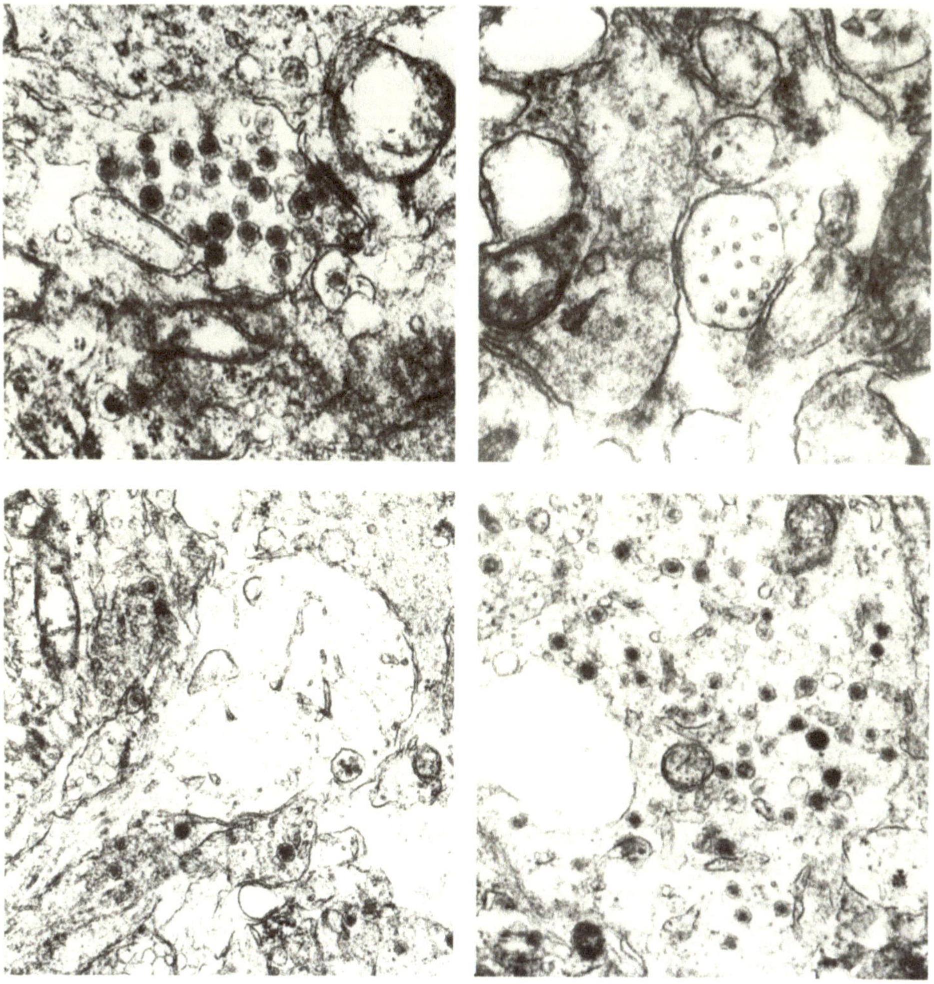

c) d)

Fig. 4 Olfactory neuroblastoma:
a) Synaptic like formation with dense core vesicles of about 1800 Å size (x 20.000).
b) Between the tumour cells, some kind of neuropil is formed; processes contain microtubules (x 18.000).
c) Bulbous expansions correspond to growing axons. Note again some microtubules (x 18.000).
d) Next to dense core vesicles, clear vesicles and intermediate forms are found (x 18.000).

the condition, that they morphologically represent those tumours, which constitute the problems of neurosurgery i. e. the supratentorial gliomas, astrocytomas, oligodendrogliomas, glioblastoma.

In experiments with resorptive carcinogens however, the diagnosis of gliomas, oligodendrogliomas, mixed gliomas and polymorphic gliomas as well as those of ependymomas were made. The latter diagnosis depended especially upon the observation of some repetitive patterns within those tumours (fig. 5 a). But the existence of this group of ependymoma or glioependymoma was not well substantiated. Different observations such as analysis of early stages of tumour growth, in vitro and transplantation experiments and others, were best interpreted, if one was dealing rather with gliomas than with ependymomas. Some have even expressed the view, that these tumours may be derived from oligodendroglial cells [12, 13]. There seems to be no doubt, that early stages of tumour growth may be supependymal (fig. 5 b) and are mostly oligodendrogliomas (fig. 5 c). The development of immunohistological methods, expecially the PAP-staining for glial fibrillary acid protein, has enabled us to analyse the cellular composition of very early stages of growth of these tumours. Our own findings are, that in the early stages of an growth they are in fact, either oligodendrogliomas or subventricular tumours containing cells derived from the interfascicular oligodendroglia and subependymal astrocytes (fig. 5 d). This shows, that experimental tumours, produced by resorptive carcinogens are presumably glial and, if histologically anaplastic, are certainly comporable with "supratentorial gliomas" in man.

This may suffice to make clear how new techniques and new developments may influence old questions. All the above-mentioned findings have led to new aspects concerning cytogenetic concepts and in this development, of course no end is in sight.

On the other hand, the need for unification, common agreement and a sound basis for understanding is also increasing. Let us mention solely the development of image processing methods which depict human brain tumours in a way familiar to neuropathologists. This forces the neuroradiologist to rely upon what the neuropathologist tells him and this should not be confusing. The second remark concerns the theme of the meeting for which this introduction is meant. Treatment of brain tumours has become much more sophisticated during recent years, but that does not mean that it has become much more effective, however for different lesions, there is an increasing pattern of possible intervention, amongst others chemotherapy or combined chemotherapy. This again demands a common and comparable concept of brain tumours in order to be able to compare the effectiveness of such schemes. In this context there is a last point, namely the stereotactic approach of otherwise inoperable deep seated brain tumours. This stereotactic approach is usually followed by interstitial irradiation and preceeded by sampling of very small pieces of tissue, which have to be analysed cytologically in the operation room by the neuropathologist. This method may come increasingly into use, yet diagnostic criteria are not commonly known and clearly established in neuro-oncology. There is no doubt, that the cytological diagnosing of smear preparations (fig. 6) has to be done according to the rules of established histological classification. These of course have to be standardised.

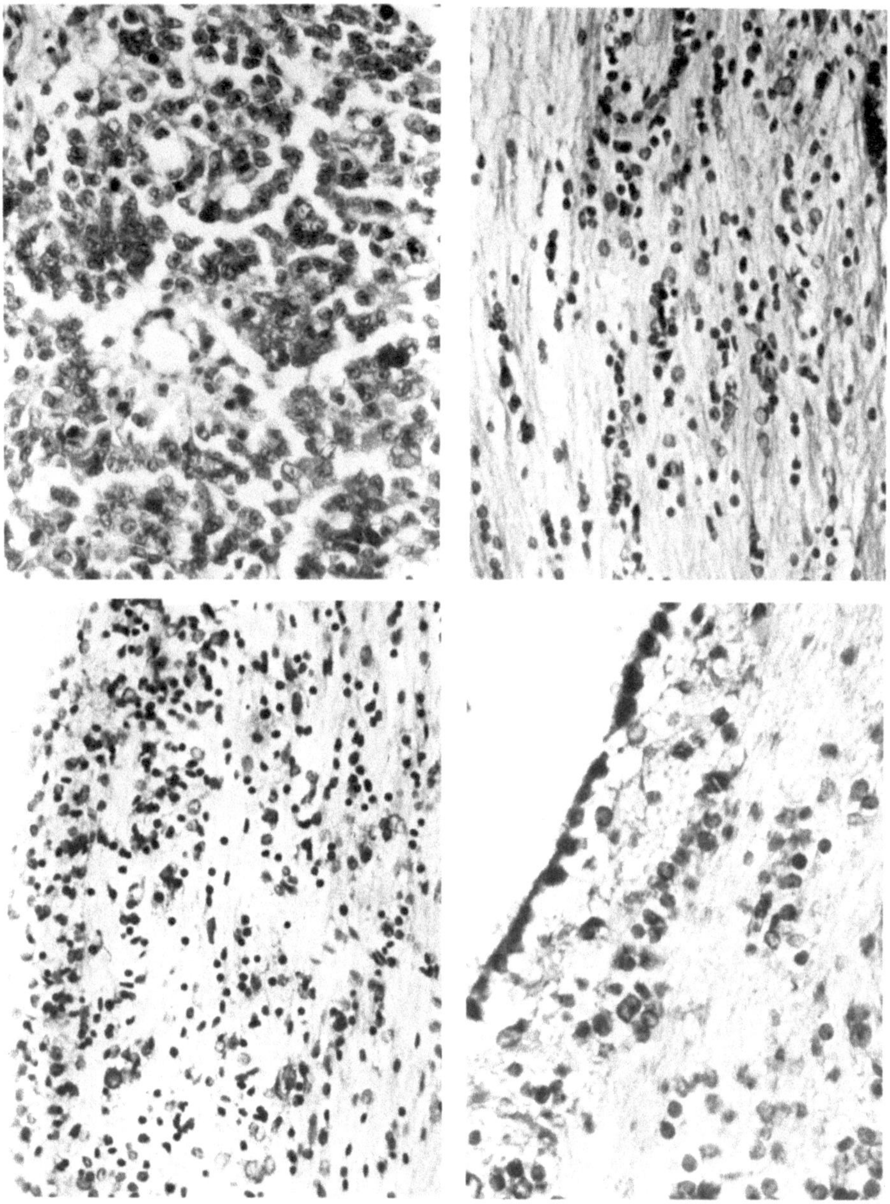

a) b) c) d)

Fig. 5 Cytogenetic derivation of experimental CNS-tumours produced by Ethylnitrosourea transplacentally:

a) Perivascular and repetitive pattern in transplanted cerebral tumour, considered to be evidence of ependymal derivation.
b) Small (micro) tumour made up by cells of the interfascicular glia within the white substance.
c) Subventricular growth of tumour showing two cell types with clearly distinguishable nuclear size.
d) Next to the ependyma, a loose net of GFAP containing astrocytes is followed by layers of oligodendroglial/astrocytic mixed population.
a) Cresylviolet (x 250); b–d) GFAP; b, c) (x 125); d) (x 250).

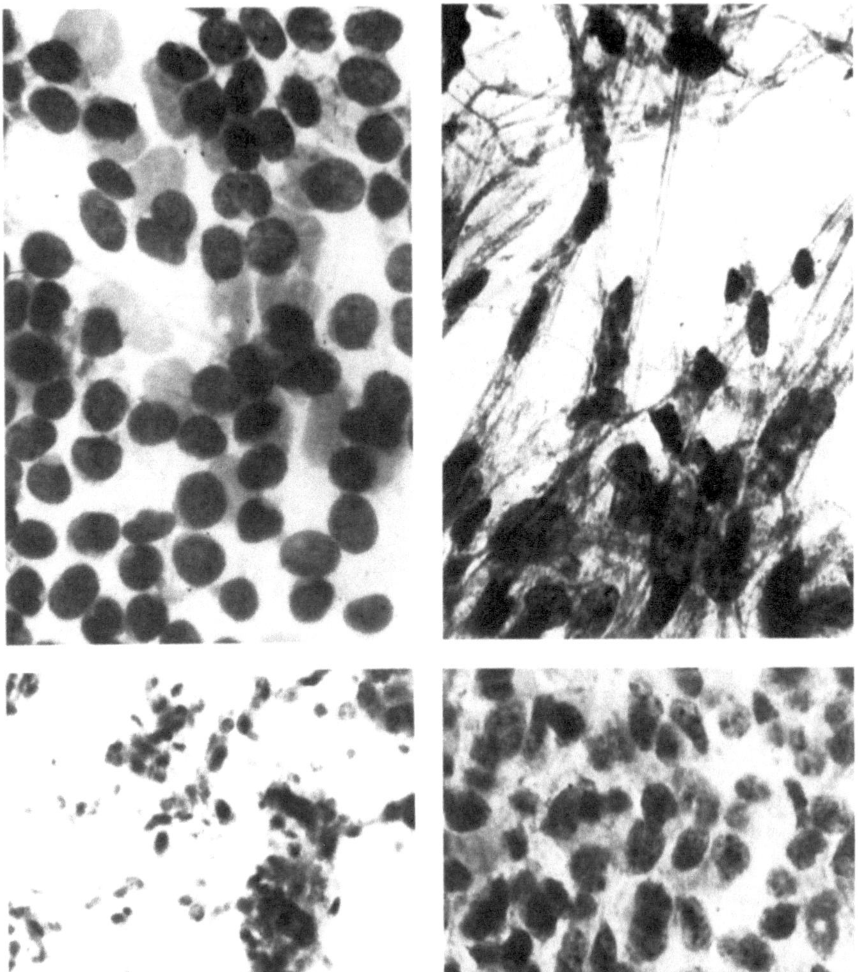

a) b)

c) d)

Fig. 6 Smear preparations of brain tumour biopsies:

a) Epithelial cells of pituitary adenoma; equal cell size, no mitoses, Cytoplasm often visible.

b) Fibrillary appearance of astrocytoma.

c) Whorl formation in meningioma.

d) Mitotic figures are diagnostic for malignant gliomas, such as anaplastic astrocytoma. (All methylene blue, x 600.)

Conclusions

These considerations lead to the conclusion, that first all approaches have their inherent rationale; none of them can easily be discarded. Second, within the single approaches, knowledge is accumulating and views are changing. No classification seems possible with continuously changing concepts. Third, any classification means preservation of the essential and disregard of the accidental and individual. Therefore, the best way for unification seems to consist in some kind of political compromise.

This has been achieved in the classification of the World Health Organisation. Different centres and different schools were grouped around a reference centre and debated about diagnoses during some years of work and in two plenary sessions. The resulting classification has no doubt some shortcomings and misunderstandings, but it has been well accepted, especially by neurosurgeons and neuroradiologists.

It is not the aim of this contribution to show and comment on all the rubrics of the WHO "Histological typing of Central Nervous System Tumours" [23]. A few remarks may be sufficient:

Most of the groups were given one or more grades, which correspond widely to the grading of Zülch. These grades are meant to give an indication of the presumable

Table 5 Classification and grades of human intracranial tumours

Tumour	Grade I benign	Grade II	Grade III	Grade IV malignant
Angioblastoma	++			
Craniopharyngioma	++			
Pituitary adenoma	++	+		
Meningioma	++		+	
Neurilemmoma	++		+	
Choroid plexus papilloma	++		+	
Gangliocytoma	++	+	+	
Pineocytoma	++	+		
Ependymoma	+	+	+	
Pilocytic astrocytoma	++		+	
Astrocytoma		++	+	
Oligodendroglioma		++	+	
Glioblastoma				++
Medulloblastoma				++
Germinoma				++
Sarcoma				++

Explanation: ++ usual and + exceptional grade of malignancy.
Concise scheme of diagnoses and grades showing the central role of supratentorial gliomas.

clinical evolution of the tumour bearer after operation. This grading therefore will be especially valuable for the clinician.

One of the shortcomings is the fact that glioblastomas were put together into one group with the medulloblastoma and not with tumours of glial origin. However, just the fact of the attribution of grades shows that glioblastoma may very well be considered to be in one common evolution with tumours of glial derivation. Thus even this unnecessary separation does not contradict the most probable common derivation of glial tumours.

For the frequent and important tumours, one could use an abbreviation of the rather differentiated classification of the WHO, which in addition puts the group of supratentorial gliomas together. This scheme (tab. 5) has the advantage, that all glial neoplasms forming some continuous evolution are grouped together. They comprise pilocytic astrocytoma, former polar spongioblastoma, benign astrocytoma and oligodendroglioma, less benign or more malignant intermediate forms and glioblastoma multiforme, as the malignant tumour of supratentorial site. In the same time, there is a continuous increase from the younger to the old. However, the first group of pilocytic astrocytoma does not belong entirely to the supratentorial group. Nevertheless, it plays a role in our context as the glioma of the thalamus or periventricular region.

We thus come back to the start. Supratentorial gliomas are not considered to be a clear cut entity from the neuropathologists view point, but stand for the whole group of tumours of glial origin which present problems of treatment and management for neurosurgeons.

References

[1] Bailey, P.: Histological atlas of gliomas. Arch. Path. **4** (1927) 871–921.

[2] Bailey, P.: Further notes on the cerebellar medulloblastomas. The effect of Roentgen radiation. Amer. J. Path. **6** (1930) 125–135.

[3] Bailey, P.: Intracranial tumours. Thomas, Springfield 1933.

[4] Bailey, P., H. Cushing: A classification of the tumors of the glioma group on a histogenetic basis with a correlated study of prognosis. J. E. Lippincott Comp., Philadelphia, London, Montreal 1926.

[5] Bailey, P., H. Cushing: Die Gewebsverschiedenheit der Gliome und ihre Bedeutung für die Prognose. G. Fischer, Jena 1930.

[6] Berger, L., H. Luc, H. Richard: L esthesioneuroepitheliome olfactif. Bull. Ass. Franc. Cancer. **13** (1924) 416–421.

[7] Bergstrand, H.: Über das Gliom in den Großhirnhemisphären. Virchows Arch. path. Anat. **287** (1933) 797–822.

[8] Bergstrand, H.: Weiteres über sogenannte Kleinhirnastrozytome. Virchows Arch. path. Anat. **299** (1937) 725–739.

[9] Hassoun, J., D. Gambarelli, F. Grisoli, et al.: Esthesioneuroepithelioma, a true neurosensorial tumor. Acta Neuropathol. (Berl.) **55** (1981) 77–80.

[10] Hortega, Del Rio, P.: Estructura y systematisacion de los gliomas y paragliomas. Arch. esp. Oncol. **2** (1932) 411–677.

[11] Kernohan, J. W., R. F. Mabon, H. J. Svien, et al.: A. simplified classification of the gliomas. Symp. on a new simplified concept of gliomas. Proc. Mayo Clin. **24** (1949) 71–75.
[12] Mandybur, T. I., M. M. Alvira: Ultrastructural findings in so-called ependymal rat tumors induced by transplacental administration of ethylnitrosourea (ENU). Acta Neuropathol. 57 (1982) 51–58.
[13] Mennel, H. D.: Transplantation of tumors of the nervous system induced by resorptive carcinogens. I. Histological investigation of intracerebrally transplanted tumors of the central nervous system. Neurosurg. Rev. **1** (1978) 123–131.
[14] Müller, J.: Über den feineren Bau und die Formen krankhafter Geschwülste. Berlin 1838.
[15] Nabeshima, S., T. S. Reese, D. Landis, et al.: Junctions of the meninges and Marginal Glia. J. Comp. Neurol. **164** (1975) 127–169.
[16] Pearse, A. G. E.: The APUD-cell concept and its implications in pathology. Path. Annu. **9** (1974) 27–41.
[17] Penfield, W.: Principles of the pathology of neurosurgery, chapt. VI, p. 303–347. Nelson + Sons, New York 1927 (Suppl. 1932).
[18] Pick, L., M. Bielschowsky: Über das System der Neurome und Beobachtungen an einem Ganglineurom des Gehirns nebst Untersuchung über die Genese der Nervenfasern in "Neurinomen". Z. ges. Neurol. Psychiat. **6** (1911) 391–437.
[19] Ringertz, N.: "Grading" of gliomas. Acta path. microbiol. scand. **27** (1950) 51–64.
[20] Roussy, G., Ch. Oberling: Atlas du cancer. Felix Alcan, Paris 1931.
[21] Russell, D. S., L. J. Rubinstein: Pathology of tumours of the nervous system. Edward Arnold (Publishers) Ltd., London 1959.
[22] UICC, (Uni Internationalis Conta Cancrum): Illustrierte Tumor-Nomenklatur. Springer-Verlag, Berlin – Heidelberg – New York 1965/1969.
[23] WHO: "Histological typing of the Central Nervous System Tumors" International histological classification of tumors. Geneva 1979.
[24] Zülch, K. J.: Biologie und Pathologie der Hirnsgeschwülste, Handbuch der Neurochirurgie, vol. III, Springer-Verlag, Berlin – Göttingen – Heidelberg 1956.
[25] Zülch, K. J., W. Wechsler: Pathology and classification of gliomas. Progr. in Neurol. Surg., vol. II, p. 1–84, S. Karger, Basel – New York 1968.
[26] Zülch, K. J., A. L. Woolf: Classification of brain tumors. Report of the Internat. Symposion at Cologne 1961. In: Acta neurochir. (Wien), Suppl. 10 (1964).

Remarks on classification and "grading" (Brief communication)

O. Stochdorph

The term glial tissue embraces a number of glial cells which are not always sharply divided from each other, but can exhibit transitional forms. Even in fully differentiated tissue not all the cells can be classified with certainty. Those cells of an ill defined cell type and undifferentiated are very frequent in tumour tissue, characterised by a mixed population next to fields of different grades of differentiation. A scheme of classification which does not consider the undifferentiated cell types and the mixed histology within the same tumour is too rigid and simulates reality. The classification of tumours accepted by the WHO has the disadvantage that the number of glial cell types listed has remained static since 1930 and has not incorporated the knowledge of later years, such as the tanycytes as a glial type. A subdivision of the classification of gliomas considers the growth pattern. Just in exceptional cases can this be compared to the invasive growth of cancer. A high degree of cytological differentiation is accompanied by a peculiar local spread, causing ill defined separation between areas of proliferation and their surroundings. The interior of the tumour exhibits the picture of hyperplasia and not the emergence of transformed cells. Glioblastoma is in itself not a tumour in its own sight, as the WHO wants one to believe, but an extreme case of diffusely growing glioma. – Marked anaplasia is always the sign of reduced differentiation and forcasts an unfavourable outcome. The degree of anaplasia can be expressed in stages, corresponding to a given type of tumour, but the use of the word 'grading' of the neuropathologist Zülch can be misleading.

Problems in the histological grading of human gliomas

F. Gullotta

The most important point in morphological classification of gliomas concerns today not so much their nomenclature but their *grading*. Recently the WHO has proposed a classification suggesting for *supratentorial gliomas* a three-stage grading which begins not with grade I but with grade II (only pilocytic astrocytoma of brain stem, cerebellum and spinal cord has been regarded as grade I). With this suggestion, the scale of malignancy has been displaced one position higher [6, 10]: the consequence of this will be that semimalignant tumours (earlier grade II) are now classified as grade-III and consequently placed on par with the true anaplastic gliomas. This will lead to misinterpretations of the results of treatment, because the postoperative survival time of patients with these grade III gliomas will be clearly longer than before – and this will be regarded as a success of (radio-/chemo-/immuno-) therapy.

According to the WHO classification, grade III gliomas are anaplastic, t. i. malignant, tumours. But this is the very point: how reliable are histological criteria in evaluating the biology of the tumour? It is generally known that mitoses, cell polymorphism, micronecroses, vascular proliferations etc. are typical signs of malignancy. Their qualitative identification is not difficult, even for the inexperienced pathologist. Greater problems however are encountered in the biological interpretation of these changes and in the consequent estimation of the tumour's growth rate. This evaluation is dependent not only upon the experience of the neuropathologist, but also on the part of the tumour biopsied and in particular on the size of the specimen. In every glioma cellular atypias can occur, that have little or nothing to do with malignancy. Their focal appearance only in one circumscribed tumour area is not necessarily representative for the whole tumour; furthermore, they can also be just an expression of degenerative changes. This is very common in human brain tumours which cannot be compared with experimental gliomas; in animals, experimentally produced gliomas will become progressively malignant and therefore the above mentioned morphological changes can be correctly evaluated as chronological criteria of malignancy. This is not always the case in the human. It is for instance a well known fact that malignant astrocytomas or oligodendrogliomas can display a postoperative survival time which clearly contrasts with their histological "malignancy".

Hence the question: what is a malignant glioma? Obviously a glioblastoma – but also an anaplastic astrocytoma or oligodendroglioma. However do anaplastic astrocytomas and oligodendrogliomas behave biologically like glioblastomas? Obviously not, or certainly not always, as we were able to demonstrate ten years ago through a follow-up examination of 1500 patients bearers of supratentorial astrocytomas, which had been classified into *4 biological grades* [4]. Eleven out of 320 grade III astrocytomas (3%) showed a postoperative survival time of more than three years. The same was observed in oligodendrogliomas [7]: eight out of 22 grade III oligodendrogliomas showed a longer postoperative survival time than expected.

These examples prove that there are malignant (anaplastic) gliomas which by themselves take a slower course than glioblastomas. Their common grouping together with glioblastomas (as it will happen with the WHO-grading) therefore seems questionable in regard to the evaluation of survival time. If the bearers of the anaplastic gliomas of our papers [4, 7] had been treated with chemotherapy, their unusual longer postoperative survival time would certainly have been credited as the result of the treatment.

An incorrect evaluation of the biological behaviour of a glioma is generally due to the overestimation of the morphological factors mentioned above – mitoses, capillary proliferations, necroses, cell polymorphism etc. Such incorrect evaluation is particularly frequent in oligodendrogliomas. In these tumours some foci suggestive of "anaplasia" are frequently seen (high cellularity, large nuclei, giant cells, endothelial buddings). Their exact biological value can however be assessed only upon consideration of the morphological changes present in neighbouring tissue areas. Very often they are regressive in origin or consist of local, small cell clones, just detected in a growing stage (oligodendrogliomas and pilocytic astrocytomas of brain stem usually grow in pousseés, with large rest pauses). It would be erroneous to generalize the biological meaning of these single foci to the whole tumour, classifying it as an "anaplastic" one. Every neurosurgeon has treated at least one patient with an "anaplastic" oligodendroglioma, who in spite of this malignancy has survived longer than expected, irrespective of the postoperative therapy given.

The presence of giant cells can in particular lead us astray. Giant cells are not rare in oligodendrogliomas; these gliomas are hence labelled "polymorphic" and considered high malignant. The survival time of these patients is however usually longer than that of patients with glioblastomas. Giant cells are often degenerative in origin, expecially if the tumour as a whole does not show any further signs of rapid growth, or when they are coupled with lymphocytic infiltration. In 1980 we called attention to some gliomas with plenty of giant cells [3], the benign course of which was in contrast to their "malignant" histology. Such tumours may be easily mistaken for giant-cell glioblastomas or sarcomas, especially if insufficient material is examined. Cell polymorphism and giant cells are finally usually seen in gliomas invading the leptomeninges. They are therefore mistakenly thought to be highly malignant, whereas they are usually slow-growing tumours with regressive changes. Typical examples of this are frequently seen in pilocytic astrocytomas of the optic nerves or of the cerebellum.

Wrong diagnoses can also occur in cell *isomorphic* tumours and this is often the case in ependymal tumours which are mistaken for small-cell sarcomas or, in the cerebellum, for medulloblastomas. Such a mistake occurs very frequently with subependymomas.

As extensively discussed elsewhere [2], many glioblastomas and "anaplastic" gliomas with an unusual long survival time are indeed tumours whose histology had been misinterpreted on the basis of degenerative cell changes. Furthermore, scepticism is justified in evaluating glioblastomas occurring in patients under 40 years of age or in "anaplastic" gliomas and glioblastomas of the cerebellum and brain stem [1].

The prognostic value of any histological grading is fundamentally impaired due to the fact that such categorization can only be correctly applied in the one and the same tumour group. The biological behaviour of a grade II (or III) astrocytoma does not correspond necessarily to that of a grade II (or III) oligodendroglioma. The prognosis of a brain tumour is dependent not only on its histological structure, but also on its location. A somewhat reliable grading can therefore be performed by summing up the data available on the histological appearance and the location/extension of the tumour; and it has a true prognostic significance only in supratentorial gliomas. In fact, despite lower histological malignancy, deep-seated growths such as midline gliomas carry an unfavourable prognosis because of their location. *Hence in evaluating the postoperative course, clinicians must analyse not grade II or III gliomas as a whole, but the single groups (astrocytomas; oligodendrogliomas; brain stem tumours; glioblastomas) and this also in relation to the age of the patient (under/over 40–50 years).*

My critical remarks will be answered with the objection, that there are selective methods nowadays which permit an exact identification of tumour cells, and therefore of tumour types. So for instance, the immunocytochemical demonstration of GFAP, a protein which is generally considered to be astrocyte-specific, whereas, as recently demonstrated by us [5, 9] it is in reality *glia*-specific. But it would be wrong to rely only on the positivity or negativity of an immunocytochemical reaction to identify a glia cell and hence a glioma. Gliomatous cells are morphologically, biochemically and immunocytochemically different from normal glial cells. We cannot therefore expect GFAP to be exactly positive or negative in the same way as it is in normal, non-neoplastic cells. This reaction can furthermore give pseudo-positive (false) results, if GFAP from degenerated cells is phagocytosed by neoplastic non-glial elements [5, 9]. The interpretation of these findings, especially in small biopsies, has hence to be performed with extreme caution. We must avoid making *cytological* diagnoses, as will happen if we focus our attention only on the positivity or negativity of a single cell, disregarding the whole structure of the tumour. Employing these new "cyto-specific" methods there is the risk of repeating the mistakes of subjective interpretation obtained with silver impregnations. (It is very funny to see how many former critics of metal impregnations, especially in the USA, are now enthusiastically working with GFAP!)

In fact it must not be forgotten that in each glioma we are confronted with at least three cell populations: 1. the true neoplastic, 2. the reactive and 3. the degenerating cell population – and this usually consists of originally normal, neoplastic and reactive cells. We are dealing with closely interwoven elements, whose morphology deviates from the norm; they are "atypical" and their exact identification is very difficult and often purely subjective. We must therefore classify a glioma not on the basis of its cell population alone, but also according to its manner of growth, to its vascularisation and in regard to its location. These simple old criteria seem to be forgotten nowadays, but they are still valid, and there is absolutely no reason for discarding them.

A last point has to be stressed with small biopsies it is often very difficult to classify a glioma and even more difficult to do a grading. In these cases, every pathologist, having a three-stage classification available, will be inclined to "worsen" the diagnosis. In doubtful cases, to be on the safe side and according to the WHO grading, he will make a diagnosis of grade III glioma. This has already been emphasized by Schiffer [8].

Morphologists must remember that a misinterpretation of the grading will have consequences in the clinical evaluation of the follow-up – not for the single case, but for the tumour group to which the patient belongs, and therefore for the evaluation of therapy employed in this group. The results of treatment can only be correctly evaluated if histological diagnoses are right. Otherwise one is in danger of drawing incorrect conclusions, and even accepting results, which have hardly anything to do with the treatment given.

References

[1] Ferbert, A., F. Gulotta: Remarks on catamnesis of cerebellar astrocytomas. This book, p. 111.

[2] Gullotta, F.: Morphological and biological basis for the classification of brain tumours. With a comment on the WHO-classification 1979. In: Adv. a. Techn. Standards in Neurosurgery (ed. by H. Krayenbühl). *Vol. 8* (1981) 123–165.

[3] Gullotta, F., L. Casentini, J. Neumann: Giant cell gliomas of temporal lobe. Acta neurochir. (Wien) 54 (1980) 25–31.

[4] Gullotta, F., G. Kersting, R. Wüllenweber: Recurrences of gliomas. A comparative clinical and morphological study with a note on the histological grading of astrocytomas. Modern Aspects of

Neurosurgery, *Vol. 3*. Excerpta Medica Amsterdam, Intern. Congr. Ser. Nr. 287, (1973) 116–121.

[5] Gullotta, F., E. Schindler, R. Schmutzler, et al.: GFAP in brain tumour diagnosis. Possibilities and limitations. Paper presented at the IXth European Congress of Pathology, Hamburg 1983. Abstract in: Path. Res. Pract., 178 (1983) 129.

[6] Gullotta, F., R. Wüllenweber: Das Grading der Gliome unter Berücksichtigung der WHO-Klassifikation. In: Klinische Neurochirurgie (ed. by H. Dietz, R. Wüllenweber). Vol. 2. In press. Thieme, Stuttgart.

[7] Neumann, J., I. Kimpel, F. Gulotta: Das Oligodendrogliom. Klinischer Verlauf in Bezug zum histologischen Grading. Neurochirurgia 21 (1978) 35–42.

[8] Schiffer, D.: Problems of brain tumour classification. In: Multidisciplinary aspects of brain tumor therapy (Paoletti, Walker, Butti, Knerich, eds.), pp. 47–54. Elsevier/North Holland Biomedical Press, Amsterdam – New York – Oxford.

[9] Schindler, E., F. Gullotta: Glial Fibrillary Acidic Protein in medulloblastomas and other embryonic tumours of children. Virchows Archiv (Path. Anat.) 398 (1983) 263–275.

[10] Stochdorph O.: Klassifikation der Hirngeschwülste. In: Computertomographie intrakranieller Tumoren (Kazner, Wende, Grumme, Lanksch, Stochdorph, eds.), pp. 1–16. Springer, Berlin 1981.

Comparative aspects of spontaneous gliomas in animals
(Brief communications)

M. Vandevelde, R. Fankhauser, H. Luginbühl

Spontaneous tumours of the nervous system have been reported in a number of species and of all classes but detailed studies are available only in domestic animals. Brain tumours in dogs have been rarely reported, apart from brachycephalic races. In these dogs, a relatively high incidence of brain tumours occurs of neuro-ectodermal and mesenchymal origin.

Morphologically the various gliomas in the dog are comparable to those occuring in man. However, gliomas of dogs show little differentiation microscopically and immuno-cytochemically. It is therefore difficult to relate them to the classifications of human tumours. In animals, only objective and usually pre-terminal data (e. g. epileptiform fits) are known, while growth rates are unknown. Similarly a therapy is missing and data on tumour re-growth or therapeutic management are not available.

The clinical diagnosis of brain tumours in dogs is based on the clinical history and on localizing symptoms. Apart from examining the CSF, angiography, EEG, CT are only occasionally applied and for these reasons no objective data available.

Cell-mediated immune response during progressive glioma growth*

Th. Bilzer, D. Stavrou

The relationships between the brain, the developing glioma and the immune system are still poorly understood. In the normal brain, the absence of a conventional lymphatic drainage and the presence of tight-junctioned endothelia of most brain capillaries largely separate the parenchyma from the peripheral blood and the immune system. An effective barrier prevents the entry of antibodies and effector cells into, and the shedding of antigens from the brain, mediating an extraordinary immunologic status. This barrier seems to get lost during malignant glioma growth [2, 6, 24].

Malignant glioma growth is accompanied by abnormal angioplasia and destruction of blood vessels in the brain tissue involved. Dysfunction or disruption of the intercellular junctions between the endothelial cells of tumour-associated capillaries may thus alter the relationship between the brain and the immune system. Evidence suggests, that in glioma bearers macromolecular material passes through the insufficient blood-brain barrier to induce humoral and cell-mediated immune reactions.

Lymphocytic infiltration in perivascular regions within and/or around malignant brain tumours has been characterized as a frequent event [19]. Moreover, other cellular components like macrophages [8, 9] and polymorphonuclear leucocytes [13] have been found to participate in the antiglioma response. The precise function of these cells still remains speculative.

Following the initial report of Ridley and Cavanagh [14] describing an overall 65% incidence of cellular infiltrations in autopsy material, other investigators have performed studies to specify these cells and to determine their incidence and significance [4, 11]. Stavrou et al. [17] have disclosed that the majority of lymphocytes within the perivascular cuffs in gliomas represent T cells, which generally are believed to play a central role in the host reaction. In some brain tumours cytotoxic cells are widely represented in the cellular matrix of the neoplasm [11].

* This work was financially supported by the C. Bohnewand Fund for Cancer Research of Munich University, Munich.

Palma et al. [11] and Brooks et al. [4] have shown, that individuals with significant infiltrations of round cells in the tumour survive longer than those lacking evidence of such response. Furthermore, a positive correlation has been observed between the magnitude of mononuclear infiltrates in histological sections of experimental gliomas and the immunologic response [22]. These reactions have been postulated to represent host response to glioma and to be a detectable counterpart of the lymphocytic infiltration observed in brain tumours [14].

Other investigators, however, have reported that even intra-cerebral responses in glioma bearers are likely to be inadequate [1]. Among others, peripheral lymphocytes from glioma patients were found to be equally reactive with cultured autologous tumour cells or adult and fetal glial cells, suggesting that the cell-mediated response against the glioma was neither specific nor effective [23]. In those studies, a major limiting factor for the investigation of specific cell-mediated responses has to be seen in the lack of identifiable glioma-associated antigens (GAAs). In more detailed studies, analysis of surface antigens of human [7, 12, 16] and experimental [3, 18, 19, 21] gliomas by use of polyclonal and monoclonal sera as well as lymphocytic effector cells indicated the presence of different GAAs, which in both, autologous and syngeneic system were capable of eliciting a significant but variably strong immune response.

Specificity of cellular reactions was affirmed by testing lymphocytes against a panel of different target cells, taken from early culture passages. Autogeneic and syngeneic glioma cells and brain cells of various differentiation as well as allogeneic tumour cells of types both, related and unrelated to the tumour were tested. Specificity was further confirmed by different absorption procedures on appropriate cells. Under such requirements, glioma-specific lymphocyte reactions could be observed in nearly 85% of a series of patients with glial tumours [7, 12] and regularly in all experimental neural tumours [20].

However, experimental and clinical investigations on neural tumours have shown that in the course of malignant glioma growth the host's immunocompetence becomes generally impaired, often inversely paralleling the extend of neoplastic disease [2, 6, 24]. A variety of immunological dysfunctions were manifested, such as (a) inability to respond to common recall skin-tests, (b) impaired *in vitro* cellular reactivity to mitogens, (c) reduced *in vitro* T cell reactivity, (d) presence of serum blocking factors and (e) functional lymphocyte abnormalities (for review see [5]).

Factors responsible for the deterioration of immune functions are in discussion [15]: (a) intrinsic defects which render the lymphocyte incapable of normal responsiveness, (b) shifts in lymphocytic subpopulations towards a population unable to maintain immunocompetence, and (c) generation of humoral and/or cellular suppressor mechanisms.

Taking into account all variables accompanying neoplastic growth immunologic reactions against brain tumours could best be studied and manipulated in syngeneic experimental animals. A promising approach to the elucidation of glioma-specific cellular responses has been made by artificially increasing the immunogenicity of glioma cells by coupling them with trinitrophenyl groups [25]. T cells from rats sensitized with trinitrophenylized cells were detected to be significantly more cytotoxic to glioma target cells than those from untreated rats or rats sensitized with modified fetal, newborn or adult brain cells [3]. Immunocompetence in individual

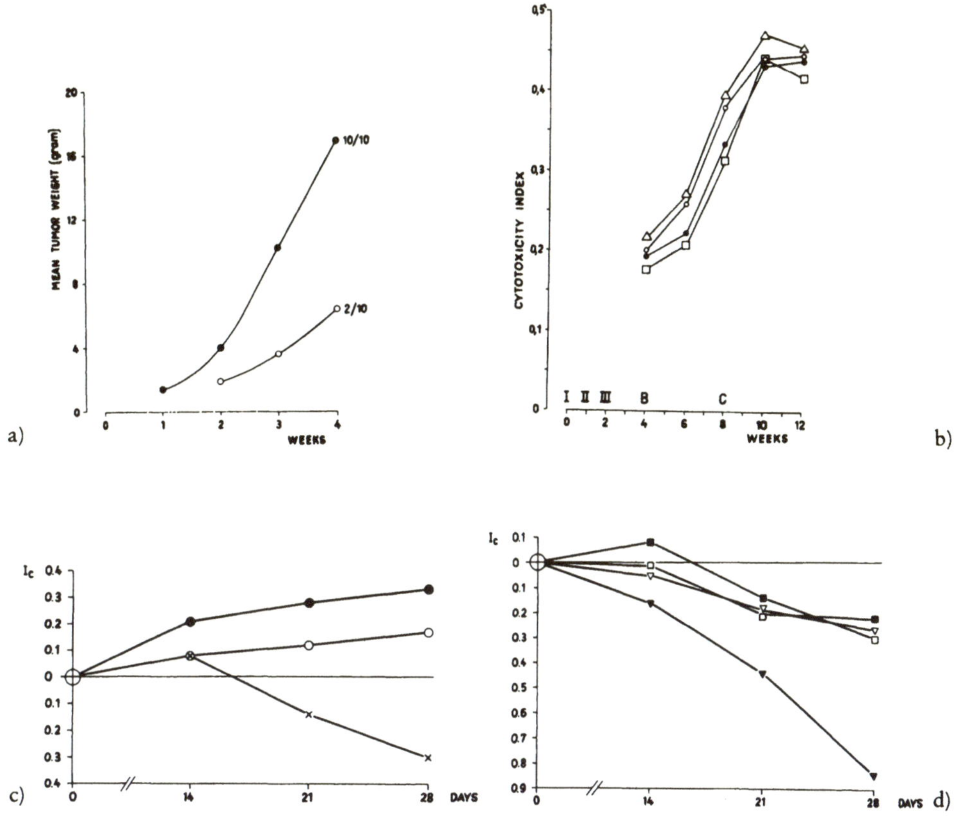

Fig. 1a–d Comparison of *in vivo* and *in vitro* data from glioma-bearing and glioma-immunized syngeneic rats. a) Glioma growth in normal rats (●———●) and in rats immunized with modified glioma cells (○———○) after challenge with native glioma cells. Tumour incidences are shown on the right. b) Cytotoxicity of T cells from glioma-immunized rats against different glioma cell lines. I, II, III: Immunization (10^6 glioma cells + trinitrobenzene sulfonic acid), B: Booster (10^6 glioma cells), C: Challenge (10^7 glioma cells). c) Cytotoxicity of T cells from rats with progressively growing gliomas (×———×) and tumour-free rats, immunized with modified (●———●) and native (○———○) glioma cells. I_c: Cytotoxicity Index. d) Cytotoxicity of peripheral blood (▽———▽), spleen (■———■), lymph node (□———□) and tumour-infiltrating (▼———▼) lymphocytes from glioma-bearing rats. I_c: Cytotoxicity Index.

animals under definite conditions has been sequentially evaluated *in vitro* by means of microcytotoxicity-assay, colony inhibition assay, conjugate formation test and differential counting of T cells. *In vitro* data were correlated to tumorigenicity and glioma growth patterns in immunized and non-immunized animals. After challenge with different syngeneic glioma lines immunized rats show distinctly lower tumour incidences and longer latency periods than controls (fig. 1 a). T cells from immunized rats cross-react with the different syngeneic glioma lines (fig. 1 b) but not with control target cells.

Progressively growing gliomas reactivity shows an overall decrease, moreover a complete loss of reactivity (fig. 1 c), and occasionally a switch-over to a stimulation of glioma target cell proliferation *in vitro*.

Another major observation is the reduced responsiveness of glioma-infiltrating lymphocytes in comparison with lymphocytes of other origin (fig. 1 d) [19]. Significant decline of reactive properties also occurs in immunized rats after tumour growth had taken place. This is not accompanied by a significant reduction of T cells in spleen and peripheral blood.

It has been suggested that the origin of immunologic impairment lies in a specific interaction between the immune system and the glioma [3]. Lymphocytes of different sites have been found either to inhibit or to enhance tumour cell proliferation, whereby the functional activities of the lymphocytes seem to depend on the stage of tumour progression [10]. It remains obscure, how these differences relate to immunosuppression and onset of neoplastic disease. In the course of progressive glioma growth several subtile cellular interactions may emerge, potentially protecting the tumour against immunologic defense.

References

[1] Albright, L., J. A. Seab, A. K. Ommaya: Intracerebral delayed hypersensitivity reactions in glioblastoma multiforme patients. Cancer **39** (1977) 1331–1336.

[2] Appuzzo, M. L. J., M. S. Mitchell: Immunological aspects of intrinsic glial tumors. J. Neurosurg. **55** (1981) 1–18.

[3] Bilzer, Th., D. Stavrou, E. Dahme, et al.: Cell-mediated immune response in rats immunized with chemically modified syngeneic glioma cells. Monitoring by in vivo parameters and in vitro immune cytolysis. Anticancer Res. **2** (1982) 345–354.

[4] Brooks, W. H., W. R. Markesbery, G. D. Gupta: Relationship of lymphocyte invasion and survival of brain tumor patients. Ann. Neurol. **4** (1978) 219–224.

[5] Cravioto, H.: Immunology of human brain tumors. In: The Hdb. of Cancer Immunology (H. Waters, ed.). Garland STPM Press, New York – London 1978.

[6] Darling, J. L., N. R. Hoyle, D. G. T. Thomas: Self and nonself in the brain. Immunol. Today **2** (1981) 176–180.

[7] Levy, N. L.: Specificity of lymphocyte-mediated cytotoxicity in patients with primary intracranial tumors. J. Immunol. **121** (1978) 903–315.

[8] Morantz, R. A., G. W. Wood, M. Foster, et al.: Macrophages in experimental and human brain

tumors. Part 1: Studies of the macrophage content of experimental rat brain tumors of varying immunogenicity. J. Neurosurg. **50** (1979) 298–304.

[9] Morantz, R. A., G. W. Wood, M. Foster, et al.: Macrophages in experimental and human brain tumors. Part 2: Studies of the macrophage content of human brain tumors. J. Neurosurg. **50** (1979) 305–311.

[10] Mule, J. J., J. W. Forstrom, E. George, et al.: Production of T-cell lines with inhibitory or stimulatory activity against syngeneic tumors in vivo: A preliminary report. Inter. J. Cancer **28** (1981) 611–614.

[11] Palma, L., N. Di Lorenzo, B. Guidetti: Lymphocytic infiltrates in primary glioblastomas and recidivous gliomas. Incidence, fate and relevance to prognosis in 228 operated cases. J. Neurosurg. **49** (1978) 854–861.

[12] Rainbird, S., G. Allwood, A. Ridley: Lymphocytemediated cytotoxicity against gliomas. Brain **104** (1981) 451–464.

[13] Ridley, A.: Antilymphocytic serum and tumor transplantation in the brain. Acta Neuropathol. (Berl.) **19** (1971) 307–317.

[14] Ridley, A., J. B. Cavanagh: Lymphocytic infiltration in gliomas: Evidence of possible host resistance. Brain **94** (1971) 117–124.

[15] Roszman, Th. L., W. H. Brooks, L. H. Elliott: Immunobiology of primary intracranial tumors: VI. Suppressor cell function and lectin-binding lymphocyte subpopulations in patients with cerebral tumors. Cancer **50** (1983) 1273–1279.

[16] Schnegg, J. F., A. C. Diserens, S. Carell, et al.: Human glioma-associated antigens detected by monoclonal antibodies. Cancer Res. **41** (1981) 1209–1213.

[17] Stavrou, D., A. P. Anzil, W. Weidenbach, et al.: Immunofluorescence study of lymphocytic infiltration in gliomas. Identification of T-lymphocytes. J. Neurol. Sci. **33** (1977) 275–282.

[18] Stavrou, D., M. Hulten, A. P. Anzil, et al.: The humoral antibody response of rats immunized with chemically modified syngeneic brain cells and glioma cells. Int. J. Cancer **26** (1980) 629–637.

[19] Stavrou, D., Th. Bilzer, A. P. Anzil, et al.: Reactivity of tumor-infiltrating, blood, spleen and lymph node lymphocytes against syngeneic glioma target cells. Anticancer Res. **1** (1981) 125–134.

[20] Stavrou, D., Th. Bilzer, M. Hulten, et al.: Immunological aspects of experimental brain tumors. Anticancer Res. **2** (1982) 151–156.

[21] Stavrou, D., Ch. Süss, Th. Bilzer, et al.: Monoclonal antibodies reactive with glioma cell lines derived from experimental brain tumors. Eur. J. Cancer Clin. Oncol. **19** (1983) 1439–1449.

[22] Tho, B. H., E. P. G. Guli: In vitro immunoreactivity against ethylnitrosourea-induced tumors of the nervous system in rat. Experientia **30** (1974) 1472–1473.

[23] Wahlström, T., E. Saksela, H. Troupp: Cell-bound antiglial immunity in patients with malignant tumor in the brain. Cell Immunol. **6** (1973) 161–170.

[24] Wikstrand, C. J., D. D. Bigner: Immunobiologic aspects of the brain and human gliomas. A review. Am. J. Pathol. **98** (1980) 517–567.

[25] Zänker, K. S., D. Stavrou, M. Hulten, et al.: The influence of various chemicals on the surface structure and the antigenicity of syngeneic glioma cells. Anticancer Res. **1** (1981) 101–107.

Application of immunohistological techniques to the diagnosis of gliomas

H. Goebel, M. Schlie, R. Moll

Introduction

Gliomas comprise astrocytomas of various types and anaplasia, oligodendrogliomas, ependymomas and glioblastomas. Neuronal tumours such as medulloblastomas, neuroblastomas and gangliocytomas represent another group of primary neuroectodermal neoplasms.

Immunohistological studies on these tumours have so far largely been confined to the demonstration of the glial fibrillary acidic protein (GFAP), while antigens of neuronal and oligodendroglial cells have chiefly been documented in normal, well differentiated cells during research. Thus, this presentation is more or less confined to a report on our diagnostic experience with GFAP.

GFAP is an acidic protein, considered to be the subunit protein of the 8–10 nm filaments type, specific for astrocytes. In other cell types, intermediate filaments are composed of other subunit proteins, namely, desmin in muscle fibres, vimentin in fibroblasts, prekeratin in epithelial cells and neurofilament proteins in neuronal cells.

Material and methods

Over the past four years, we have investigated intracranial and intraspinal neoplasms of various origin [5].

While immunofluorescent demonstration of GFAP is possible [1], the use of the peroxidase – antiperoxidase technique [16] to demonstrate GFAP has been developed as the routine method employed in formalin fixed and paraffin embedded tissue sections.

Results

GFAP-positive cells could be documented in several types of astrocytomas, such as fibrillary astrocytoma, gemistocytic astrocytoma, anaplastic astrocytoma, glioblastoma and gliosarcoma. In the latter neoplasm, the mesenchymal parts are in strong negative contrast to the positively reacting astrocytic areas (fig. 1). Neoplastic giant cells in glioblastomas may or may not be GFAP-positive. Non-GFAP giant cells in such malignant gliomas may be either too anaplastic, though of astrocytic origin, to have produced GFAP, or they are derived from a non-astrocytic lineage. GFAP is usually more strongly demonstrated in the cytoplasm than in neoplastic astrocytic processes.

If the astrocytoma has grown outside the CNS parenchyma, the diagnosis of such biopsied areas may be difficult without documentation of GFAP.

If glial tissue is displaced in a hamartomatous fashion, outside the CNS, for instance in a nasal glioma, or in meningomyeloceles, identification of such islands of astrocytes by the GFAP technique is important.

Uptake of extracellular GFAP by non-astrocytic (or also astrocytic?) cells has been discussed [2], but ought to be proven by adequate electron microscopic studies. Our own preliminary studies in tissue culture of astrocytes outgrown from fetal spinal cords suggest that astrocytes are capable of phagocytosis and that GFAP may be incorporated into macrophages.

As GFAP is present in gemistocytic astrocytes, it is impossible to distinguish between reactive astrocytes around a nonglial tumour, for instance lymphoma (figs. 2, 3) and neoplastic gemistocytes of a gemistocytic astrocytoma. Then, cytological and non-immunohistological criteria become essential for differentiation. The homogeneous central part of Rosenthal fibres of astrocytes, for instance in Alexander's disease [4], about a craniopharyngioma, the tumour cells of which are themselves GFAP-negative, or of a pilocytic astrocytoma, for instance of the cerebellum, is GFAP-negative, while the parent astrocytic process is GFAP-positive. In less differentiated astrocytomas such as astrocytoma, glioblastoma or diffuse gliomatosis, the non-reacting neoplastic cells are thought to be too undifferentiated to have produced detectable amounts of GFAP. The more sensitive method of immunohistological biotinylation, which allows higher dilution of the primary antiserum, may reveal numerically more anaplastic astrocytes producing GFAP than the number of neoplastic astrocytes demonstrated by the PAP technique.

Ependymomas may reveal GFAP-positive cells that send their processes towards vessels forming perivascular rosettes, while oligodendrogliomas lack GFAP-positive cells, unless they are mixed with neoplastic astrocytes as in a mixed oligo-astrocytoma.

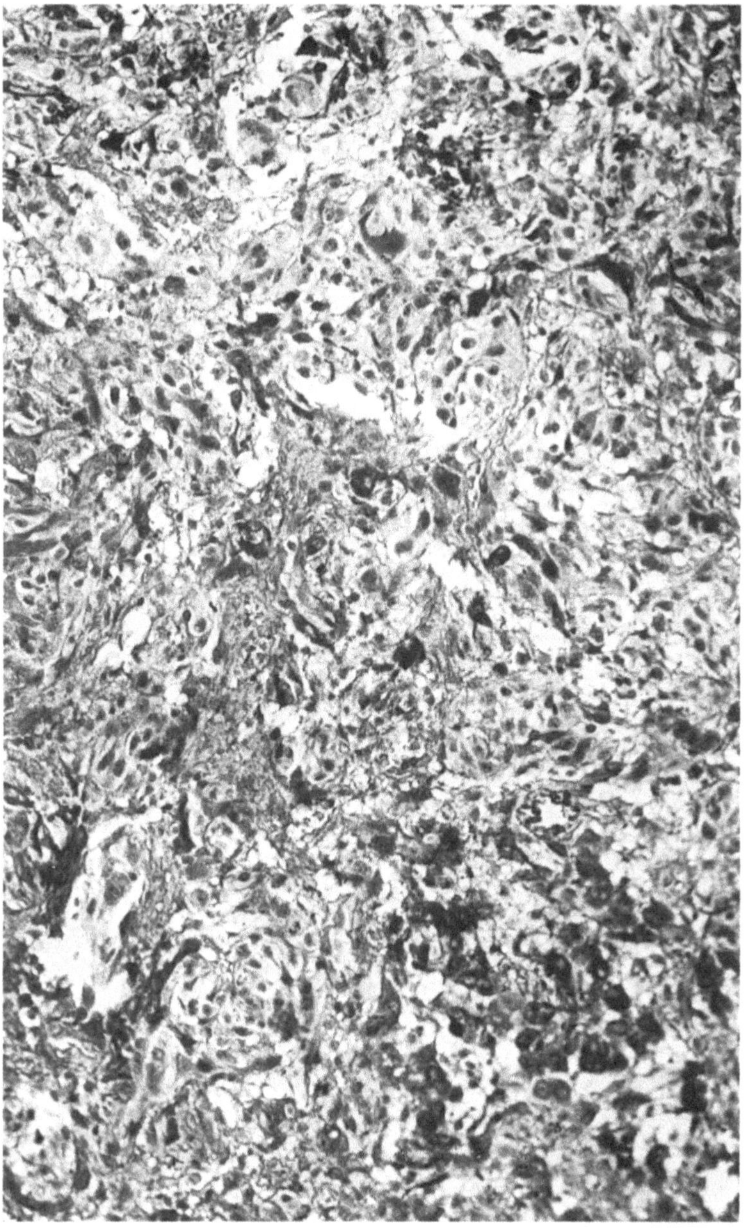

Fig. 1 There are scattered neoplastic GFAP-positive astrocytes (dark) among numerous non-reacting mesenchymal cells of proliferated vessels. Gliosarcoma, (x 260).

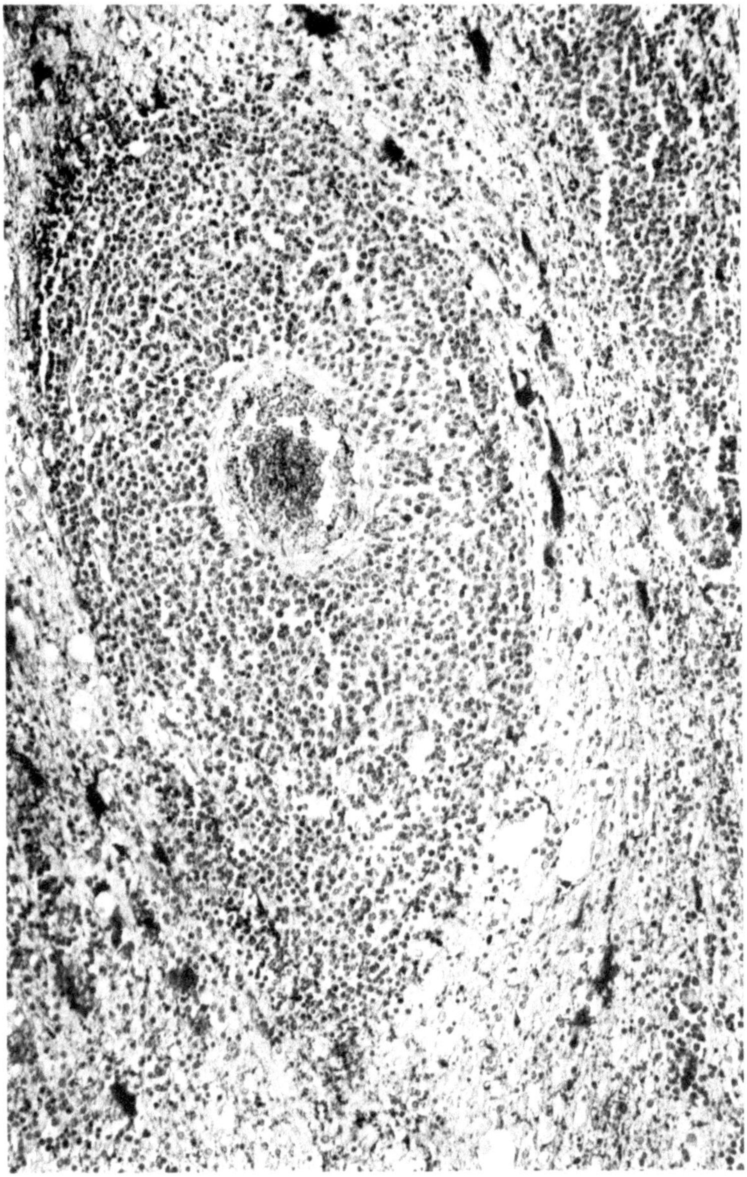

Fig. 2 Numerous reactive GFAP-positive astrocytes around a dense perivascular infiltrate. Lymphoma (x 178).

In addition to being an important diagnostic aid in individual tumours, the use of the GFAP immunohistological technique has provided new insight into the nature of tumours as haemangioblastomas in which GFAP-positive cells have been found incorporated, sometimes as stromal cells [8], the xantho-astrocytoma [9] or astrocytomas predominantly spreading in the subarachnoid space.

Differentiation of immature neuroectodermal tumours along an astrocytic line, as in medulloblastomas [12] or pineocytomas [6] have furnished scientific and diagnostic data based on the presence of GFAP in the neoplasms.

The GFAP technique has also provided evidence that neoplastic cells regarded as oligodendrocytes may be transformed into astrocytes [11], and that neoplastic astrocytes may mimic epithelial cells [10].

The medulloblastomas we have studied so far, both of the childhood and adult varieties, have exhibited few GFAP-positive cells. Such cells have been recorded by others [12, 15] and have been regarded as either evidence of glial differentiation of neoplastic cells, or as reactive astrocytes [15]. When GFAP-positive cells are located within the subarachnoidal compartment of a medulloblastoma, they may safely be considered neoplastic cells, differentiated along an astrocytic line. Likewise, neuroblastomas may contain GFAP-positive astrocytes. Neuronal tumours may contain other cytological markers such as vimentin in the gangliocytoma, or neurofilaments [17] or enolase [3] in neuroblastomas.

Conclusion

Immunological demonstration of GFAP has now been proved as a very valuable diagnostic aid in neuropathological oncology, firmly ensconced in many neuropathology laboratories throughout the world. The following aspects appear of particular relevance in the employment of immunohistology to demonstrate GFAP:

1. In unequivocal astrocytomas, the degree of differentiation, as well as the extent of anaplasia may be recognised more easily, as the presence and amount of GFAP in a tumour largely correlates to the degree of its differentiation [14].
2. Exophytically growing astrocytomas may be distinguished from primarily extra-CNS neoplasms.
3. Mixed tumours containing neoplastic astrocytes enable localisation of such astrocytic tumour cells, but immunhistological demonstration of the other cellular components is still deplorably inadequate.
4. Complete absence of GFAP in an intra- or extra-cerebral tumour largely rules out an astrocytoma, the most common glioma of the brain (fig. 3).

While GFAP is the most widely known antigenic marker in neuropathology, others such as the factor VIII, for instance in tumours of vascular origin, neurofilament proteins in primary neuronal tumours, enolase in neuronal tumours and myelin basic protein and myelin associated glycoprotein of oligodendrocytes are other antigenic markers of non-astrocytic cells which will most probably become available for diagnostic use in the near future.

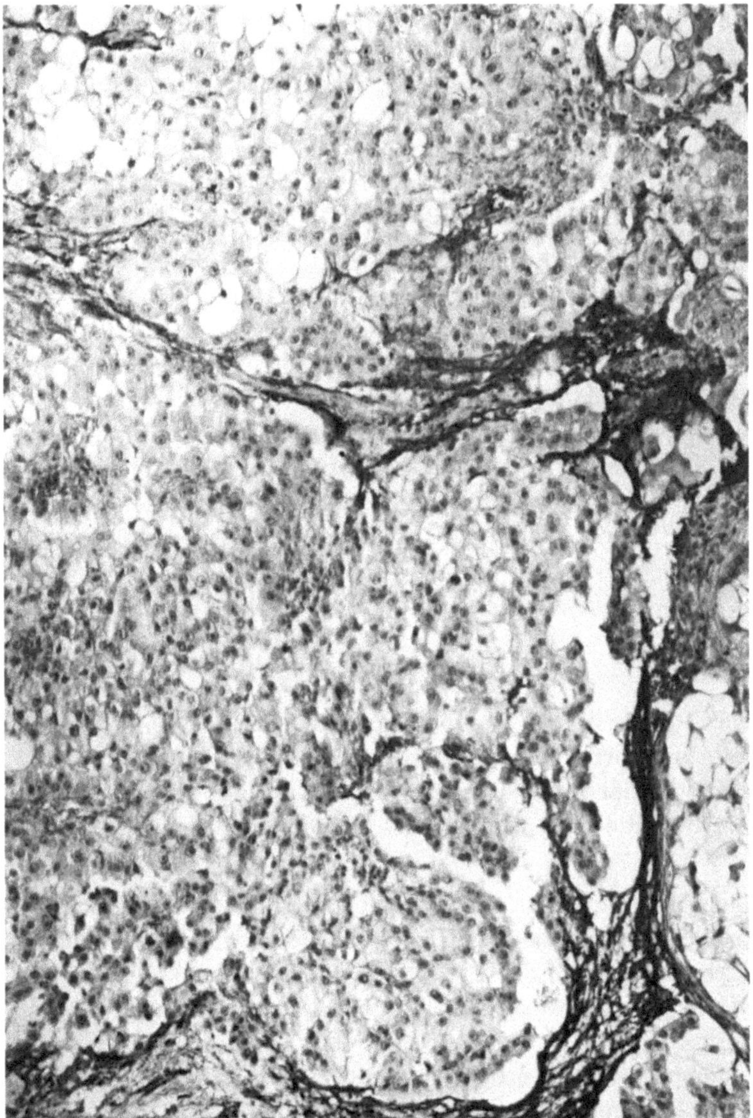

Fig. 3 GFAP-negative epithelial cells of metastatic carcinoma are surrounded by GFAP-positive processes (dark) of reactive astrocytes (x 125).

Another intermediate filament protein, vimentin, characteristic of mesenchymal cells and tumours derived thereof, may also be present in meningiomas [13] and in immature neoplasms such as the ganglioneuroma [7].

Summary

The glial fibrillary acidic protein is now the most commonly employed antigenic marker in neuro-oncology. It identifies reactive and neoplastic, though differentiated astrocytes, thus demonstrating the degree or lack of anaplasia in an astrocytoma, the extra-cerebral growth of astrocytomas, the presence of neoplastic astrocytes in mixed gliomas and the differentiation along an astrocytic line in certain neuronal tumours, enabling diagnostic exclusion of astrocytoma in GFAP-negative intra- or extra-CNS neoplasms.

Other antigenic markers are factor VIII, neuro-filaments of nerve cells and myelin basic protein, as well as myelin associated glycoprotein of oligodendrocytes, the use of which is still largely at an experimental stage.

References

[1] Chronwall, B. M., P. E. McKeever, P. L. Kornblith: Glial and nonglial neoplasms evaluated on frozen section by double immunofluorescence for fibronectin and glial fibrillary acidic protein. Acta Neuropathol (Berl. **59** (1983) 283–287.

[2] De Armond, S. J., L. F. Eng, L. J. Rubinstein: The application of glial fibrillary acidic (GFA) protein immunohistochemistry in neurooncology. Path. Res. Pract. **168** (1980) 374–394.

[3] Dhillon, A. P., J. Rode, A. Leatham: Neurone specific enolase: an aid to the diagnosis of melanoma and neuroblastoma. Histopathology **6** (1982) 81–92.

[4] Goebel, H. H., G. Bode, R. Caesar, et al.: Bulbar palsy with Rosenthal fiber formation in the medulla of a 15-year-old girl. Localized form of Alexander's disease? Neuropediatrics **12** (1981) 382–391.

[5] Goebel, H. H., M. Schlie, G. Bode, et al.: Die immunhistologische Darstellung des Gliafaserproteins in der neuropathologischen Tumordiagnostik. Pathologe **3** (1982) 164–167.

[6] Herrick, M. K., L. J. Rubinstein: The cytological differentiating potential of pineal parenchymal neoplasms (True pinealomas). Brain **102** (1979) 289–320.

[7] Kahn, H. J., H. Yeger, R. Baumal, et al.: Categorization of pediatric neoplasms by immunostaining with antiprekeratin and antivimentin antisera. Cancer **51** (1983) 645–653.

[8] Kepes, J. J., S. S. Rengachary, S. H. Lee: Astrocytes in hemangioblastomas of the central nervous system and their relationship to stromal cells. Acta Neuropathol. (Berl.) **47** (1979) 99–104.

[9] Kepes, J. J., L. J. Rubinstein, L. F. Eng: Pleomorphic anthoastrocytoma: A distinctive meningocerebral glioma of young subjects with relatively favorable prognosis. Cancer **44** (1979) 1839–1852.

[10] Kepes, J. J., K. H. Fulling, J. H. Garcia: Adenoid elements in glial component of gliosarcoma. A histologic feature imitating metastatic mucus producing adenocarcinoma. A review of five cases. J. Neuropath. Exp. Neurol. **41** (1982) 377.

[11] Meneses, A. C. O., J. J. Kepes, N. H. Sternberger: Astrocytic differentiation of neoplastic oligodendrocytes. J. Neuropath. Exp. Neurol. **41** (1982) 368.

[12] Merkel, K. H. H., M. Zimmer, W. Wahlen, et al.: The usefulness of immunocytological demonstra-

tion of glial fibrillary acidic protein for diagnostic problems of cerebral tumours. In: D. Voth, P. Gutjahr, C. Langmaid (eds.) Tumours of the Central Nervous System in Infancy and Childhood, pp. 58–61. Springer, Berlin, Heidelberg, New York 1982.
[13] Ramaekers, F. C. S., J. J. G. Puts, O. Moesker, et al.: Antibodies to intermediate filament proteins in the immunhistochemical identification of human tumours: an overview. Histochem. J. **15** (1983) 691–713.
[14] Rubinstein, L. J.: "Tumors of the Central Nervous System", Supplement. Atlas of Tumor Pathology, pp. 21–30. Armed Forces Institue of Pathology, Washington, D. C.
[15] Schindler, E., F. Gulotta: Glial fibrillary acidic protein in medulloblastomas and other embryonic CNS tumours of children. Virchows Arch. (Pathol. Anat.) **398** (1983) 263–275.
[16] Sternberger, L. A.: Immunocytochemistry, 2nd edn. Wiley and Sons, New York, Chichester, Brisbane, Toronto 1979.
[17] Trojanowski, J. Q., V. M. Y. Lee: Anti-neurofilament monoclonal antibodies: Reagents for the evaluation of human neoplasms. Acta Neuropathol. (Berl.) **59** (1983) 155–158.

Acknowledgements

We are grateful to Lawrence F. Eng, Ph. D, Veterans Administration Hospital, Paolo Alto/CA, for generously providing antiserum against GFAP.

Flow cytometry and micronucleus formation in brain tumours*

D. van Beuningen, C. Streffer, M. Bamberg, A. Rebmann, W. Klug

Introduction

Cell proliferation kinetics especially the position of cells in the cell cycle at the time of treatment, can have great importance for the success of the therapy. By means of flow cytophotometry it is possible to determine the percentage of cells in the different phases of the cell cycle. Furthermore it is possible to determine the DNA content of aneuploid G_1-phase peaks, if the tumour contains aneuploid tumor cells.

The degree of aneuploidy and the distribution of cells in the cell cycle seem to have a prognostic significance. Tribukait et al. [8] found in urinary bladder carcinomas a relationship between the occurrence of aneuploid cell populations, histological grading and cytological findings. Olszewsky et al. [6] saw a higher proportion of S-phase cells in medullary carcinomas of the breast than in papillary or well differentiated carcinomas. Atkin [1] reported, that nuclear DNA content of uterine cervix carcinomas is related to prognosis and radiosensitivity. On the other hand Meyer et al. [5] found no evidence, that colorectal carcinoma can be divided into cell kinetic subsets. Therefore it seemed of interest, to determine if similar relationships exist in brain tumour.

The second test, which was used in the current studies, was the micronucleus test [4]. Micronuclei are chromatin fragments, which can be seen in the cytoplasm. They are also called karyomeres. They occur spontaneously or in a higher degree after treatment with cytotoxic agents, for instance after radiotherapy. A direct relationship between cell death and micronucleus formation could be found in a human melanoma cell line [3]. A cell, which has formed one micronucleus, is unable to survive. The spontaneous micronucleus formation was measured in untreated brain tumours. This factor could be seen as a measure of the spontaneous cell loss in the tumours. Thus, it seems to be possible to measure the cell renewal and the cell loss in tumours by using these two methods. In this way it could be possible, to determine the cell

* This work has been supported by the Deutsche Forschungsgemeinschaft, Sonderforschungsbereich 102, Projekt D 3.

turnover – an important factor for the success of a radio- or chemotherapy – of each individual tumour. This could be helpful in considering the biological characteristics of different tumours with regard to an improvement in the tumour treatment.

Material and methods

50 astrocytomas grade II to IV were measured. It was not possible to determine all factors in each tumour, therefore a discrepancy for the values of S-phase cells and micronuclei exists. The mean age of the patients with astrocytomas grade II was 34 years (n=9, range 17–46 years) and with astrocytomas grade II/III, III to IV 56 years (n=41, range 37–73 years). Tumour fragments, obtained by biopsy or operation (Neurochirurgische Klinik und Poliklinik des Universitätsklinikum Essen-Gesamthochschule, Direktor: Prof. Dr. med. W. Grote), were minced by scissors and rubbed through a gauze (44 mesh/cm^2). During the rubbing the minced tumour was rinsed with ice-cold Tris-EDTA-buffer (0.1 M pH 7.5). The buffer was washed off by centrifuging and the cells were fixed with ice-cold ethanol (96%). From the same cell suspension flow cytophotometry analysis and micronucleus test were performed. For flow cytophotometry the cell nucleus suspension was prepared by treatment with RNase and pepsin. The suspension was stained with ethidium bromide. The DNA content of the cells was analysed using a rapid flow cytophotometer (ICP 22, Phywe). The position of the peak of normal diploid (2N) cells in the histogram was determined by non-proliferating peripheral human lymphocytes.

For the micronucleus test an aliquot of the cell suspension was fixed on a slide, treated with RNase and stained with ethidium bromide. The micronuclei were scored under a fluorescence microscope (excitation 450 nm, emission 540 nm). The cells were classified in groups with 0, 1, 2, 3, 4 and 5 and more micronuclei. In the present paper only cells without micronuclei are indicated. The histological diagnosis was performed in the "Institut für Neuropathologie des Universitätsklinikum Essen-Gesamthochschule, Direktor: Frau Prof. Dr. med. L. Gerhard".

Results

In figure 1 the DNA content of the astrocytomas is shown. From 50 tumours 47 could be measured. 26 astrocytomas (55%) had a DNA content according to diploid cells (2 N), 18 (38%) had a DNA content which is tetraploid (4 N), only three tumors (6%) had cells with a DNA content about 3 N. This distribution of the DNA content is remarkable and seems to be a characteristic of astrocytomas (also of oligodendrogliomas, not presented here), that they contain mainly diploid or tetraploid tumour cells. In comparison to the primary brain tumours the position of

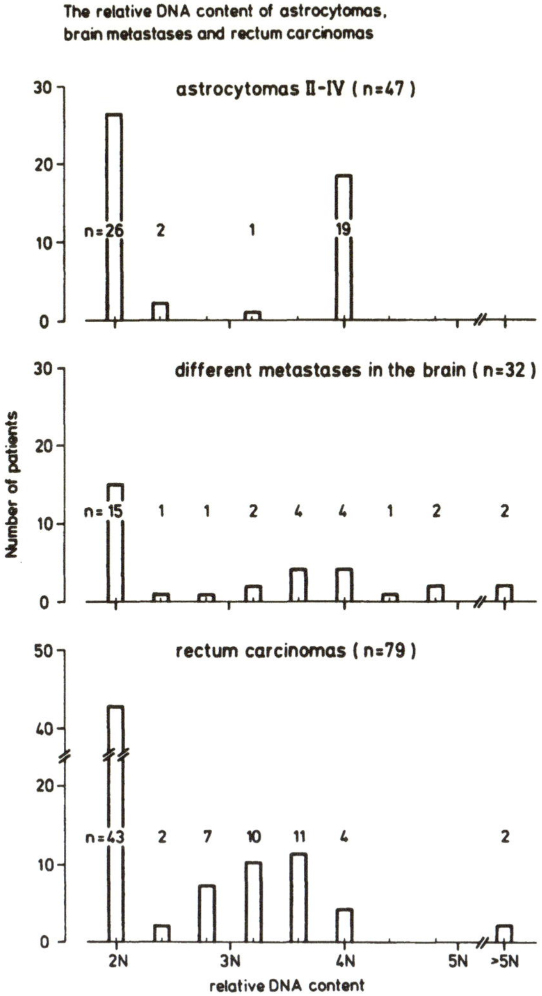

Fig. 1 The DNA content of $G_{1/0}$-phase cells in astrocytomas, brain metastases and rectal carcinomas.

pseudodiploid G_1-phase peak of brain metastases or primary rectum carcinomas is much more variable. In brain metastases we found only 12% tetraploid cell lines and in rectum carcinomas only 5%.

In table 1 the percentage of the S-phase cells of diploid and tetraploid astrocytomas is shown. The tetraploid tumour cells have a significantly higher number of S-phase cells than the diploid tumour cell lines.

In table 2 the formation of micronuclei in diploid and tetraploid astrocytomas is shown. There is no significant difference in the micronucleus formation between diploid (2 N) and tetraploid (4 N) tumour cells.

Table 1 Percent of S-phase cells

all astrocytomas	diploid astrocytomas	tetraploid astrocytomas
n = 40	n = 26	n = 17
$\bar{x} = 17.5 \mp 9.0$	$\bar{x} = 14.2 \mp 6.3$	$\bar{x} = 23.7 \mp 10.2$
$\tilde{x} = 15.5$	$\tilde{x} = 13.0$	$\tilde{x} = 22$
range: 5–51	5–29	11–51

In figure 2 the attempt is made to relate the micronucleus formation to the number of S-phase cells. The median values of the tables 1 and 2 are also plotted in this graph. The astrocytomas are separated into the groups grade II, grade III and grade IV. Of eight astrocytomas in grade II six tumours have tetraploid cells, a high proliferation and a low micronucleus formation. This behaviour seems to be characteristic for astrocytomas in grade II, if one compares these findings with those from astrocytomas in grade III and IV. Here one sees tumour cells, which have a great variability in S-phase cells and micronucleus formation. Although all tumours have the histological diagnosis "astrocytomas grade III" each tumour differs in the number of S-phase cells and in the formation of micronuclei.

Discussion

The degree of ploidy represents a measure for the number of chromosomes in tumours [2]. Astrocytomas and also oligodendrogliomas (not presented here) have either a near diploid or a near tetraploid chromosome number with a few exceptions. In this respect they differ from other tumours such as rectal carcinomas or brain metastases. It seems, that mainly glial cell clones with diploid or tetraploid chromosome numbers are able to develop as primary brain tumours. Other tumour cell clones as in rectal carcinomas do not show this feature. The biological background of this phenomenon is unknown until now, but these findings could be helpful for the histological diagnosis.

Tetraploid astrocytomas have a higher proliferation than diploid astrocytomas. Similar results have also been reported from urinary bladder tumours [8]. The average

Table 2 Percent of cells without micronuclei

cell astrocytomas	diploid astrocytomas	tetraploid astrocytomas
n = 49	n = 25*	n = 18*
$\bar{x} = 80.3 \mp 12.4$	$\bar{x} = 80.3 \mp 9.4$	$\bar{x} = 80.2 \mp 16.3$
$\tilde{x} = 82.5$	$\tilde{x} = 81$	$\tilde{x} = 85.5$
range: 43–98	63–96	43–98

* In some cases the micronuclei could be measured but not the DNA content.

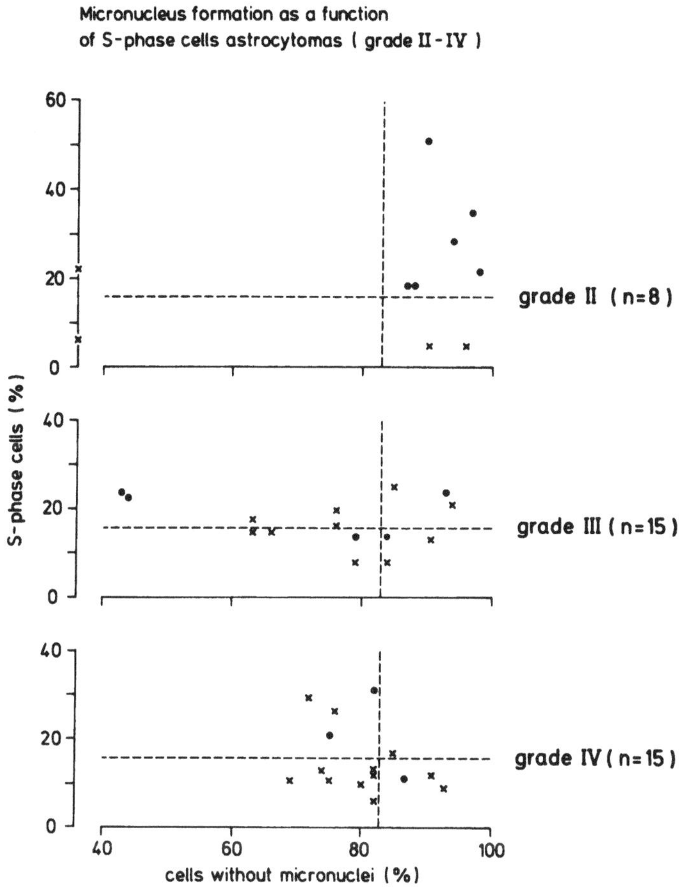

Fig. 2 Micronucleus formation as a function of S-phase cells.
In the upper part: astrocytomas grade II;
in the middle part: astrocytomas grade III;
in the lower part: astrocytomas grade IV.
• tetraploid cells; x diploid cells.
Abscissa: cells without micronuclei (%)
Ordinate: S-phase cells (%)

cell loss (micronucleus formation), however is similar in diploid or tetraploid tumours. This would mean, that tetraploid tumours have greater growth rates than diploid tumours. From the experimental view point this tendency should have an influence on the therapeutic success and on the prognosis, but it is too early to answer this question, because the number of patients is too small. However, from the first complete follow up studies of patients with astrocytomas grade IV one can see, that six of ten patients have a longer survival than the mean one. These six patients have tumours with a lower proliferation than the other four patients.

The astrocytomas grade II seem to have other characteristics. They have mainly a tetraploid DNA content, a very high proliferation and a low cell loss. The survival of these patients is relatively long (in this study some patients have survived for up to 25 months so far). These characteristics of astrocytomas II can be useful in underlining the histological findings. For instance, we found in two oligodendrogliomas – these tumours have a relative low proliferation – tetraploid cells with a high proliferation and a low cell loss similar to astrocytomas grade II. From the histological examination these two oligodendrogliomas had an astrocyte component. All these factors are common for certain groups of astrocytomas. On the other hand, especially with regard to astrocytomas grade III to IV, great differences in the proliferation and the cell loss are observed in spite of the fact that the histological diagnosis is the same. Some tumours have a high proliferation and a low cell loss and vice versa. This fact shows, that each tumour is an individual *per se*. The follow up of these patients will show if it is possible to correlate these findings with the clinical data and to give help to the clinician and pathologist. The first results, reported here, are encouraging.

Summary

In 50 untreated astrocytomas the DNA content was measured by flow cytometry and micronuclei were counted. These two investigations could give some information about the cell turnover in these tumours. With a few exceptions the astrocytomas had either a diploid (2 N) or a tetraploid (4 N) DNA content in contrast to other tumours. Tetraploid cells had a higher proliferation than diploid cells, but the micronucleus formation was about the same in the two groups. Astrocytomas grade II had mainly tetraploid cells with a high proliferation and a low micronucleus formation (cell loss). Astrocytomas grade III to IV differed widely with regard to the proliferation and cell loss, although the histological diagnosis was the same. In this way it might be possible to determine the cell turnover for each individual tumour. This could be a step towards selecting specific treatment for each tumour. We intend to correlate these particular findings with the clinical follow-up. Our initial results are reported.

References

[1] Atkin, N. B.: Nuclear size in carcinoma of the cervix: its relation to DNA content and to prognosis. Cancer **17** (1964) 1391–1399.

[2] Atkin, N. B., G. Mattinson, M. C. Baker: A comparison of the DNA content and chromosome number of fifty human tumours. Brit. J. Cancer **20** (1966) 87–101.

[3] Van Beuningen, D., C. Streffer, G. Bertholdt: Mikronukleusbildung im Vergleich zur Überlebensrate von menschlichen Melanomzellen nach Röntgen-, Neutronenbestrahlung und Hyperthermie. Strahlentherapie **157** (1981) 600–606.

[4] Heddle, J. A.: A rapid in vivo test for chromosomal damage. Mutat. Res. **18** (1973) 187–190.

[5] Meyer, J. S., P. G. Prioleau: S-phase fractions of colorectal carcinomas related to pathologic and clinical features. Cancer **48** (1981) 1221–1228.

[6] Olszewski, W., Z. Darzynkiewicz, P. P. Rosen, et al.: Flow cytometry of breast carcinoma: II. Relation of tumor cell cycle distribution to histology and estrogen receptor. Cancer **48** (1981) 985–988.

[7] Streffer, C., D. Van Beuningen, M. Molls: Possibilities of the micronucleus test as an assay in radiotherapy. 2nd International Meeting on Radio-Oncology 21.–23. 5. 1981 in Baden bei Wien. IAEA, Vienna 1981, in press.

[8] Tribukait, B., P. L. Esposti: Quantitative flowmicrofluorometric analysis of the DNA in cells from Neoplasms of the urinary bladder: Correlation of aneuploidy with histological grading and the cytological findings. Urological Research **6** (1978) 201–205.

Comparative impulsecytophotometric DNA investigations of glioblastomas, oligodendrogliomas and astrocytomas*

A. Ahyai, O. Spoerri, M. Blech, F.-W. Spaar

Introduction

Microspectrophotometric DNA evaluation is often used to qualify tumours. From a technical point of view, the most essential advance achieved is the fact that the DNA content and distribution in a large number of cells in suspension can be investigated quite quickly by means of flowcytometry [2, 3, 7]. The amount of DNA in cell nuclei is generally determined by the fluorescence intensity. The values obtained by a multiplier system can be recorded graphically, and the resulting histogram can then provide information on the quantitative values of DNA. Thus, variations in the DNA content both in the cell population and the stages of cell cycle can be identified. Normally, the DNA curve demonstrates a high, thin single peak (so-called 2c peak), i.e. as long as all the investigated cells only have a diploid number of chromosomes, in which case the 2c peak must be estimated at 100%. If additional peaks appear, these can also reach 100% provided the corresponding amounts are measured in relation to the diploid nuclei.

Depending upon their position, multiple peaks can show variations in their DNA content due to additional cells, which, for instance, can belong to pathological tetraploid or heteroploid cell populations. Solid tumours with a slight malignancy distinguish themselves by predominantly diploid histograms, whereas those of anaplastic tumours are often polyploid and aneuploid. Investigations of tumours of the CNS have been repeatedly carried out, although presenting diverse results regarding the correlation between histological classification and DNA evaluation [4–6, 8, 9, 11–14]. It was the intention of this investigation to determine in gliomas and glioblastomas whether or not there is any correlation between their DNA distribution and the extent of their histologically classified anaplasia.

---

* Supported by Deutsche Forschungsgemeinschaft grant Sp 168/2.

Methods

We investigated 38 tumours both directly after operative removal and in cell cultures. There were 37 brain tumours, and one was a case of spinal astrocytoma. Cell nucleus extraction and DNA staining was performed with ethidium bromide in accordance with the methods of Dittrich and Göhdes [3]. The impulse photocytometer was an ICP 11 from Phywe Inc., Goettingen. Immediately after surgical removal of the tumour tissue, the cell cultures were prepared and cultivated from a minimum of four to a maximum of 28 days, on average 1–3 weeks. At different time-intervals , the histograms of the freshly operated material were compared with those of their respective cell cultures.

Results

Altogether, we determined the DNA patterns of 21 glioblastomas, eight oligodendrogliomas and nine astrocytomas. The glioblastomas are shown in table 1. Here five types of tumour were found determined by their DNA distribution. The first group consists of five tumours, which histologically exhibit severe cell polymorphy and profuse cell division. They are characterized by extraordinary polyploidy combined with a regular pathological increase of the s-phase section. A typical example is the first case which involved left temporal glioblastoma in a 64-year-old man

Table 1 FCM DNA distribution in glioblastomas (21 cases)

Type of histogram	No. of cases	G1 area*	G2 + M area* (% = max. 2c value)	S-phase*
1. polyploid	5	21.2–87.5% 31–100%	100% 6.2–100%	4.8–8.9% 3–16%
2. distinct tetraploid (reduction in TC)	7	6.2–100% 86.5–100%	29–100% 30–43%	3.3–7.5% 4.3–10.2
3. diploid-tetradiploid	4	100% 100%	13.3–21% 13.2–19%	4–9.9% 4.5–13.2%
4. diploid-hyperdiploid	3	99–100% 15–99%	2.1–4.2% 4–4.9%	1.1–2.1% 4–4.9%
5. diploid-near-diploid	2	99–100%	1.3–18.2%	2.1–17.1%

* Top figure = operation tissue
Bottom figure = tissue culture

(fig. 1a). An extreme tetraploidy can be seen reaching the maximum of 100%. Even its octaploid duplication value has a peak of 16.1%. On the contrary, the number of diploid cells has been forced down to 36%. An additional peak in the hypertetraploid area by 6c shows that this tumour is aneuploid. This is analogically confirmed, at least during the first two weeks, in the cell culture. In the second group of seven glioblastomas, a typical surplus tetraploidy between 29% to a maximum of 100% occurs. Moreover, a certain duplication rhythm may appear in the tissue culture, which further fortifies the pathological curve development. The histograms of the first case in this series show, in both the operated tissue and the cell culture, such an extreme tetraploidy with a tendency to octaploid duplication and, simultaneously, an increased s-phase (fig. 1b). The third group consists of four glioblastomas showing an intense diploid DNA distribution with relatively moderate tetraploidy. The s-phase is, in part, greatly increased both in the operated tissue and during the first week of cell cultivation, which can certainly be assessed pathologically. Histologically, this group demonstrates particularly abundant polycaryocytes with oval, medium-sized nuclei, and their forms are not as bizarre as they usually are in the case of giant cell glioblastoma multiforme. Group four, with three tumours, has a diploid-hyperdiploid DNA pattern, the additional peaks in the operated tissue varying greatly between 12.2–98%. In the cell culture in one case, an enormous increase in the hyperdiploid part of primary 38.2% up to 100% can be observed and thus be regarded as a characteristic of this tumour (fig. 1c). Another case in this group, concerns a rare tumour combination of a subarachnoid sarcoma and a glioblastoma, which had developed in the neighbouring cerebral substance. The DNA distribution of the remaining two cases reveals near-diploid histograms with an additional peak before each 2c peak, but also shows, in part, other cell populations with a pathologically increased DNA content. These cases could not be assessed as pathological as obviously as those in other groups could.

In the case of the *oligodendrogliomas*, first of all, three sub-groups were formed corresponding to a 4-stage grading scale. In table 2, the cases are classified according to increasing histological anaplasia, from grade I–III. The first well-differentiated tumours belong to grade I and demonstrate a diploid DNA pattern with the regular 4c peak, which remains completely stable in the tissue cultures. In contrast to this finding, are two oligodendrogliomas of grade II, i.e. on the bounds of grade III, whose histograms obviously indicate already abnormal DNA relations, one in the form of hyperdiploidy and the other in the form of an increased 4c peak. The hyperdiploid tumour had a peak of 29% in channel 39/40, which disappeared during the cell cultivation (fig. 2a). This incident can probably be assessed as an artefact, as, at the same time, a enormous growth of fibroblasts was observed in the cell culture. Histologically, there was no doubt that this was a case of an oligodendroglioma grade II. As far as this is possible in such an individual case, one could conclude that even some histologically still quite well-differentiated oligodendrogliomas can in-

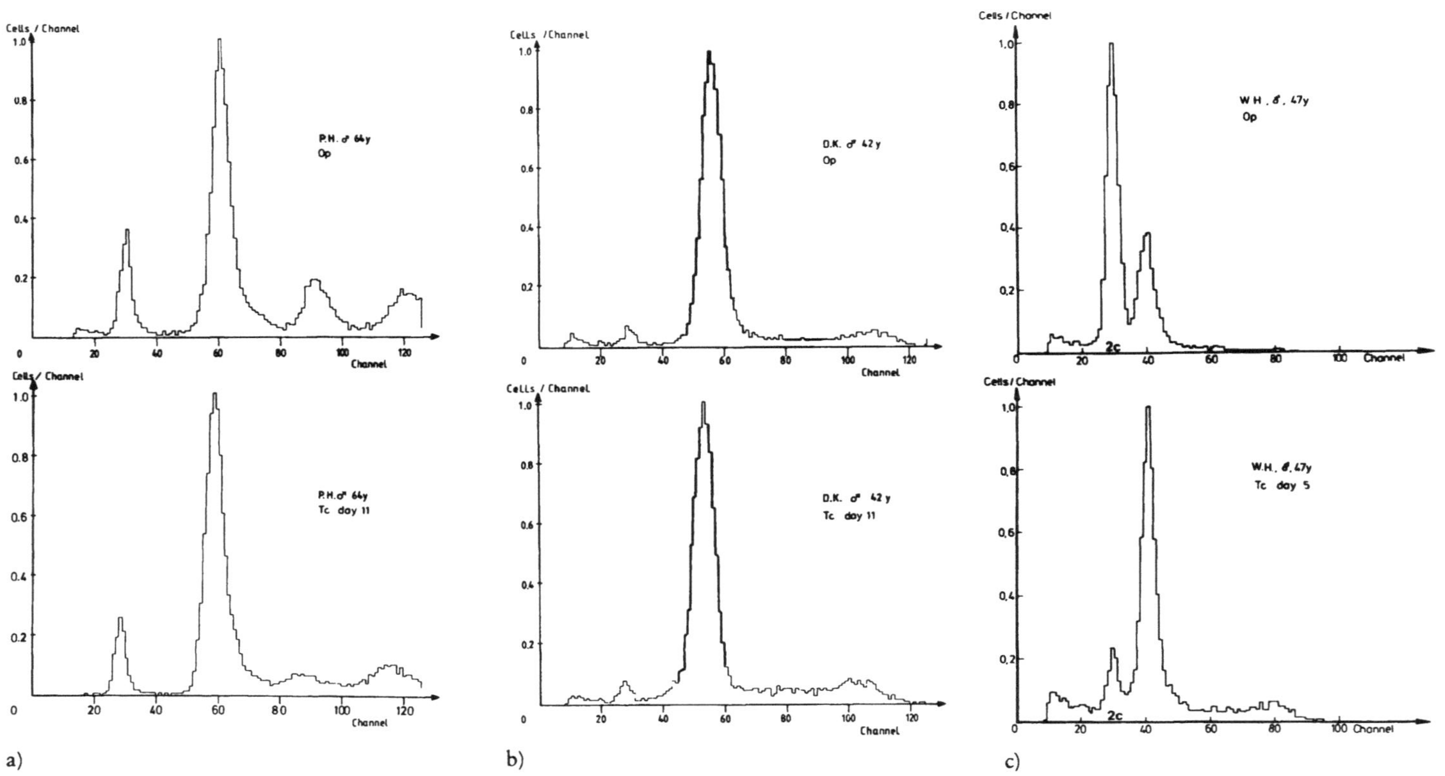

Fig. 1 a) Glioblastoma showing a constant "polyploid" DNA distribution pattern, both after surgical removal (above) and *in vitro* on day 11 in the tissue culture (below).
b) Glioblastoma (derived from a 3-year-old oligodendroglioma) showing an extreme "primarily tetraploid" DNA pattern (above), which is even more stable in the tissue culture on day 11 (below).
c) Glioblastoma showing a diploid-hyperdiploid histogram. In the tissue culture the diploid cells have clearly decreased, whilst the hyperdiploid cells have increased from primarily 38.2% to 100% (below).

Table 2 FCM DNA distribution in oligodendrogliomas (8 cases)

Type of histogram	Grade of malignancy	No. of cases	G1 area*	G2 + M area* (% = max. 2c value)	S-phase*
1. diploid	I	2	100% 100%	1–2.6% 2.5%	1–1.5% 2.5%
2 a: diploid-hyperdiploid	II	1	100% 100%	3.4% 6.2%	 2%
b: diploid with increased proliferation	II–III	1	100% –	6% –	2% –
3. diploid-tetraploid	III	4	100% 100%	15–42.4% 16.1–48.2%	3.8–6.1 % 3–7.2%

* Top figure = operation tissue
Bottom figure = tissue culture

volve abnormal changes in their DNA distribution and, thus, already distinguish themselves clearly from the oligodendromas in group I. The third sub-group concerns the last four cases in the table. Their DNA histograms are, without doubt, markedly pathological which is most evident during cell cultivation. Here, a considerable expansion and increase of the 4c peak up to 48% simultaneously connected with an abnormal s-phase partly extending into the area of the 4c peak and well above the standard value, is typical (fig. 2b). Microscopically, these tumours are always of grade III, and their histograms also remain stable in their tissue cultures. At least, the last mentioned group yields evidence that, within the class of various stages of oligodendrogliomas, karyograms can demonstrate fundamental differences, which are obviously in proportion to the extent of anaplasia. To supplement this, a case from the glioblastoma group is stressed, in which a histologically grade I oligodendroglioma had been operated on three years previously. At the second operation, it was a dedifferentiated grade IV tumour, i.e. a glioblastoma with a polyploid DNA histogram, typical of a high grade glioma after malignant transformation.

Table 3 summarizes nine *astrocytomas*, in which a relation to the extent of morphological anaplasia could also be recognised: The first four were pilocytic astrocytomas of the cerebellum. Like other benign neoplasms, they once again show a purely diploid DNA distribution. In the tissue cultures, a relative increase of the 4c peak occurs, probably as an expression of a certain increase in the cells due to a more optimal growth, as the milieu of the culture medium is apparently more favourable for metabolism. A tumour of the cerebrum and a spinal astrocytoma of grade I–II are situated in second place. These two cases also have completely diploid histograms. Conversely, in serverely anaplastic astrocytomas up to grade III, certain abnormal, if not extreme, curve developments are found. This particularly applies to the three

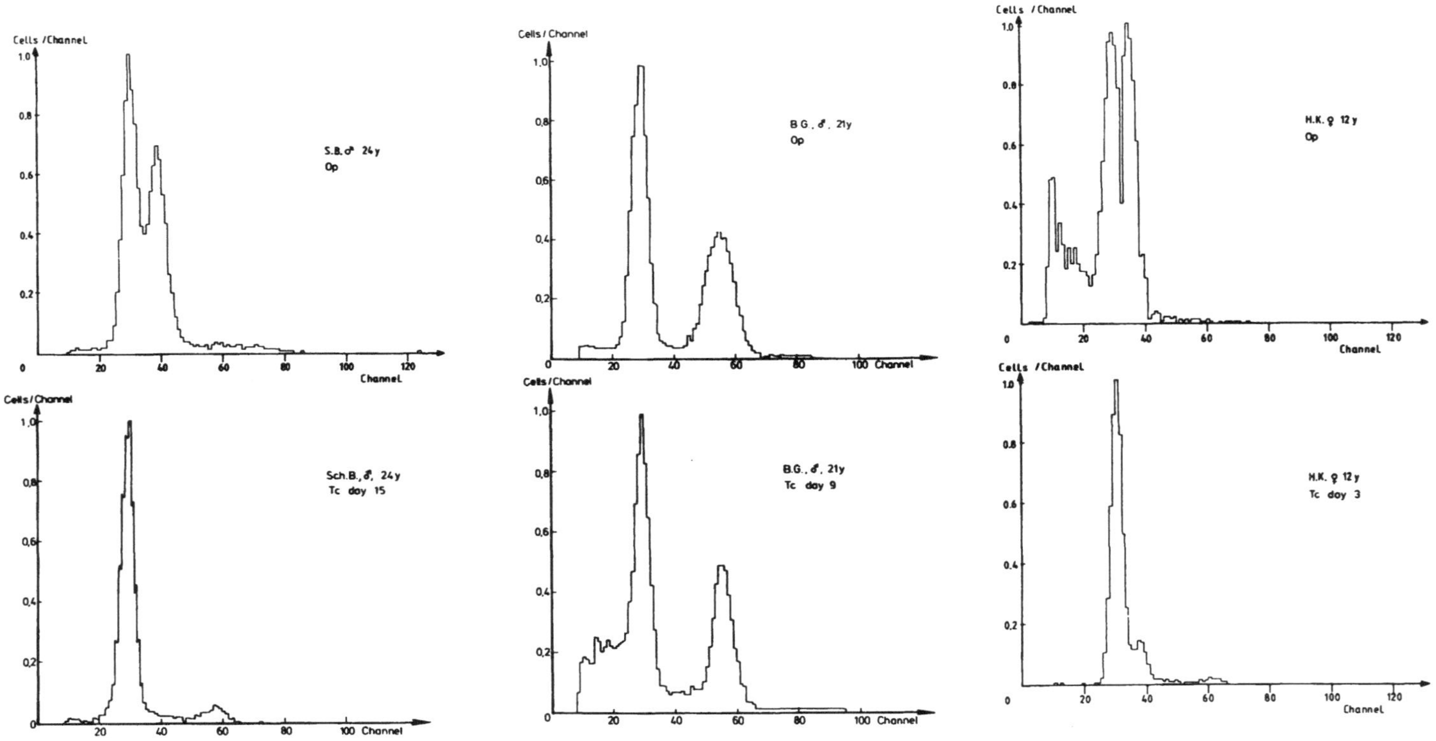

a) b) c)

Fig. 2 a) Oligodendroglioma II presenting hyperdiploid DNA histogram from well-differentiated tumour biopsies (above). The formation of a small 4c peak on day 15 in the tissue culture, could indicate proliferation activity as was documented by the growth occurring for over 2 weeks in the tissue culture (below).

b) Oligodendroglioma III confirming the DNA pattern as being "diploid-tetraploid with a clearly elevated s-phase" (above). The same pattern can also be seen in the tissue culture on day 9, which corresponds to the microscopic anaplasia found in several parts of the tumour.

c) Cerebral astrocytoma II/III: a diploid-hyperdiploid DNA distribution (above), can also be seen in the tissue culture on day 3.

Table 3 FCM DNA distribution in astrocytomas (9 cases)
(4 cerebellar, 4 cerebral and 1 spinal astrocytoma)

Type of histogram	Grade of malignancy	No. of cases	G1 area*	G2 + M area* (% = max. 2c value)	S-phase*
1. diploid (increasing cell proliferation in TC)	I	4	100% 100%	3–4.5% 5.1–8.2%	0.5–1% 1–1.5%
2. diploid	I–II	2	100%	0–2.9%	1.1–2%
3. diploid-hyperdiploid	II–III	1	100% 100%	1% 2%	3% 1.2%
4. diploid with increased 4c	III	2	100% 100%	6.2–7% 4.5%	2.5–3–1 % 3%

* Top figure = operation tissue
Bottom figure = tissue culture

cases in the last two columns of the table. Essentially, hyperdiploidy and changes in the 4c area occur, which reflect a specific growth activity of the macroglia, especially since cells are often simultaneously evident in the s-phase (fig. 2c).

Discussion

As yet, there are relatively few investigations on brain tumours to be found in the literature. However, the results of those that do exist are not uniform. This also applies to individual studies on the DNA evaluation of tumour cells in tissue cultures [9, 12]. Lehman and Krug's [11] results from eight glioblastomas were difficult to define, as a distinct polyploid DNA pattern was only present in two cases. Analogous to our studies, all these tumours had an increased s-phase section. The sharp demarcation between glioblastomas and anaplastic astrocytomas was not indicated, since polyploidy with extensive hypertetraploidy occurred in both groups. In several continued tissue culture specimens of two benign astrocytomas and six malignant glioblastomatous tumours, Kawamoto et al. [9] confirmed that the occurrence of cells with an augmented DNA content can quite often be explained by their degeneration *in vitro*. The disturbing effect of trypsinisation in DNA histograms can also play a role in the technical handling of cell cultures. In our procedure, however, we did not use trypsinisation in the tissue cultures. In their tissue cultures of glioblastomas, Mørk and Laerum [12] found an unsystematic change in the DNA distribution. However, as they used long-term cultures with repeated passages, one could assume that this was due to the difficult predictable effects of selection on the individual cell components or clones of the respective preparations. The advantage of primary cell cultivation renders the immediate observation and control of the tumour cell's behaviour in vitro possible. The DNA patterns of the primary cell cultures generally remained stable. There was only, an occasional, more or less, levelled off curve development of the cells investigated by flow cytometry. Analogous to Kawamoto et al. [10], who differentiated three types in a study of 11 glioblastomas, we have discerned, on investigating 21 glioblastomas, at least four preliminary subtypes each according to the underlying DNA pattern. The first polyploid and the second tetraploid group are not only characterized by their distinctly marked tetraploidy but also by their duplication rhythm in the octaploid area. The third group is somewhat analogous to the type 2 indicated by Kawamoto with moderate tetraploidy but a distinctly augmented s-phase. Our fourth subgroup and our last two cases are characterized by hyperdiploid or near-diploid DNA patterns respectively which are difficult to interpret. They appear, however, to differ from Kawamoto's [10] prototypes and need to be further elucidated.

Regarding the oligodendrogliomas, we only found a purely diploid DNA distribution in two tumour cases with a differentiation grade of I–II. Reports in the literature, in which it is stated that oligodendrogliomas quite generally show no abnormalities impulse photocytometrically [1], can by no means be confirmed, as a hyperdiploid occured even in our oligodendrogliomas of grade II–III. This supports the view that, in no way, do the relatively well-differentiated oligodendrogliomas have to be uniform in composition. As for the oligodendrogliomas with high malignancy of grade III, a correlation with the pathological curve deviations and histological anaplasia was confirmed in all cases. Quite similar, was the behaviour of the astrocytomas, whose pilocytic and relatively well-differentiated forms showed no specific deviations up to grade II. If the histological anaplasia is increased, they present a stronger tendency to proliferation and an aneuploid curve development.

Summary

In 38 brain tumours a distinct correlation between the extent of the histological dedifferentiation and the occurrence of the pathological DNA distribution pattern was found. With *astrocytomas* and *oligodendrogliomas*, the well-differentiated tumours of grade I–II normally have purely diploid DNA histograms. On the other side severely anaplastic forms of grade II–III already show distinct pathological changes. This applies in all cases to grade IV, i.e. the transitions to glioblastoma.

As the types of pathological curves remained constantly identifiable in the primary cell cultures for up to three weeks, they were quite certainly free of artefacts.

In the *glioblastomas*, distinct disturbanced in DNA distribution plus the stages of the cell cycle could be identified quickly and safely using flowcytometry. The curves are, however, non-uniform. There were 3–4 different sub-types (as found by Kawamoto et al. [10], whose special cytological correspondence still remains to be elucidated.

However, the results of flow cytophotometry can, in our opinion, provide substantial help in the determination of the prognosis of individual tumours, especially those transitional cases which are difficult to classify. Thus, they can contribute essential support for diagnostic assessment of glial tumours.

References

[1] De Reuck, J., H. Roels, H. van der Elcken: Cytophotometric DNA determination in human astroglial tumors. Histopathol 3 (2) (1979) 107–115.

[2] Dilla, M.A. van, T.T. Trujillo, P.F. Mullancy, et al.: Cell microfluorometry: A method for rapid fluorescence measurement. Science **163** (1969) 1213–1214.

[3] Dittrich, W., W. Göhde: Impulscytophotometrie bei Einzelzellen in Suspensionen. Z. Naturforschung **24b** (1969) 360–361.

[4] Frederiksen, P., E. Reske-Nielsen, P. Bichel: Flow cytometry in tumours of the brain. Acta Neuropath **41** (1978) 179–183.

[5] Frederiksen, P., P. Bichel: Sequential flow cytometric analysis of the single cell DNA content in recurrent human brain tumours. Flow cytometry **IV** (1980) 398–402.

[6] Hoshino, T., N. Kazuhiro, B.W. Charels, et al.: The distribution of nuclear DNA from human brain-tumor cells. J. Neurosurg. **49** (1978) 13–21.

[7] Kamentsky, L.A., M.R. Melamed, H. Derman: Spectrophotometer: New instrument for ultrarapid cell analysis. Science **150** (1965) 630–631.

[8] Kawamoto, K., F. Herz, R.C. Wolley, et al.: Flow cytometric analysis of the DNA distribution in human brain tumors. Acta Neuropathol. (Berl) **46** (1979) 39–44.

[9] Kawamoto, K., F. Herz, R.C. Wolley, et al.: Flow cytometric analysis of the DNA content in cultured human brain tumor cells. Virchows Arch. B. Cell. Path. **35** (1980) 11–17.

[10] Kawamoto, K., T. Nishiyama, Y. Ikeda, et al.: Flow cytometry studies of human brain tumors – Part I: Human malignant brain tumors. No Shinkei Geka. **8** (1980) 723–728.

[11] Lehman, J., H. Krug: Flow-through fluorocytophotometry of different brain tumors. Acta Neuropathol. (Berl) **49** (1980) 123–132.

[12] Mørk, S.J., O.D. Laerum: DNA distribution in human gliomas in vivo and in vitro. Acta Patho. Microbiol. Scand. A. Suppl. **274** (1980) 403–406.

[13] Mørk, S.J., O.P. Laerum: Modal DNA Content of human intracranial neoplasm studied by flow cytometry. J. Neurosurg. **53** (1980) 198–204.

[14] Müller, W., D. Afra, R. Schröder: Supratentorial recurrences of gliomas: Morphological studies in relation to time intervals with oligodendrogliomas. Acta Neurochir. (Wien) **39** (1978) 15–25.

Repair of O^6-alkylguanine in cellular DNA: significance for tumour induction and chemotherapy

O. D. Wiestler, A. E. Pegg, P. Kleihues

Reaction of aliphatic alkylating agents with DNA

Carcinogenic, mutagenic and chemotherapeutic alkylating agents react at a number of nucleophilic sites in DNA bases [29]. The biological consequences of such base alterations are diverse and include gene amplification, genetic rearrangements and stable point mutations during cell replication [37]. Compounds reacting predominantly at ring N-atoms are in general weakly carcinogenic, but strongly cytotoxic, whereas agents that preferentially alkylate oxygen positions (e.g. alkylnitrosoureas, dialkylnitrosamines, dialkyl-aryltriazenes) usually have a considerable carcinogenic potential [29]. The affinity of ethylating compounds and higher aliphatic homologues for oxygen atoms is considerably stronger than that of methylating agents.

Role of O-alkylated DNA bases in mutagenesis and carcinogenesis

Alkylating carcinogens have been shown to interact with all exocyclic oxygens in DNA bases, i.e. O^6 of guanine, O^2 of cytosine, O^2 and O^4 of thymine. All these O-alkyl derivatives may interfere with hydrogen bonding between the complementary DNA strands. *In vitro* studies revealed that miscoding during the following DNA synthesis cycle is most likely to result from alkylation at O^6 of guanine (fig. 1; [1, 40]) and O^4 of thymine but less frequently if at all from O^2-methylthymine and O^2-methylcytosine. There is increasing evidence that O^6-alkylation of guanine is responsible for point mutations in Bacteria and Chinese hamster cells [26, 27]. "Adaptation" of *E. coli* strains to N-methyl-N'-nitro-N-nitrosoguanidine (MNNG) is linked to an increased capacity to enzymically remove O^6-methylguanine from their DNA [18, 35]. However, it has also been postulated that lesions other than O^6-alkylguanine may contribute to mutagenesis and carcinogenesis in mammalian cells [15].

O^6-alkylguanine repair

N3- and N7-alkylguanines are spontaneously lost from DNA by chemical depurination with half lives ranging from approximately 26 h (N3-alkylguanine) to 155 h (N7-alkylguanine). O^6-alkylguanines are chemically stable, but can be enzymically

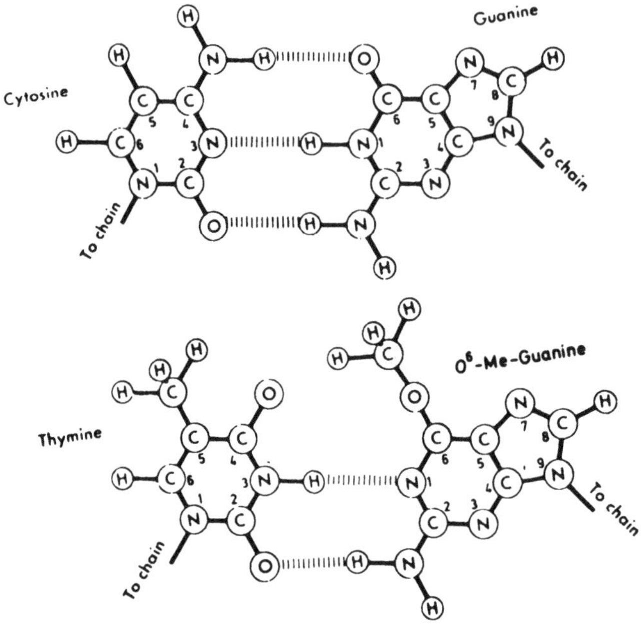

Fig. 1 Interference in the O^6-alkylation of guanine with hydrogen bonding between complementary DNA strands leads to mispairing (G-T transition) during DNA replication.

removed by the action of a protein termed O^6-alkylguanine-DNA alkyltransferase (O^6-AT) which transfers the alkyl group to a cystein residue contained in its sequence [22, 28, 31, 33, 34]. This reaction restores the guanine in the DNA but inactivates the alkyltransferase. Therefore, O^6-methylguanine can be rapidly repaired until the available O^6-AT molecules are used up. Additional characteristics of this DNA repair system are:

- The enzyme acts not only on methyl adducts but also on O^6-ethylguanine and higher aliphatic homologues of O^6-methylguanine and on adducts formed by chloroethylnitrosoureas [12, 24, 42].
- The alkyltransferase prefers double-stranded DNA as substrate [31]. It acts much more slowly on single-stranded or partially depurinated DNA but no repair activity was observed with RNA or monomeric O^6-alkyldeoxyribonucleotides. The rate of reaction depends on the extent of alkylation of the DNA substrate.
- Repair of O^6-alkylguanine occurs by a similar mechanism in *E. coli*, rat liver, human liver and other mammalian tissues [8, 11, 13, 25, 28, 30, 32]. The enzyme isolated from *E. coli* is a monomer of molecular weight 18 000, the acceptor site and the catalytic site being contained within the same molecule. The transmethylase in rodent and human cells has an apparent mol.wt. of 22.000.
- The enzyme is inactivated during the reaction since the cystein acceptor site is not regenerated. The repair system for O^6-methylguanine can, therefore, be over-

loaded with high doses of alkylating compounds and probably requires de novo synthesis of the alkyltransferase molecules.

- In *E. coli*, exposure to low concentrations of MNNG and related methylating agents induces the repair system for O^6-methylguanine [35]. This *adaptive response* largely protects against the mutagenic effects of subsequent doses. The DNA alkyltransferase activity can be increased in rat liver by pretreatment with low doses of hepatocarcinogenic and hepatotoxic agents [5, 31]. This induction has also been observed after partial hepatectomy [34] and after whole body irradiation [36] in rats, but not in mice [23], hamsters and Mongolian gerbils [2].
- The amount of O^6-AT present in mammalian tissues varies with the species and the cell type. All human tissue extracts investigated so far exhibited substantially higher activities than equivalent extracts prepared from rodents (tab. 1). Considerable differences in the amount of activity extractable from various organs were noted. Enzyme fractions isolated from liver had the highest activity in both humans and laboratory rodents [30, 34], with kidney having an intermediate activity and brain the lowest. Even within the same organ striking differences exist in the alkyltransferase activity obtained from different cell types: rat hepatocytes have 4–12 fold higher levels than non-parenchymal liver cells [39].

Persistence of O^6-alkylguanine *in vivo*: possible role in experimental neuro-oncogenesis

If alkylation of DNA is a crucial event in the initiation of malignant transformation, one may expect that the extent of this reaction in different organs correlates with the location of tumours in carcinogenicity studies. Such a relationship has been demonstrated for the induction of intestinal, pulmonary and esophageal tumours by methylating carcinogens in rats [20], but no correlation was found with tumour models affecting other tissues. In contrast, target organs often showed a lower initial extent of DNA modifications than non-target organs. Therefore, it was postulated that the persistence of promutagenic DNA bases would carry a greater risk of malignant transformation than their initial level in cellular DNA.

Evidence for a differential repair capacity of various tissues was first demonstrated for the neuro-oncogenic alkylnitrosoureas. It was found that O^6-ethylguanine produced by a single injection of ethylnitrosourea (ENU) into 20-day old rats was removed from DNA of the brain, which was the target organ, at a much slower rate than from DNA of the liver, a low risk organ in this model [16]. Similarly, O^6-methylguanine produced by a single dose of methylnitrosourea (MNU) to adult rats persisted considerably longer in brain DNA than in other organs, 25% of the initial concentration still being detectable six months after injection of the carcinogen. When MNU was given in weekly doses (10 mg/kg each), O^6-methylguanine was found to accumulate in target tissue DNA (brain) to a much greater extent than in kidney, spleen and intestine. A preferential accumulation of O^6-methylguanine also occurred in cerebral DNA after multiple doses of dimethylphenyltriazene (DMPT), a compound which initially caused much higher levels of alkylation in liver and kidney [5].

These data seemed to indicate that nervous system-specific carcinogenesis by alkylating agents results from a deficient capacity for DNA repair in the brain. However, such a correlation was not always found. Mice, although as deficient as rats in the repair of O^6-methylguanine in cerebral DNA rarely develop nervous system tumours [4]. After a single dose of MNU to Mongolian gerbils, 40% of the initial concentration of O^6methylguanine in cerebral DNA was still present after six months [19], but so far, attempts to induce nervous system tumours in this species have completely failed, with the exception of neural crest-derived cutaneous melanomas. This suggests that the formation and persistence of O^6-alkylguanine may constitute a necessary, but not a sufficient event for malignant transformation of neuroectodermal cells.

In contrast to laboratory rodents, the human brain contains significant amounts of the O^6-AT (tab. 1). In view of the lack of correlation with species specificity in laboratory animals, it is, however, hardly justifiable to conclude from this finding that there is a resistance of the primate nervous system towards neuro-oncogenic alkylnitrosoureas.

Prolonged persistence and/or accumulation of O^6-methylguanine has further been found to be associated with tumour induction in rat kidney [27], colon [38], breast [7] and urinary bladder [6] but no comparative studies have been performed on species with different susceptibility to malignant transformation at these sites.

Possible role of O^6-alkylguanine repair in chemotherapy

Chloroethylnitrosoureas are chemotherapeutic drugs, which produce crosslinking of DNA strands [12, 21]. Binding of a chloroethylgroup to the O^6-position of guanine by these agents may, in a second step, be followed by a slow reaction of the chlorethyl substituent with other nucleophilic sites and thus cause DNA interstrand or intrastrand crosslinks (fig. 2).

A number of cultured human brain tumour cell lines have been shown to be deficient in the capacity to remove O^6-alkylguanine adducts from their DNA and these cells have little or no detectable alkyltransferase activity [9, 10, 14]. This could indicate that such tumours are particularly sensitive to alkylating agents which react at the O^6-site in DNA. Similarly, normal human cells may be particularly susceptible to the toxic effects of alkylating agents if they lack the O^6-AT. Since rodent brain had the lowest activity of all rodent tissues investigated, we tested human brain samples and a selection of human brain tumours for this activity [41].

Table 1 Levels of O^6-alkylguanine-DNA alkyltransferase in rat and human tissues

Tissue	Alkyltransferase activity (fmol/mg protein) Rat (mean)	Human (mean and range)
Liver	86	873 (411–1795)
Regenerating liver	494	N.M.
Lung	29	122 (41–194)
Colon	21	261 (135–413)
Oesophagus	54	217 (184–283)
Brain	15	76 (37–122)
Kidney	41	N.M.

From Pegg, A. E., 1984 [34].
N.M., not measured.

All of the normal human brain samples and all of the brain tumours were found to contain O^6-alkyltransferase (tab. 2). The mean activity of the normal brain was 76 ± 39 fmol O^6-methylguanine removed/mg protein with a 3.3 fold variation (37–122) of the individual values. These individual variations are not unexpected within the genetically diverse human population. Some of the brain tumours had considerably higher AT levels than the normal brain samples, but the mean activity for the 23 tumour samples was only slightly higher (117 ± 98). The tumours varied from 21–458, a 22 fold range. Surprisingly, meningiomas and neurinomas i.e. benign tumors of mesodermal and Schwann cell origin exhibited the highest O^6-AT activity of all samples tested.

Contrary to certain speculations that some human tumours may lack the alkyltransferase, all of the brain tumours studied contained this protein. In fact, most (with the exception of some gliomas), had higher levels than the normal tissue, although there was much variation from one sample to another. These results are in contrast to reports on the alkyltransferase activity in cultured human tumour cell lines. About 20% of such lines had the mer⁻ phenotype which is associated with the loss of the enzyme activity and 8 out of 23 brain tumour-derived lines were mer⁻ [10]. It appears

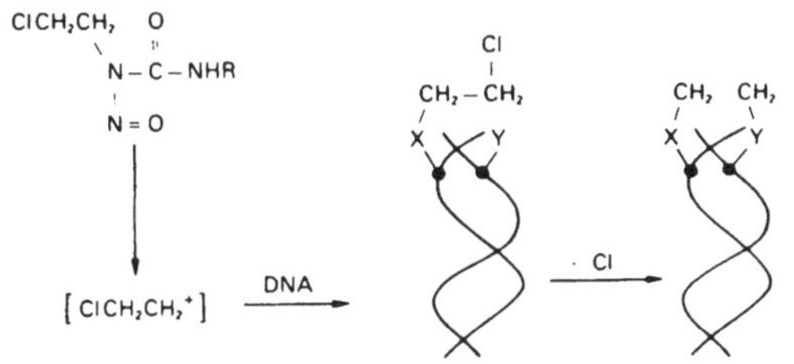

Fig. 2 Proposed two step-mechanism of DNA crosslink formation by chloroethylnitrosoureas. X and Y are nucleophilic sites on opposite DNA strands. (Redrawn from [21].)

Table 2 O^6-alkylguanine-DNA alkyltransferase activities in human brain samples

Sample	O^6-Alkylguanine-DNA alkyltransferase activity (fmol/mg) Individual samples	Mean ± S. D.
Normal brain*	37, 53, 93, 122	76 ± 39
Fibrillary astrocytoma	75, 67	
Cerebellar astrocytoma	59	69 ± 25
Pilocytic astrocytoma	38	
Oligodendroglioma	26	29 ± 3
Anaplastic oligodendroglioma	30, 31	
Medulloblastoma	119	
Neurinoma	78, 130, 222	143 ± 73
Haemangioblastoma	76	
Meningioma	96, 183, 198, 249, 458	207 ± 123
Malignant meningioma	99, 167	
Metastasis (melanoma)	21, 88	72 ± 35
Metastasis (carcinoma)	84, 96	

* Brain and brain tumour samples were obtained during neurosurgical intervention. Normal brain samples (4 specimens) consisted of peritumoral tissue, which had to be removed to gain access to the tumour. From Wiestler et al., 1984 [41].

unlikely that this high deficiency-rate can exist in the primary tumour since none of the 23 samples studies here were deficient. This discrepancy may be due to cellular heterogeneity of the brain tumours, which are usually composed of cell populations with different morphological and functional properties. It is also possible that the mer^- phenotype arises during culture of the malignant lines.

The levels of O^6-AT activity may be related to the sensitivity of the cells to chloroethylnitrosoureas (CNU, CCNU, BCNU and others) since an initial event in crosslinkformation by these agents involves attack at the O^6-position. The relatively low amount of the alkyltransferase present in the brain may render this tissue more susceptible to such chemotherapeutic drugs. Although the tumours had comparable or higher levels than the normal brain, their rate of cell division is considerably greater and these cytostatic agents are more toxic towards dividing cells. However, it is clear that the basis for the successful use of nitrosoureas as treatment for brain tumours is unlikely to be a deficient O^6-alkylguanine repair [3].

Conclusions

1. Carcinogenic, mutagenic and chemotherapeutic alkylating agents react with DNA at a number of sites including the O^6-position of guanine. The guanine-O^6-alkylation interferes with hydrogen bonding between complementary DNA bases and causes stable point mutations (G-T transitions) during DNA synthesis.
2. O^6-Alkylguanine is enzymically repaired by an O^6-alkylguanine-DNA alkyltransferase which transfers the alkylgroup to a cystein residue contained within its sequence and restores the guanine in DNA. This enzyme has been isolated from *E. coli* and from several rodent and human tissues.
3. O^6-Alkylguanine repair-deficiency of the rat brain may be an important factor contributing to the neuro-oncogenic effect of alkylnitrosoureas in this species.
4. Binding of a chloroethyl group to the O^6-position of guanine by chloroethylnitrosoureas (CNU, CCNU, BCNU) can, in a second step, be followed by a slow reaction of the alkyl group with nucleophilic sites in the same or in the opposite DNA strand and thus cause intrastrand or inter-strand crosslinks. Rapid repair of the initial O^6-alkylated base prevents crosslinking and confers resistance to mutagenicity and cell killing by CNU and related cytostatic nitrosoureas.
5. The O^6-AT levels of the human brain are considerably greater than those reported for the rat brain, but were significantly less than the activities found in human liver and other human tissues.
6. O^6-AT was found in both normal human brain samples and in a variety of brain tumours with most tumours having higher levels than the normal brain. All 23 tumour samples examined had alkyltransferase activity in contrast to published data, which show that about 35% of human brain tumour cell lines grown in culture were repair-deficient. This discrepancy may be due to the cellular polymorphism of cerebral neoplasms but also indicates that complete loss of the O^6-repair enzyme is not a common feature in human brain tumours. Therefore, the basis for the successful use of nitrosoureas in the treatment of brain tumors is unlikely to be an alkyltransferase-deficiency.

References

[1] Abbott, J.P., R. Saffhill: DNA synthesis with methylated poly (dC-dG) templates: evidence for a competitive nature to miscoding by O^6-methylguanine. Biochim. Biophys. Acta **562** (1979) 51–61.

[2] Bamborschke, S., P.J. O'Connor, G.P. Margison, et al.:
DNA methylation by dimethylnitrosamine in the Mongolian gerbil (Meriones unguiculatus): indications of a deficient, noninducible hepatic repair system for O^6-methylguanine.
Cancer Res. **43** (1983) 1306–1311.

[3] Bodell, W.J., M.R. Rosenblum: Removal of O^6-methylguanine in 9L cells sensitive and resistant to BCNU. J. Cell. Biochem., **Suppl. 7B** (1983) 197–200.

[4] Buecheler, J., P. Kleihues: Excision of O^6-methylguanine from DNA of various mouse tissues following a single injection of N-methyl-N-nitrosourea. Chem. Biol. Interact. **16** (1977) 325–333.

[5] Cooper, H.K., E. Hauenstein, G.F. Kolar, et al.: DNA alkylation and neuro-oncogenesis by 3,3-Dimethyl-1-phenyl-triazene. Acta neuropathol. **43** (1978) 105–109.

[6] Cox, R., C.C. Irving: Selective accumulation of O^6-methylguanine in DNA of rat bladder epithelium after intravesical administration of N-methyl-N-nitrosourea. Cancer Lett. **3** (1977) 265–270.

[7] Cox., R., C.C. Irving: O^6-methylguanine accumulates in DNA of mammary glands after administration of N-methyl-N-nitrosourea to rats. Cancer Lett. **6** (1979) 273–278.

[8] Craddock, V.M., A.R. Henderson, S. Gash: Nature of the constitutive and induced mammalian O^6-methylguanine DNA repair enzyme. Biochem. Biophys. Res. Commun. **107** (1982) 546–553.

[9] Day, R.S., C.H.J. Ziolkowski, D.A. Scudiero, et al.: Human tumor cell strains defective in the repair of alkylation damage. Carcinogenesis **1** (1980) 21–32.

[10] Day, R.S., D.A. Scudiero, M.R. Mattern, et al.: Repair of O^6-methylguanine by normal and transformed human cells. Proc. Am. Ass. Cancer Res. **24** (1983) 335–337.

[11] Demple, B., A. Jacobsson, M. Olsson, et al.: Repair of alkylated DNA in E.coli: physical properties of O^6-methylguanine-DNA methyltransferase. J. Biol. Chem. **257** (1982) 13776–13780.

[12] Erickson, L.C., G. Laurent, N.A. Sharkey, et al.: DNA crosslinking and monoadduct repair in nitrosoureatreated human tumour cells. Nature **288** (1980) 727–729.

[13] Foote, R.S., S. Mitra, B.C. Pal: Demethylation of O^6-methylguanine in a synthetic DNA polymer by an inducible activity in Escherichia coli. Biochem. Biophys. Res. Commun. **97** (1980) 654–659.

[14] Foote, R.S., B.C. Pal, S. Mitra: Quantitation of O^6-methylguanine-DNA methyltransferase in HeLa cells. Mutation Res. **119** (1983) 221–228.

[15] Fox, M., J. Brennand: Evidence for the involvement of lesions other than O^6-alkylguanine in mammalian cell mutagenesis. Carcinogenesis **1** (1980) 795–798.

[16] Goth, R., M.F. Rajewsky: Persistence of O^6-ethylguanine in rat brain DNA: Correlation with nervous system-specific carcinogenesis by ENU. Proc. Natl. Acad. Sci. **71** (1974) 639–643.

[17] Hora, J.F., A. Eastman, E. Bresnick: O^6-methylguanine methyltransferase in rat liver. Biochemistry **22** (1983) 3759–3763.

[18] Karran, P., T. Lindahl, B. Griffin: Adaptive response to alkylating agents involves alteration in situ of O^6-methylguanine residues in DNA. Nature **280** (1979) 76–77.

[19] Kleihues, P., S. Bamborschke, G. Doerjer: Persistence of alkylated DNA bases in the Mongolian gerbil (Meriones unguiculatus) following a single dose of methylnitrosourea. Carcinogenesis **1** (1980) 111–113.

[20] Kleihues, P., R.M. Hodgson, C. Veit, et al.:
DNA modification and repair in vivo: towards a biochemical basis of organ-specific carcinogenesis by methylating agents. In: Organ and species specificity in chemical carcinogenesis. (R. Langenbach, S. Nesnow, J.M. Rice, eds.), pp. 509–528. Plenum Press, New York–London 1983.

[21] Kohn, K.W.: Interstrand cross-linking of DNA by 1,3–bis (2-chloroethyl)-1-nitrosourea and other 1-(2-haloethyl)-1-nitrosoureas. Cancer Res. **37** (1977) 1450–1454.

[22] Lindahl, T.: DNA repair enzymes. Ann. Rev. Biochem. **51** (1982) 61–87.

[23] Maru, G.B., G.P. Margison, Y.-H. Chu, et al.: Effect of carcinogens and partial hepatectomy upon the hepatic O^6-methylguanine repair system in mice. Carcinogenesis **3** (1982) 1247–1254.

[24] Mehta, J.R., D.B. Ludlum, A. Renard, et al.: Repair of O^6-ethylguanine in DNA by a chromatin fraction from rat liver: Transfer of the ethyl group to an acceptor protein. Proc. Natl. Acad. Sci. **78** (1981) 6766–6770.

[25] Myrnes, B., K.E. Giercksky, H. Krokan: Repair of O^6-methylguanine residues in DNA takes place by a similar mechanism in extracts from HeLa cells, human liver, and rat liver. J. Cell. Biochem. **20** (1983) 381–392.

[26] Newbold, R.F., W. Warren, A.S.C. Medcalf, et al.: Mutagenicity of carcinogenic methylating agents is associated with a specific DNA modification. Nature **283** (1980) 596–599.

[27] Nicoll, J.W., P.F. Swann, A.E. Pegg: Effect of dimethylnitrosamine on persistence of methylated guanines in rat liver and kidney DNA. Nature **254** (1975) 261–262.

[28] Olsson, M., T. Lindahl: Repair of alkylated DNA in *Escherichia coli*: Methyl group transfer from O^6-methylguanine to a protein cystein residue. J. Biol. Chem. **255** (1980) 10569–10571.

[29] Pegg, A.E.: Formation and metabolism of alkylated nucleosides: possible role in carcinogenesis by nitroso compounds and alkylating agents. Adv. Cancer Res. **25** (1977) 195–267.

[30] Pegg, A.E., M. Roberfroid, C. von Bahr, et al.: Removal of O^6-methylguanine from DNA by human liver fractions. Proc. Natl. Acad. Sci. **79** (1982) 5162–5165.

[31] Pegg, A.E., L. Wiest, R.S. Foote, et al.: Purification and properties of O^6-methylguanine-DNA transmethylase from rat liver. J. Biol. Chem. **258** (1983) 2327–23333.

[32] Pegg, A.E., L. Wiest: Regulation of O^6-methylguanine-DNA methyltransferase levels in rat liver and kidney. Cancer Res. **43** (1983) 972–975.

[33] Pegg, A.E.: Formation and removal of methylated nucleosides in nucleic acids of mammalian cells. Recent Results Cancer Res. **84** (1983) 49–62.

[34] Pegg, A.E.: Properties of the O^6-alkylguanine-DNA repair system of mammalian cells. IARC Sci. Publ. (1984, in press).

[35] Schendel, P.F., P.E. Robins: Repair of O^6-methylguanine in adapted Escherichia coli. Proc. Natl. Acad. Sci. **75** (1978) 6017–6020.

[36] Schmerold, J., O.D. Wiestler: Unpublished observation.

[37] Singer, B., J.T. Kuśmierek: Chemical mutagenesis. Ann. Rev. Biochem. **52** (1982) 655–693.

[38] Swenberg, J.A., H.K. Cooper, J. Buecheler, et al.: 1,2-dimethylhydrazine-induced methylation of DNA bases in various rat organs and the effect of pretreatment with disulfiram. Cancer Res. **39** (1979) 465–467.

[39] Swenberg, J.A., M.A. Bedell, K.C. Billings, et al.: Cell-specific differences in O^6-alkylguanine DNA repair activity during continuous exposure to carcinogen. Proc. Natl. Acad. Sci. **79** (1982) 5499–5502.

[40] Toorchen, D., M.D. Topal: Mechanisms of chemical mutagenesis and carcinogenesis: effects on DNA replication of methylation at the O^6-guanine position of dGTP. Carcinogenesis **4** (1983) 1591–1597.

[41] Wiestler, O., P. Kleihues, A.E. Pegg: O^6-alkylguanine-DNA alkyltransferase activity in human brain and brain tumors. Carcinogenesis (1984, in press).

[42] Zlotogorski, C., L.C. Erickson: Pretreatment of normal human fibroblasts and human colon carcinoma cells with MNNG allows chloroethylnitrosourea to produce DNA interstrand cross-links not observed in cells treated with chloroethylnitrosourea alone. Carcinogenesis **4** (1983) 759–764.

Escape phenomenon of glioma cells to allogenic lymphocytes and rhythmically altered protein synthesis encoded by signal transfer

K. S. Zänker, T. Lederer, A. Trappe, G. Blümel

Introduction

Tumour cells can protect themselves *in vitro* and *in vivo* against immune assault by various mechanisms. They may secrete non-specific or anti-inflammatory factors or may shed tumour-specific antigens on their surface [3, 7]. In this report we focus our interest on a further mechanism, which can prevent immune effector cells from establishing membrane contact with tumour cells *in vitro*, in so doing, inhibits lymphocyte-mediated spontaneous cytolysis. A similar phenomenon has already been described [1], but for human glioma cells it does not seem to have been previously reported. Our findings might be of interest in elucidating the mechanism of immune escape and tumour heterogeneity with regard to spontaneous cell-mediated lysis and hierarchically controlled protein biosynthesis. Preliminary experiments with cloned glioma cells, which escaped spontaneous cell-mediated cytotoxicity, showed that these cloned cells are able to control the rate of protein biosynthesis within their vicinity by signal transfer.

Materials and methods

A human glioma cell line was established from a tumour located in the left cerebral hemisphere. Primary and secondary cultures were maintained in Medium 199 supplemented with 20% fetal calf serum and pen/strep at 37° C in an atmosphere of 5% CO_2 in air. The glioma cells were propagated *in vitro* by splitting the cells at a ratio of 1:3 twice a week. To 10^5 glioma cells growing in hydrophilic Petriperm® dishes, a 100-fold excess on cell number of normal peripheral lymphoid cells was added and incubated under standard conditions overnight. The cultures were then examined by phase-contrast microscopy (Diavert, Zeiss) for glioma cells forming a halo, into which no lymphoid cells penetrated. These cells were picked up by gentle agitation with a micropipette and transferred into Costar wells with a micropipette manipulator. One cell was seeded into each well and 20μl of conditioned Medium 199 supplemented with 20% human serum (AB, Rh^+, Seromed, Berlin,) were added; the medium was changed when the clones reached semiconfluence.

Chemical signals which can mediate coordinate functioning of neighbouring cells were studied from the parental and clonal lines. Five hundred μl of ultrasound soluble material (USSM) prepared from different takings, and 20μl ^{75}Se-Met were added to various target cell cultures. The one hour incorporation rate of ^{75}Se-Met into TCA-precipitable material (protein) was measured in various target cells. In a different set of experiments, the stimulation of protein synthesis by USSM, derived from the clonal lines, was approached on a spectrum of allogeneic cell lines and the values obtained compared with the native cells (omitting USSM).

All cell cultures used were routinely established from tissue specimens freshly obtained from the operation theatre and raised as stated elsewhere [8]. Natural killer cell activity was determined as described recently [9]. The single cells of the parent glioma line as well as the derived clones were tested for their colony formation ability in soft agar [2].

Results

After co-culturing the parental line for more than 4 hours, 5–15% of the mass culture cells prevented lymphcytes from approaching the cell membrane by forming a transparent halo (fig. 1A). This proportion increased to 60–75% in the clonal line, which concomitantly expanded clonogenicity from 0.2% to about 3.0%. Figure 1B shows the typical morphology, as observed four days after incubation, of the cluster/colony transition. The very compact and sharply outlined appearance of the clusters, formed by the cloned, highly NK-resistant glioma cells is characteristic. After 10 to 14 days the clusters developed gradually into colonies of about 100 to 200 cells each.

Plots of Met-incorporation vs time revealed sinusoid characteristics of augmented or reduced rates of protein synthesis in relation to control values. USSM from the parent glioma cell line was able to stimulate protein biosynthesis within acceptor cells during a certain, but periodic phase, lasting 9 to 14 hours (fig. 2); the cell cycle time for the major fraction of the parental line was determined by 25 to 30 hours. USSM prepared from the clonal line showed a significant augmentation of protein biosynthesis in rat osteoblasts, human breast cancer cells and, to some extend on a second glioma cell line, derived from an astrocytoma. No response was obtained using cells from a lung cancer patient (fig. 3).

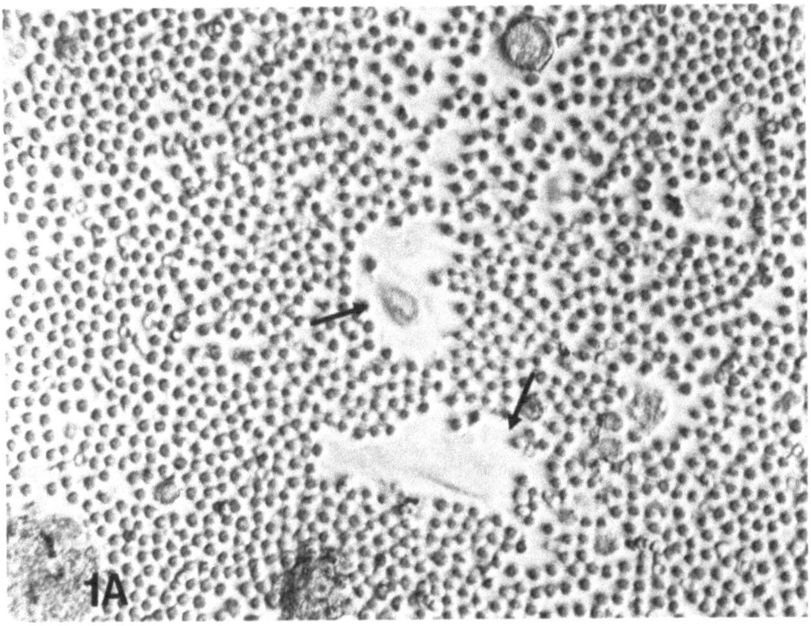

Fig. 1A Cells in a glioma mass culture, eluding lymphoid cell attack. Note the halos (↗) formed by distinct cells even in cultures overcrowded with lymphoid cells. x 410 Phase contrast.

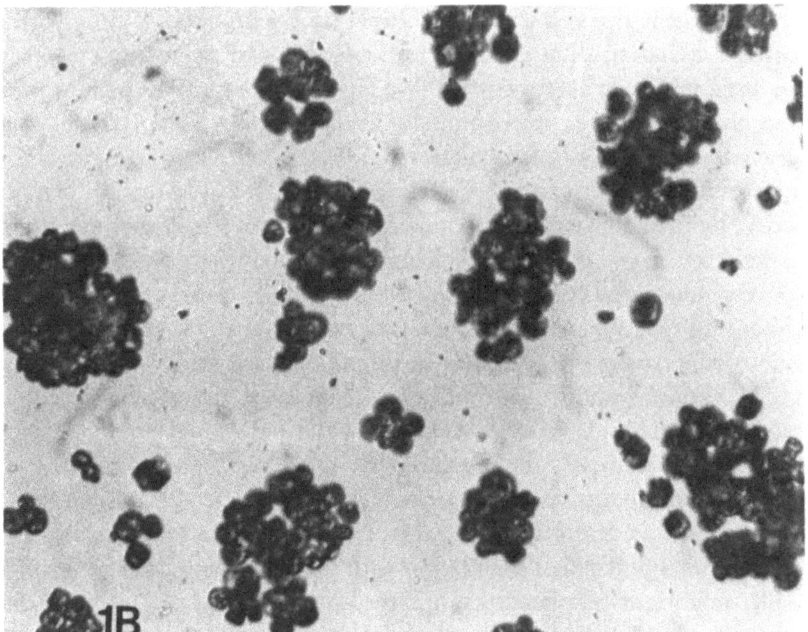

Fig. 1B Colony formation of cloned glioma cells which prevented membrane contact to lymphoid cells. Four days incubation feature of early clusters. x 320 Phase contrast.

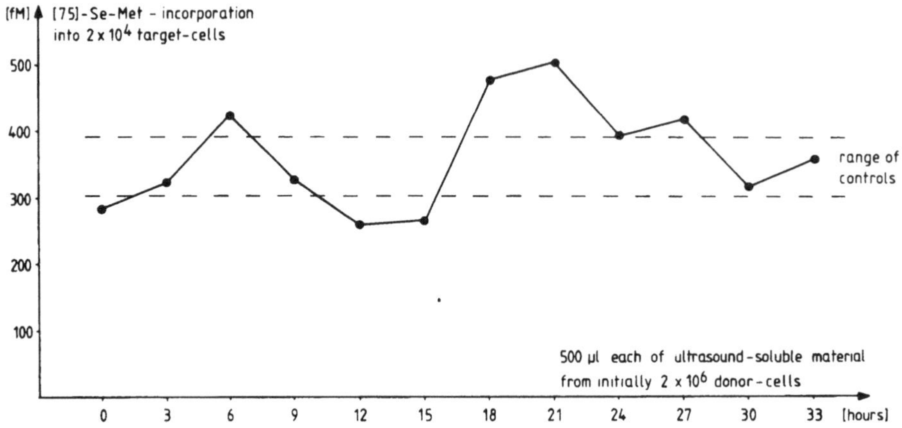

Fig. 2 Sequence of protein biosynthesis induced/inhibited in the glioma target cell culture by USSM prepared from different takings of the log-phase growing homologous donor cell line.

Discussion

Tumours are not uniform entities populated by cells with similar properties, but are highly heterogeneous and contain multiple subpopulations of cells with different properties, including differences in responsiveness to the various measures commonly used in cancer treatment [6]. We have described here some properties of a human glioma cell line, where tumour subpopulations in polyclonal populations influenced each other's behaviour in regard to regulating protein biosynthesis and escape from lymphocytes attack. For example, if a particular therapy were to kill the majority, but not all, of the subpopulations in a polyclonal tumour, the surviving subpopulation may be rendered phenotypically more resistant to NK-cells and, moreover, induce and control the rate of protein biosynthesis within the vicinity of neighbouring cells [4]. At present we lack information about several fundamental questions concerning the evolution of cellular diversity and escape phenomena to killing by various natural (host defense mechanisms) and applied assaults (clinical therapy). However, experiments suggest that in polyclonal tumour some form of "interaction" is occurring on the ground of controlling protein biosynthesis between the constituent clonal subpopulations, which is not restricted to a single homologous tumour cell line as demonstrated in figure 3. The finding that tumour cell variants emerge within a polyclonal population with low susceptibility for NK-cells has potentially important implications for therapeutic practice. The question arises whether the phenotypic diversification of the residual tumour burden surviving an initial treatment program (single or multiple modalities) can be blocked by treatment with a series of additional modalities applied in rapid succession [5].

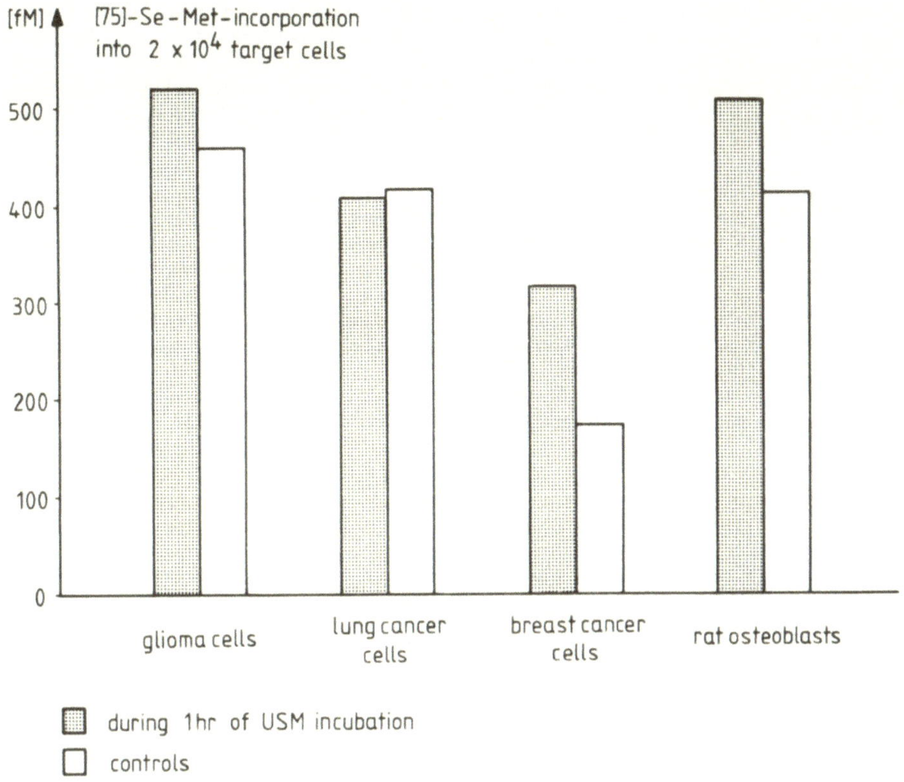

Fig. 3 Influence of USSM prepared from the clonal line (escape from lymphoid cell-tumour cell contact) on allogeneic and xenogeneic (rat) target cells in respect of modifying protein biosynthesis.

Summary

A proportion of cells from an established culture of a human astrocytoma showed inpenetrable translucent halos which might influence their susceptibility to NK lysis. Experiments performed on this assumption revealed that cloned tumour cells forming a halo were not the primary target for NK lysis. Moreover, NK-resistant glioma cells were able to control the rate of protein biosynthesis within their vicinity by signal transfer in homologous and allogeneic cell lines; the signals seemed to be rhythmically pulsed within the cell cycle time.

References

[1] McBride, W.H., J.B. Bard: Hyaluronidase-sensitive halos around adherent cells. Their role in blocking lymphocyte-mediated cytolysis. J. Exp. Med. **149** (1979) 507–515.

[2] Hamburger, A.W., S.E. Salmon: Primary bioassay of human tumour stem cells. Science **197** (1977) 461–463.

[3] James K.: The influence of tumour cell products on macrophage function *in vitro* and *in vivo*: A review. In: The Macrophages and Cancer (K. James, W.H. McBride and A.E. Stuart, editors and publishers), p. 225. Edinburgh 1977.
[4] Lederer, T., K.S. Zänker, G. Blümel: Rhythmical alteration of protein synthesis in log-phase growing clonogenic tumour cells encoded by signal transfer. Abstr. Commun. 15th Europ. Biochem. Soc. Meet. (1983) 219.
[5] Poste, G.: Cellular heterogeneity in malignant neoplasms and the therapy of metastases. Ann. N.Y. Acad. Sci. **397** (1982) 34–48.
[6] Poste, G., I.J. Fidler: The pathogenesis of cancer metastasis. Nature **283** (1980) 139–146.
[7] Prager, M.D., F.S. Baechtel: Methods for modification of cancer cells to enhance their antigenicity. In: Methods in Cancer Research (H. Busch, ed.), Vol. 9, pp. 339–400. Academic Press, New York 1973.
[8] Zänker, K.S., D. Stavrou, G. Blümel: Fibrin degradation products, produced by glioma cell-associated fibrinolysis and the partial inhibition of cell growth and migration in tissue culture. Cell. and Mol. Biol. **25** (1980) 387–394.
[9] Zänker, K.S., A. Trappe, G. Blümel: *In vitro* resistance of cloned human glioma cells to natural killer activity of allogeneic peripheral lymphocytes. Br. J. Cancer **46** (1982) 617–624.

Microscopical investigations on cell death in experimental gliomas in rats

T. Hürter

Introduction

Tumour growth is a result of cell growth, mitosis and cell death. All these processes are intermingled, and the aim of chemotherapy is the alteration of the relation between them.

It is the purpose of this investigation to describe the morphological alterations, which take place during the degeneration of neoplastic brain cells. Studies were carried out with intracerebrally implanted gliomas in rats, which are known to be a good model for the study of malignant human brain tumours [4, 7, 9, 11]. Reconstruction was done by comparing cells at different states of regression. Special attention was paid to the intracellular digestive apparatus, which is known to play an important role in cell degradation [1, 3, 11, 13].

Methods

For these investigations a cultured glioma cell clone (RGl 2.2) was implanted in BD-IX rat brains (for details see [8]) by intracerebral injection. After the development of neurological signs, the rats were perfused through the heart by phosphate-buffered glutaraldehyde. Brain slices were postfixed in osmiumtetroxide, dehydrated in ethanol and embedded in araldite. Ultra-thin slices were cut with the Om U 3 microtome (Reichert) and investigated with a EM 200 (Philips) microscope.

Results

Vital tumour cells exhibit an irregular shape with filiform processes. Their cytoplasm is poorly structured. Ribosomes are found both free and attached to cisterns of the endoplasmic reticulum. Cells often exhibit large vacuoles (lysosomes) with granular content. In addition, there are pinocytotic vesicles and a Golgi-apparatus, consisting of vesicles and dictyosomes. The nucleus is mostly found in the centre of the cells, while mitochondria are dispersed all over the cytoplasm.

First signs of cell degeneration are vacuoles (fig. 1) containing irregular shaped membranes and particles. Their content is derived from organelles of the cells, for heterophagocytosis of this material does not take place.

With increasing degeneration, there are disruptions of the inner mitochondrial membrane adding other vacuoles to the autophagic vacuoles. In addition further development leads to a vacuolic deformation of the endoplasmic reticulum (fig. 2) leaving sparse filamentous or granular cytoplasm between them.

In the next stage there are disruptions of the vacuole membranes and the nuclear envelope. The osmiophilic material has been highly reduced when compared with earlier stages.

At the end of degeneration (fig. 3), tumour cells can be located in autophagic vacuoles of macrophages. At that time they are mostly still covered by a cell membrane. In this way cellular debris can be degradated.

Discussion

Cell death of the rat glioma cell clone RGl 2.2 starts with the appearance of autophagic vacuoles. This autophagy cannot be demonstrated in vital cells, where lysosomes are involved in the digestion of serum proteins [4, 5, 6]. Autophagic

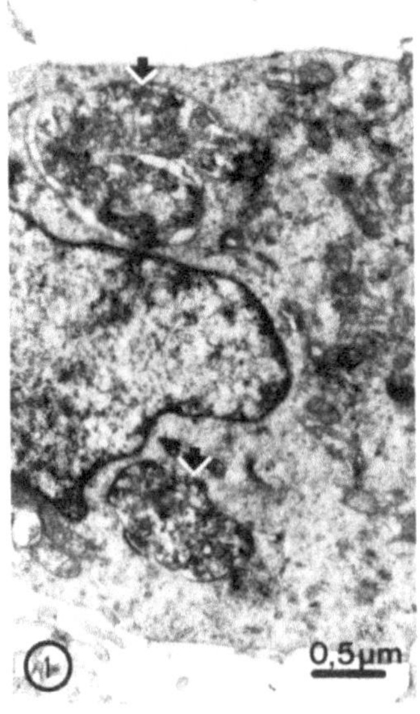

Fig. 1 The tumour cell exhibits two autophagic vacuoles, which are filled with membranes and other cellular debris (arrows).

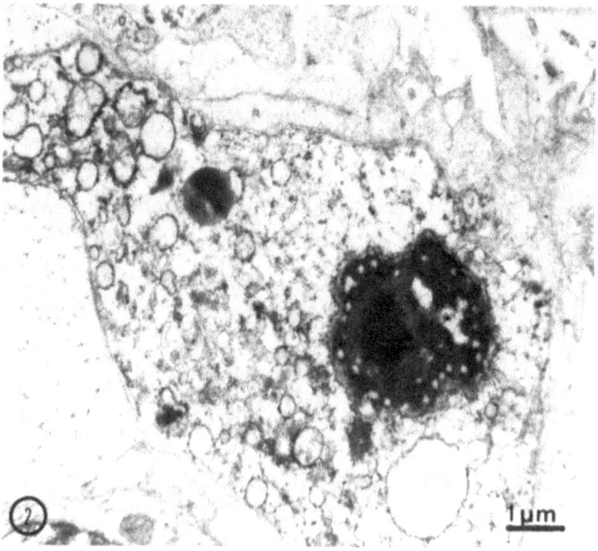

Fig. 2 The cytoplasmic organelles show vacuolic degeneration. The nucleus has undergone shrinkage.

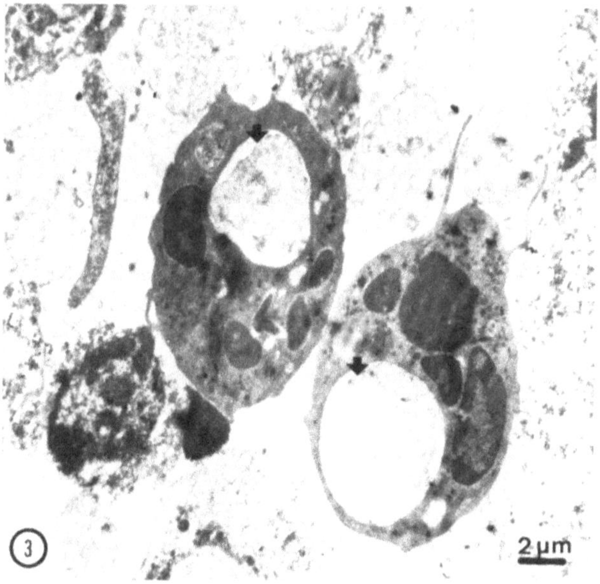

Fig. 3 Two macrophages have ingested the cellular debris of tumour cells by their heterophagic vacuoles (arrows).

vacuoles therefore mark a process of autolysis, which is well known to occur in other cells under physiological and pathological circumstances [1, 3, 10, 12]. The following stages are marked by vacuolization of mitochondria and the endoplasmic reticulum. This indicates a degradation of organelles outside the lysosomes.

At last residues of tumour cells are ingested by macrophages, which are well known to be involved in other diseases of brain [2, 8]. The end of degeneration therefore is characterized by heterophagy, while it starts with cellular autophagy.

Abstract

The degeneration of intracerebrally implanted gliomas (cell clone RGl 2.2) into BD-IX rats has been reconstructed by electron microscopy. It begins, when autophagic vacuoles appear in the cytoplasm. The following stages are marked by a vacuolic degeneration of organelles (mitochondria, ER) outside the lysosomes. At the end cellular debris is ingested by the heterophagic vacuoles of macrophages.

References

[1] Daems, W.T.: On the role of electron microscope in the identification of lysosomes. Verh. Dtsch. Ges. Pathol. **60** (1976) 1–9.
[2] Fujita, S., T. Kitamura: Origin of brain macrophages and the nature of microglia. In: Progress in neuropathology H.M. Zimmerman, ed.), vol. 3, 1976.
[3] Hündgen, M.: Der intrazelluläre Verdauungsapparat kultivierter Hühnerherzzellen. Eine morphologische, enzymcytochemische und morphometrische Untersuchung. Zool. Jb. Anat. **94** (1975) 591–622.
[4] Hossmann, K.-A., W. Wechsler, F. Wilmes: Experimental peritumorous edema. Morphological and pathophysiological observations. Acta Neuropathol. **45** (1979) 195–203.
[5] Hossmann, K.-A., T. Hürter, U. Oschlies: The effect of dexamethasone on serum protein extravasation and edema development in experimental brain tumors of cat. Acta Neuropathol. **60** (1983) 223–231.
[6] Hürter, T., W. Bröcker, K.-A. Hossmann: Evaluation of vasogenic edema in experimental brain tumors by cathodoluminiscence and fluorescence microscopy. Histochem. **72** (1981) 249–254.
[7] Hürter, T., H.D. Mennel: Experimental brain tumors and edema in rats. 1. Histology and cytology of tumors. Acta Neuropathol. **55** (1981) 105–111.
[8] Kitamura, T.: Dynamic aspects of glial reactions in altered brains. Path. Res. Pract. **168** (1980) 301–343.
[9] Ko, L., A. Koestner, W. Wechsler: Morphological characterization of nitrosourea-induced glioma cell lines and clones. Acta Neuropathol. **51** (1980) 23–31.
[10] Langer, K. H.: Lysosomen und Heterophagie. Verh. Dtsch. Ges. Pathol. **60** (1976) 9–27.
[11] Mennel, H.D.: Short-term tissue culture observations of experimental primary and transplanted nervous system tumors. J. Neuropathol. Exp. Neurol. **39** (1980) 639–660.
[12] Pfeifer, U.: Lysosomen und Autophagie. Verh. Dtsch. Ges. Pathol. **60** (1976) 28–64.

Human glioma xenografts in nude mice: experimental model for pre-clinical chemo-radiotherapy studies

M. Bamberg, V. Budach, L. Gerhard, D. van Beuningen, H.C. Nahser,

Introduction

The five-year survival rates for high grade astrocytomas treated with radiotherapy are 0–12% and the response rates for completely irradiated recurrent gliomas with nitrosourea chemotherapy alone are 7–32% [1, 7]. In order to improve these results, new chemo-radiotherapeutic combinations, the effects of which are not predictable, need to be tested. To avoid possible harm to patients the efficacy of diverse treatment schedules must be determined from preclinical studies. The nude mouse with its genetically caused lack of thymus-derived cell mediated immune response can serve as a living "tumour-bank" as well as an ideal therapeutic model [3, 5, 6, 9]. Few groups have yet dealt with glioma xenografts in nude mice due to insufficient "take-rates"* [2, 4, 5]. Over the last two years we have successfully established three human astrocytomas grade III–IV.

Material and method

For transplantation we used 5 to 7 week-old male animals (NMRI-background), which were bred and maintained under special pathogen free (SPF) conditions in laminar air flow units. Having reached a diameter size of about 1 cm, the astrocytoma tumours, which had been successfully passaged nine times in nude mice, were excised from their subcutaneous sites, cut to pieces of about 5 mm^2 and 1 mm thickness and inserted into the right flanks of males through small incisions under sterile conditions.

Selection of strong and viable looking hosts was a prerequisite for reliable therapeutic trials. Part of the grafts was retained for the neuropathologist for section stainings and for the radiobiologist for Impulse-cyto-photo-fluorometry (ICP) – measurement of DNS-content, which is a valid method allowing the genome con-

* No. of growing transplants/total no. of grafts

stancy during subsequent tumour passages in nude mice to be checked. After a period of 2 to 3 weeks of latent phase, the inoculated tumour slices had grown to a diameter of more than 5 mm and growth curves studies were initiated. Eight to 10 mice were randomized for each treatment group. The tumour volume at the beginning of treatment was normalized as 1 and the mean changes of treated and control-animals were recorded twice weekly.

The development of a special mouse holding-system for localized irradiation of the tumour region itself was essential, which made dosimetric investigations for estimation of potential radiogenic side-effects to the mouse-body necessary, utilizing thermoluminescent dosimeters and ionisation chambers in a polystyrene phantom. The principle of the irradiation-system is a tangentially focused ^{60}Co beam, which is concentrated on the protruding subcutaneous tumour, and sparing most of the body from direct radiation by using a Lipowitz-metal-block with a central hole.

For tumour treatment three fractionation pattern have been selected: a high dosed single 19.5 Gy/day, a conventional 5 × 5.6 Gy/week and a superfractionated 8 × 3.25 Gy/day. All mice were tranquillized i.p. with a mixture containing 20% Diazepam (6.5 mg/kg body-weight) and 80% Chlorpromazine (20.0 mg/kg body-weight) ten minutes before irradiation. The chemotherapeutic agents were dissolved in aqua pro injectione or physiological saline and given i.p. We used LD_{10}-doses according to Steel to imitate the clinical dosage in patients and administered up to four courses with the following drugs: BCNU, Cyclophosphamide, DTIC, Procarbazine and Vincristine (tab. 1) [8].

Results

A low take-rate is the main obstacle in subcutaneous inoculation of high grade astrocytomas in nude mice. We found 5% take-rates for gliomas and 19% for brain metastases, which is in agreement with the observations of Bradley (5 to 12.5%) [2]. For primary establishment intracranial grafting is able to increase "rates" up to 76,0% [4]. For tumour growth measurements subsequent passages can be located

Table 1 Dosage of chemotherapy

Drug	Time Schedule (days)	Dosage ($mg \times kg^{-1}$) single	total
BCNU	1 + 2	33	66
Cyclophosphamide	1	250	250
DTIC	1, 7, 14, 21	100	400
Procarbazine	1 − 5	100	500
Vincristine	1 + 5	0.6	1.3

Table 2 Doses of radiotherapy

Fractionation scheme	Doses (Gy) single	Doses (Gy) total
single (1 × / day)	19.5	19.5
conventional (5 × / week)	5.6	28.0
superfract (8 × / day)	3.25	26.0

subcutaneously. A latent phase on average of five months was found by Bradley before a palpable tumour nodule could be detected. However, our latent phases were distinctly shorter, about two months. A follow-up of growth curves gave a homogeneous impression with doubling times of 5–7 days. The sectionstagings gave equivalent histological features in passage 2 and 7. ICP-measurements over the same period showed the constancy of the cellular DNS-content.

The different radiotherapy schemes were comparable; all caused a marked growth delay in relation to the controls and resulted in the same side effects on the skin of the mice, measured as 25% of moist desquamation in the irradiated fields in 50% of the animals (tab. 2).

Equivalent doses in relation to the aforementioned side effects appeared to result in similar tumours growth delays. The growth behavior of this brain tumour might be correlated to that of a fast proliferating tissue.

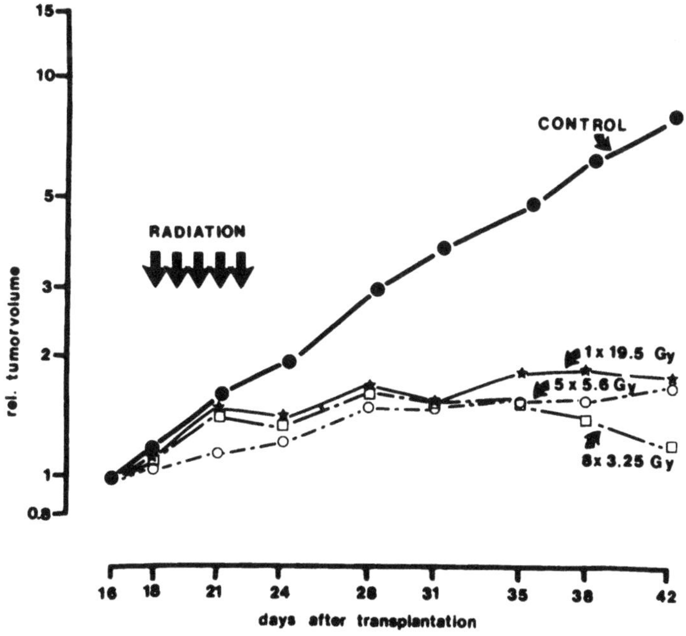

Fig. 1 Effects of different irradiation regimens.

A significant difference of the three fractionations was not seen. The follow-up of 42 days was not sufficient to show the exact growth delays. Only 8–10 weeks after beginning of treatment an increase of previously constant tumour volume was seen in the remaining mice (fig. 1).

With chemotherapy we found a growth delay of about ten days for Vincristine and 23 days for Cyclophosphamide compared to seven days for the controls (fig. 2). BCNU, DTIC and Procarbazine caused effective growth delays of more than eight weeks. Regrowth thereafter never reached the steepness as before. These results are in agreement with clinical observations for BCNU, Procarbazine, Cyclophosphamide and Vincristine. The efficacy of DTIC in tumour delay was surprising and needs further trials (fig. 3).

Summary

These preliminary results seem promising and confirm previous experience in that the xenograft reflects many properties of the *in situ* tumour in patients. As a screening method for diverse radio-chemotherapy studies as well as combined form of treatment, additional investigations on this pre-clinical tumour model could yield chances of improving tumour treatment in patients and making it more effective.

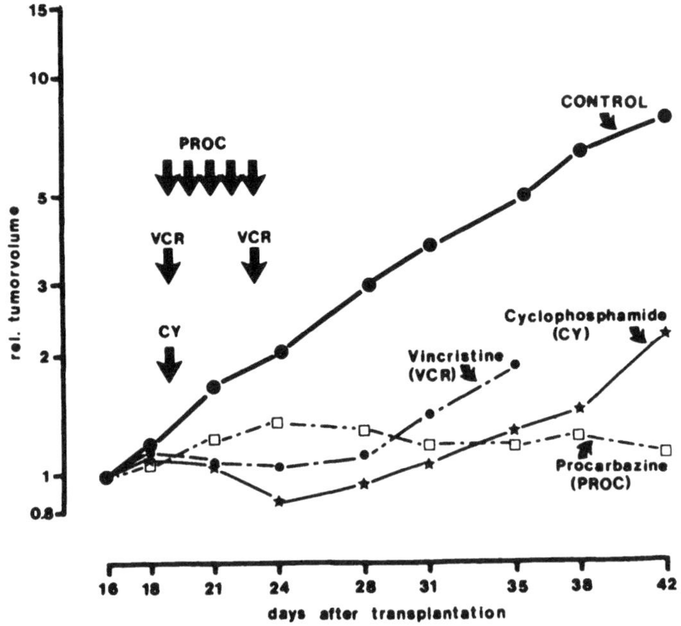

Fig. 2 Growth delay compared to treated glioma growth with i.p. administration of Cyclophosphamide, Procarbazine and Vincristine.

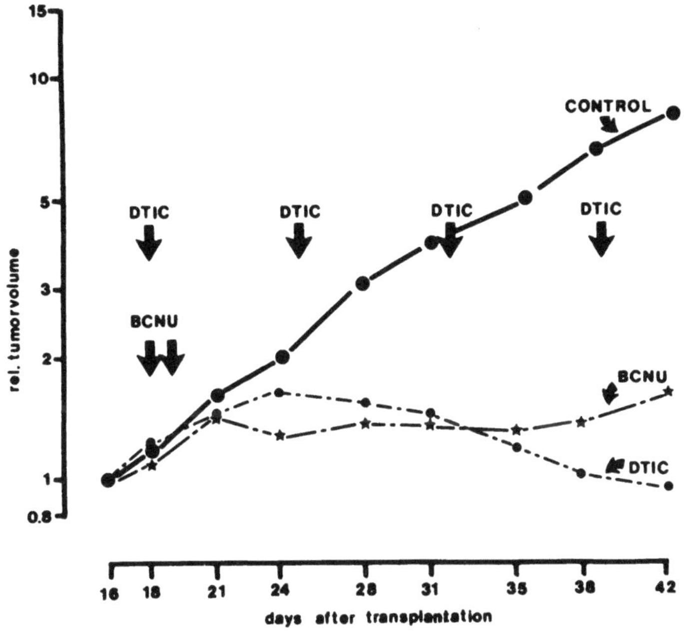

Fig. 3 Growth delay of a human glioma after administration of BCNU and DTIC.

References

[1] Bloom, H.J.G.: Intracranial tumours: response and resistance to therapeutic endeavours, 1970–1980. Int. J. Radiat. Oncol. Biol. Phys. **8** (1982) 1084–1093.

[2] Bradley, N.J., H.J.G. Bloom, A.J.S. Davies, et al.: Growth of human gliomas in immune deficient mice: a possible model for pre-clinical therapy studies. Br. J. Cancer **38** (1978) 263–272.

[3] Flanagan, S.P.: "Nude", a new hairless gene with pleiotropic effects in the mouse. Genet. Res. **8** (1966) 295–309.

[4] Horten, B.C., G.A. Basler, W.R. Shapiro: Xenograft of human malignant glial tumours into brains of nude mice. J. Neuropath. Exp. Neurol. **40** (1981) 493–511.

[5] Houchens, D.P., A.A. Ovejera, S.M. Riblet, et al.: Human brain tumour xenografts in nude mice as a chemotherapy model. Eur. J. Cancer Clin. Oncol. **19**, no. 6 (1983) 799–805.

[6] Pantelouris, E.M.: Absence of thymus in a mouse mutant. Nature **217** (1968) 370–371.

[7] Sheline, G.E.: Radiation therapy of brain tumours. Cancer **39** (1977) 873–881.

[8] Steel, G.G., V.D. Courtenay, M.J. Peckham: The response to chemotherapy of a variety of human tumour xenografts. Br. J. Cancer **47** (1983) 1–13.

[9] Wara, W.M., A. Begg, T.L. Phillips, et al.: Growth and treatment of human brain tumours in nude mice – preliminary communication. In: Proceedings of the symposium on the use of nude mice in cancer research (Houchens and Ovejera, eds.), pp. 251–256. Gustav Fischer Verlag, New York 1978.

Mononuclear infiltrates in human brain tumours – possible morphological equivalence of an immunological defence reaction

D.-K. Böker, F. Gullotta

Introduction

Lymphocytes have been recognized as effector cells in cell-mediated immune reactions. A well-known example are the lymphocytic infiltrates which are to be seen in rejected transplants. As tumours can be regarded as special forms of transplants one could suppose that lymphocytic infiltration in and around tumours might represent an attempt of immunological tumour rejection. For several carcinomas a better prognosis in the presence of such infiltrates has been shown [1, 2, 3, 4, 6, 7]. As the brain is at least partially to be regarded as an immunologically privileged site, it is interesting to see if those prognostic influences of mononuclear infiltrations are also to be found in human brain tumours. Until now there are only a few reports dealing with this topic [5, 8, 9, 10].

Material and methods

We reviewed the histological slides from 146 patients with astrocytoma grade I–III, from 199 glioblastomas and 104 patients with solitary metastases to the brain. In 77 of the latter group we had sufficient follow-up information. Perivascular infiltrates in the tumour itself and in the tumour vicinity were recorded. They were classified according to the number of vessels showing infiltrates and to the intensity of the infiltrates from ø to +++. Details have been reported elsewhere [5].

Follow-up details were mainly concerned with pre-operative steroid treatment, specific therapy and postoperative survival times of the patients.

In 67 patients a leucocyte migration inhibition test (LMI) was performed to examine a possible correlation between presence of infiltrates and cell mediated immune reactions to autologous tumour extract. For details of this technique see [5].

Results

Lymphocytic infiltrates were found in about 72% of the 449 tumours (tab. 1). They were more frequent in the more malignant types of tumour, and in metastases more frequent than in gliomas. Mostly the infiltrates were only scanty, classified as +. Only in the metastases group the ratio of ++ infiltrates was rather high. Marked infiltration, classified as +++ was only seen in 11 cases (4%).

Pre-operative steroid treatment did not severely affect the frequency of mononuclear tumour infiltration (tab. 2), at least at the doses routinely administered by us. But in a small group of glioblasoma patients (n=14) who received pre-operative steroid treatment at doses more than 200 mg of dexamethasone each, we were not able to detect any mononuclear infiltration.

The mean survival time in the group of glioma patients was longer in each therapy group in the presence of infiltrates. For detailed values see tables 3a and 3b. The same was found in patients with brain metastases: In the absence of an infiltrate mean survival time was only 3.5 months, whereas it was 10.0 months when lymphocytic infiltration was present (tab. 3c).

Table 1 Frequency of lymphocytic infiltration in astrocytomas, glioblastomas and metastases

	Lymphocytic infiltrates Ø	+	++	+++	total
Astrocytoma I	n = 46	20	3	0	69
Astrocytoma II	17	13	2	3	35
Astrocytoma III	16	21	4	1	42
Glioblastoma	65	82	48	4	199
Metastases	26	15	60	3	104
	170 = 38%	151 = 32%	117 = 26%	11 = 4%	449

Table 2 Frequency of infiltrates depending on pre-operative steroid-therapy with dexamethasone (mean total dose 90.0 mg in the 92 cases)

	Infiltrates Ø	+/++/+++
no pre-op. steroid treatment n = 211	n = 57 (27%)	n = 154 (73%)
pre-op. steroid treatment n = 92	23 (25%)	69 (74%)
n = 303	80	223

Table 3a Survival times in astrocytoma (grade I–III) patients according to therapy (Op = operation, R = radiation, C = chemotherapy, RecOp = operation of recurrent tumour) and presence or absence of infiltrates

	∅ Infiltrates		Infiltrates +/++/+++	
Op	n = 17	25.6 mths	n = 16	32.8 mths
Op, R	10	27.4	16	29.4
Op, R, C	4	16.5	3	44.6
RecOp	13	37.1	12	39.2

Table 3b Survival times in glioblastoma patients according to therapy and presence and absence of infiltrates

	∅ Infiltrates		Infiltrates +/++/+++	
Op	n = 24	4.5 mths	n = 59	6.1 mths
Op, R	8	7.6	35	10.0
Op, R, C	2	8.5	9	14.2
Op, C	1	9.0	1	6.0
	35	5.6 mths	104	8.1 mths
Op. mort.	19		41	
	54		145	

Table 3c Influence of lymphocytic infiltration in brain metastases on postoperative survival time

Infiltrates		Survival time
∅	n = 22	3.5 mths
+/++/+++	55	10.0
	77	7.7 mths

As shown in table 4 mean postoperative survival time is longer in the presence of more marked infiltrates. In our glioblastoma group, mean survival time in the absence of infiltrates is 5.6 months (n = 35), whereas it is 7.5 months in the presence of a + infiltrate (n = 62) and 8.8 months with ++ infiltrates (n = 38). The four cases with marked (+++) infiltration survived 8.4 months each.

Mean age in the total group of patients was 46.6 years. In the group without infiltrates it was 48.3 years, and in the group presenting with infiltrates 45.5 years.

All patients in this study were either free of neurological signs or were at least capable of taking care of themselves and did not need help from others.

In 67 patients a leucocyte migration inhibition test was carried out, using autologous tumour extract as antigen source. In 26 cases we found migration inhibition, show-

Table 4 Survival times in glioma patients according to intensity of infiltrates, irrespective of treatment

	Infiltrates		Survival time
Astrocytoma I	Ø	n = 22	36.4 mths
	+	14	47.8
	++	2	57.5
	+++	0	–
Astrocytoma II	Ø	11	26.7
	+	8	37.0
	++	2	11.0
	+++	1	4.0
Astrocytoma III	Ø	10	10.4
	+	11	15.1
	++	3	16.3
	+++	1	3.0
Glioblastoma	Ø	35	5.6
	+	62	7.5
	++	38	8.8
	+++	4	8.4

ing a cell mediated immunity. Detailed results in comparison to mononuclear infiltrates are given in table 5. Here it should be stressed that in 18 cases we were unable to detect cell mediated immunity despite the presence of mononuclear tumour infiltration.

Discussion

Whereas it has to be assumed that prognosis in intracranial tumours is influenced by many factors it seems to be clear that the presence of mononuclear infiltration is strongly correlated with a better prognosis. In our study age and Karnofsky grade at time of operation did not play an important role because these factors were not significantly different in the groups with and without infiltrates. Especially in the group of patients with brain metastases one has to be very careful with the interpretation of the role of lymphocytic infiltration, because the complexity of the problem

Table 5 Correlation of results of leucocyte migration inhibition test (LMI) and presence or absence of mononuclear tumour infiltration

INF Ø LMI +	INF Ø LMI Ø
4	23
INF + LMI +	INF + LMI Ø
22	18

is still greater in cancer patients than in glioma patients. But as different forms of treatment did not lead to very different survival times, and because size and localisation of the metastases were not different in both groups, the influence of lymphocytic infiltration is strongly suggestive. One can assume that infiltration will not only be present in and around the metastases but also in the primary tumour. As initially mentioned lymphocytic infiltrates are correlated to a better prognosis in several cancers. Thus, infiltration in brain metastases might also reflect a better resistance of the host to his tumour.

In the glioma group mononuclear infiltrates are found in 52% of cases. Infiltrates were seen more frequently in more malignant tumours. But a marked infiltration was only seen in 8 out of 345 gliomas. There also seems to be a correlation between intensity of the infiltrates and survival as shown in table 4. This tendency is also seen in astrocytomas, but here the numbers of cases may be somewhat small. More indicative are the figures of the glioblastoma group. Here it is interesting that the ++ group has a longer mean survival time than the +++ group. The latter consists only of four cases, but perhaps the scanty infiltration of a great number of vessels (++) is a more effective form of rejection reaction than marked, multilayered infiltration around few vessels (+++). This is in accordance with the findings of Brooks [6].

Pre-operative anti-oedematous treatment with dexamethasone seems not severely to affect the infiltrates when the total dosages are below 100 mg. But at higher dosages infiltrates seem to be eliminated. At least we could not detect any infiltration in a small group of glioblastoma patients who each received more than 200 mg of dexamethasone.

When comparing the presence of mononuclear infiltrates to the results of LMI we found relevant results, i.e. presence of infiltrates and migration inhibition, or both missing in 45 out of 67 cases, thus indicating that infiltrates are a morphological equivalent of an immunological rejection reaction. In four cases there were no infiltrates, but migration inhibition. Perhaps infiltrates would have been found if more extense histological investigation could have been performed. For the 18 cases exhibiting mononuclear infiltration without detectable cell mediated immune reactions there are two possible explanations: The *in vitro* reactivity of the lymphocytes might have been altered by preoperative steroid treatment, or the infiltrating lymphocytes are mainly suppressor cells which inhibit the immune reaction. Both explanations need further investigation. Only then might prognostic conclusions be possible from the presence of a mononuclear tumour infiltrate in an individual case. Furthermore, chemotherapy could be of special value in those cases where infiltrates consist predominantly of suppressor cells.

Summary

The histological slides of 146 astrocytomas, 199 glioblastomas, and 104 brain metastases were reviewed for the presence of mononuclear infiltration. Results were compared with follow-up data. The following conclusions are made: Lymphocytic infiltration can be found more frequently in more malignant tumours, for the total glioma group in 52% of cases. Infiltrates are in most instances only scanty. The presence of mononuclear infiltration correlates with a better prognosis of the disease. Pre-operative steroid treatment seems not to affect severely the infiltrates at low doses, but to eliminate them at high doses. A comparative study with LMI showed that in most cases the presence of infiltrates coincides with an *in vitro* detectable cell mediated immune reaction to autologous tumour extract. This indicates that infiltrates are the morphological equivalent of an immunological attempt at tumour rejection. But several cases with conflicting results stress the need for further immunocytochemical differentiation of the infiltrating lymphocytes.

References

[1] Bagshawe, K. D.: Risk and prognostic factors in trophoblasic neoplasia. Cancer **38** (1976) 1375–1378.

[2] Berg, J. W.: Inflammation and prognosis in breast cancer. Cancer **12** (1959) 714–720.

[3] Black, M. M., S. R. Opler, F. D. Speer: Structure representations in tumour-host relationship in gastric carcinoma. Surg. Gynecol. Obstet. **102** (1956) 599–603.

[4] Bloom, H. J. G., W. W. Richardson, J. R. Field: Host resistance and survival in carcinoma of the breast: A study of 104 cases of medullary carcinoma in a series of 1411 cases of breast cancer followed for 20 years. Br. Med. J. **3** (1970) 181–188.

[5] Böker, D. K.: Lymphocytic infiltration in human intracranial tumors-Morphological evidence for a host immune reaction. Comparison with the leukocyte migration inhibition test. Clin. Neuropathol. **1** (1982) 113–120.

[6] Brooks, W. H., W. R. Markesbery, G. D. Gupta, et al.: Relationship of lymphocyte invasion and survival of brain tumor patients. Ann. Neurol. **4** (1978) 219–224.

[7] Hamlin, I. M. E.: Possible host resistance in carcinoma of the breast: A histological study. Br. J. Cancer **22** (1968) 383–401.

[8] Di Lorenzo, N.; L. Palma, S. Nicole: Lymphocytic infiltration in long-survival glioblastomas: Possible host's resistance. Acta Neurochir. **39** (1977) 27–33.

[9] Maunoury, R., C. Vedrenne, J. P. Constans: Infiltrations lymphocytaires dans les gliomes humaines. Neurochirurgie (Paris) **21** (1975) 213–222.

[10] Palma, L., N. Di Lorenzo, B. Guidetti: Lymphocytic infiltrates in primary glioblastomas and recidivous gliomas. J. Neurosurg. **49** (1978) 854–861.

II General and specialised diagnostic methods for intrinsic brain tumours

Correlation between grade of malignancy of gliomas and their computer tomographic density values

W. Mauersberger

Introduction

Computer tomography is by far the most reliable examination by which an intracranial space-occupying lesion can be diagnosed with a great accuracy. Regarding this Elke [1], Kretzschmar [3] and Wende [7] have given figures which range between 92 and 98.4%. Nevertheless a specific diagnosis, even in the tumours most commonly dealt with is only possible in a very limited number of cases. Steinhoff et al. were able to establish a pre-operative histological diagnosis in only 206 cases out of 295 glioblastomas, even taking into consideration that the series included 41 cases of recurrent tumours in which a preliminary histological diagnosis was previously known. Tans and de Jongh [6] could achieve an exact diagnosis in 69% of astrocytomas which they examined by computer tomography. However, an exact diagnosis not only of the site, but also of the possible histological diagnosis of the tumor, is indispensable for the planning of the best lines of treatment, as well as for evaluation of the results.

The purpose of this study was basically to estimate the density values of gliomas of variable malignant grades in a plain scan as well as after injection of contrast medium and to check the significance of these density values in the grading of these tumours on the basis of the measurements carried out.

Material and method

A total of 111 gliomas operated on and histologically examined was investigated. The distribution of cases is shown in table 1. The number of spongioblastomas and mixed gliomas was very limited so that a statistical analysis of their results could not be achieved and consequently they were not considered in the study. All examinations were carried out by the same device (Tomoscan 200 B) with a tube capacity of 140 KV and 28 mA. All cases were examined both before and after injection of contrast medium. By regular checking of the zero point, a maximal deviation of less

Table 1 Distribution of the operated cases

Glioblastoma	40
Astrocytoma grade II*	25
Astrocytoma grade III	12
Astrocytoma grade IV	13
Oligodendroglioma grade II	14
Anaplastic oligodendroglioma	7
Cases	111

* WHO classification

than 3 HU was recorded. Lastly we estimated the density values of the whole tumour area as well as these values separately on the solid and cystic necrotic components in cases of non-uniform tumours.

Results

Astrocytoma grade II

In 25 cases examined, a hypodense picture was seen in 23 in the plain scan. Injection of contrast medium did not lead to any detectable enhancement. The average density value in the plain scan was 22 HU, the central 80% value 18–27 HU. After injection of contrast medium, the average value was 24 HU, the central 80% value showed no particular change (18–31 HU). This minimal change of values after injection of contrast medium corresponds to the normal change of brain tissue (2–3 HU) after injection of contrast medium. However the gemistocytic astrocytoma, which was described by Kazner [2] as an exception to other astrocytomas considering the fact that they showed great enhancement after injection of contrast medium, was not observed in our study.

Astrocytoma grade III

In contradiction to the previous group a great liability to develop cystic and necrotic areas in tumours of this group was seen. Injection of contrast medium resulted in an increase in density values, an observation which was not predictable in only two patients. By quantitative analysis of the solid tumour component, an average value of 26 HU in the plain scan was recorded, which was raised to 31 HU after injection of contrast medium. On the other hand, the results in the cystic and necrotic portions of the tumour showed no particular change before and after injection of contrast medium (17 and 18 HU, respectively).

Astrocytoma grade IV

CT, in this group shows a great variability in the composition of the tumour, whereby a mixed density distribution factor predominates. The solid component of these tumours showed an average density value of 31 HU in the plain scan and corresponded in its behaviour to the normal brain tissue. However, the values were increased to 39 HU after injection of contrast medium. According to density measurements, no significant difference of the values in the necrotic parts of the tumour, before and after injection of contrast medium could be demonstrated (21 and 22 HU respectively).

Glioblastoma

The absorption analysis of the whole tumour area yielded an average value of 27 HU in plain CT, where the central 80%-scope, admitted the coverage of a relatively wide spectrum between 22 and 33 HU. The relation of the solid and necrotic components of tumours in this group plays the most important role in determining the measurements. After injection of contrast medium, the average value was raised to 35 HU and the central 80% value ranged between 30 and 41 HU. The solid component showed, in the plain scan, an average density value of 29 HU, which was raised to 39 after injection of contrast medium. On the other hand, the value of the necrotic parts of the tumour did not show any change and remained unchanged at a value of 23 HU, both before and after injection of contrast medium.

Oligodendroglioma grade II

Depending on the extent of tumour calcification, density values varied greatly. The fact that injection of contrast medium did not lead to any change in the average density values of the same tumour, is very significant. The problem of differential diagnosis can crise with every tumour which does not show calcification. In this group the average value was 26 HU and after injection of contrast medium raised to 27 HU.

Anaplastic oligodendroglioma

The most common presentation of these tumours in CT is an isodense picture. The number of cases with tumour calcification is very small compared to that in grade II oligodendrogliomas. The average density values of 27 HU in these anaplastic tumours are not significantly different from the non-calcified portions of low grade oligodendrogliomas. However, after injection of contrast medium, a great increase to an average value of 40 HU was recorded.

Discussion

It is probably true to say that an increase in the morphological signs of malignancy in gliomas is practically always accompanied by rapid progress in the clinical development of the disease. Kuhlendahl [4] and Wüllenweber [8] found that, after excluding the operative mortality, the 50% survival rate probability in grade II astrocytomas was 4 years, in grade III astrocytomas 2.3 years and in grade IV astrocytomas 7 months.

Schröder [5] found that a striking similarity in the progress of the disease exists in cases of oligodendrogliomas and astrocytomas of the same malignant grade, so that no significant difference between both tumours could be proved.

The question remains unanswered as to how far CT helped us to differentiate gliomas of variable malignant grades on the basis of quantitative density measurements.

Grade II astrocytomas are seen in CT as hypodense tumours and rarely as isodense tumours with an average value of 22 HU, which showed no significant change in density value after injection of contrast medium (24 HU).

Grade III astrocytomas showed in their solid component a relatively high density value of 26 HU which jumped to 31 HU after injection of contrast medium. On the other hand, the density values of the cystic and necrotic portions of the tumour were not significantly influenced.

In grade IV astrocytomas density values in the plain scan were distinctly higher than those of grade II and III with a striking increase of these density values after injection of contrast medium. This increase in density value in grade IV astrocytomas is considered, by far the most prominent in this tumour group.

Statistically, this behaviour of astrocytomas was confirmed in the U-test. By comparing the values after injection of contrast medium in grade II and III astrocytomas "p" was found to be 0.05. By comparing the grade III and IV astrocytomas "p" was found to be 0.03 and with grade II and IV astrocytomas, "p" was found to be 0.01.

The density of the non-calcified grade II oligodendroglioma and the anaplastic oligodendroglioma in the unenhanced scan showed no significant difference (26 and 27 HU). Injection of contrast medium resulted in different responses of both groups of tumour. Whereas in grade II oligodendroglioma no change of the values was seen, there was a marked increase of the value to 40 HU in the anaplastic oligodendrogliomas.

Differentiation between the non-calcified grade II oligodendrogliomas and grade II astrocytomas on the basis of density values could not be achieved either before or after injection of contrast medium.

Both tumours could, however, be differentiated from the higher malignant grade gliomas by the lack of enhancement, a phenomenon which is always met with in higher malignant grade gliomas.

The solid component of glioblastomas showed before injection of contrast medium as well as after, no different values from those of grade IV astrocytomas although a significant difference ($p = 0.05$) in grade III astrocytomas, was noted especially after enhancement.

Non-calcified anaplastic oligodendrogliomas and glioblastomas could not be differentiated from each other on the basis of density analysis, since the average density value in the plain scan was 27 HU which suggested glioblastoma, and because the difference of 1 HU after injection of contrast medium was considered insignificant.

A difference of great significance was predicted in grade II astrocytomas especially after contrast medium injection whereby the "up" value was 0.001. Comparable values could be elicited in U-test in the non-calcified component of grade II oligodendrogliomas.

It is possible to achieve a quite clear differentiation between low grade gliomas and those of higher malignant grade and glioblastomas by means of density studies in computed tomography.

References

[1] Elke, M., U. Wiggli, R. Hünig: Praktische Gesichtspunkte zur Diagnose intracranieller Tumoren durch die Computertomographie. Radiologe **17** (1977) 157–170.

[2] Kazner, E., S. Wende, Th. Grumme, et al.: Computertomographie intrakranieller Tumoren aus klinischer Sicht. Springer-Verlag, Berlin/Heidelberg/New York 1981.

[3] Kretzschmar, K., Th. Grumme, H. Steinhoff: Der Wert der Computertomographie und Angiographie für die Diagnose supratentorieller Hirntumoren. Neuroradiol. **16** (1978) 487–490.

[4] Kuhlendahl, H., H. Milz, R. Wüllenweber: Die Astrozytome des Großhirns. Untersuchung zur Gruppierung und Prognose. Acta Neurochir. **29** (1973) 151–162.

[5] Schröder, H., W. Müller, G. Bonis, et al.: Statistische Beiträge zum Grading der Gliome. III. Astrozytome und Oligodendrogliome. Acta Neurochir. **23** (1970) 1–29.

[6] Tans, J. T. J., I. E. de Jongh: Computed tomography of supratentorial astrocytoma. Clin. Neurol. Neurosurg. **80** (1977) 156–168.

[7] Wende, S., A. Aulich, K. Kretzschmar, et al.: Die Computertomographie der Hirngeschwülste. Eine Sammelstudie über 1658 Tumoren. Radiologe **17** (1977) 149–156.

[8] Wüllenweber, R., H. Kuhlendahl, H. Miltz: Astrocytomas of the cerebral hemispheres. A review on 1500 cases. In: Proceedings German Society of Neurosurgery. Modern aspects of neurosurgery. Vol. 3, pp. 100–107. Excerpta Medica, Amsterdam 1973.

Cerebral gliomas studied with positron emission tomography

K. L. Leenders, D. G. T. Thomas, R. P. Beaney, D. J. Brooks

Introduction

The study of cerebral tissue function in man *in vivo* has become possible since the development of positron emission tomography (PET). The measurement of regional cerebral blood flow (rCBF), oxygen utilisation (rCMRO$_2$), oxygen extraction (rOER), blood volume (rCBV) and glucose utilisation (rCMRGlu) have been firmly established in our laboratory. In addition regional tissue haematocrit, pH, blood-brain barrier integrity, uptake of L-Dopa, and the binding of the dopaminergic receptor tracer methyl-spiperone are under investigation. Such measurements can readily be applied to patients with brain tumours. We will report here some of our results regarding the measurements of rCBF, rOER, rCMRO$_2$, rCBV and rCMRGlu in patients with cerebral gliomas and also the preliminary findings of the effect of dexamethasone therapy and craniotomy on these values.

Methods

Isotopes

Short lived positron emitting isotopes are used such as ^{15}O (T = 2.1 min), ^{11}C (T = 20 min) and ^{18}F (T = 110 min). A positron once emitted from a radionuclide, travels no more than a few mm in soft tissue before interacting with an electron leading to their annihilation. The energy resulting is released as two photons given off at approximately 180°. It is the coincident detection of these paired photons that form the basis of positron emission tomography.

Tomographic camera

We have used the ECAT-II tomograph (EG & G Ortec), a single slice whole body scanner, which has a spatial resolution of 17 x 17 x 16 mm (FWHM). This tomograph can make precise regional measurements of the cerebral isotope concentration throughout a tomographic slice of brain. The sensitivity is relatively low so that a scanning time of five minutes is required to obtain sufficient coincidence counts to reconstruct and quantify a tomographic image. The whole scanning procedure (two planes) has a duration of 1.5 hours to measure rCBF, rOER, $rCMRO_2$ and rCBV. If the measurement of rCMRGlu is included the duration of the investigation amounts to 2.5 hours.

Arterial cannulation

Arterial blood samples need to be taken during the scan so that the concentrations of the isotopes in the tissue can be compared with the quantity of isotopes delivered to it (i.e. the concentrations in the arterial blood). The arterial blood sampling is carried out by means of a fine gauge radial artery cannula which is inserted under local anaesthesia.

Oxygen-15 steady state technique

Measurement of rCBF is derived from the ratio of cerebral ^{15}O uptake and arterial ^{15}O activity during continuous inhalation of a trace amount of oxygen-15 labelled carbon dioxide ($C^{15}O_2$). In the lung this is rapidly converted to $H_2\,^{15}O$. After about 10 minutes a dynamic steady state of $H^{15}O_2$ is reached: the rate of arterial delivery of the tracer and its perfusion through the tissues is in equilibrium with the washout and radioactive decay. The concentration of $H^{15}O_2$ during the steady state is directly related to the perfusion of the tissue by water and is a function of rCBF.

Measurement of oxygen extraction involves tomographic measurement of ^{15}O tissue uptake during continuous inhalation of molecular $^{15}O_2$. This is transferred from the lung to the haemoglobin of the erythrocytes. Oxygen extracted by the brain is used for aerobic metabolism and the ^{15}O in the cerebral tissue is almost entirely in the form of labelled water of metabolism. This water of metabolism also includes a component from recirculating water of metabolism during attainment of the steady-state and this will contribute to the signal from the tissue. Comparison of the attenuated data of the $C^{15}O_2$ and $^{15}O_2$ uptake scans enables the fractional extraction of oxygen by the tissues to be calculated. This technique and the equations pertaining to it are described in detail elsewhere together with several applications [1–5].

The $rCMRO_2$ is calculated as the delivery of oxygen to the tissues from the relationship: $rCMRO_2 = rCBF \times rOER \times$ arterial oxygen content.

Cerebral blood volume

Regional cerebral blood volume is measured after bolus inhalation of ^{11}C-carbon monoxide. The ^{11}CO binds to the haemoglobin thereby marking the intravascular compartment and permitting the calculation of rCBV [6–8].

Measurement of cerebral glucose metabolism

Using ^{18}F-deoxyglucose (FDG), a glucose analogue, and a simplified Sokoloff model [5, 9], rCMRGlu can be measured. ^{18}FDG is administered intravenously over two minutes as a bolus, and is taken up by the brain and phosphorylated. The phosphorylated FDG is not metabolised, as in the case of normal glucose, and so is effectively trapped by the tissue. After one hour all the FDG administered is entirely in the phosphorylated form. The scan ^{18}F uptake data at this stage when combined with the integrated arterial isotope concentrations and the real glucose content of the blood, allows the regional consumption of glucose to be calculated. The assumptions to be made and the limitations of the technique have already been extensively discussed in the literature [9–11].

Results

Baseline measurements in patients with cerebral gliomas

Positron emission tomography has been used to study regional physiology not only in tumours but also the peritumoural oedema and remote 'normal' brain. Figure 1 shows an X-ray transmission CT scan of a patient with a left fronto-parietal metas-

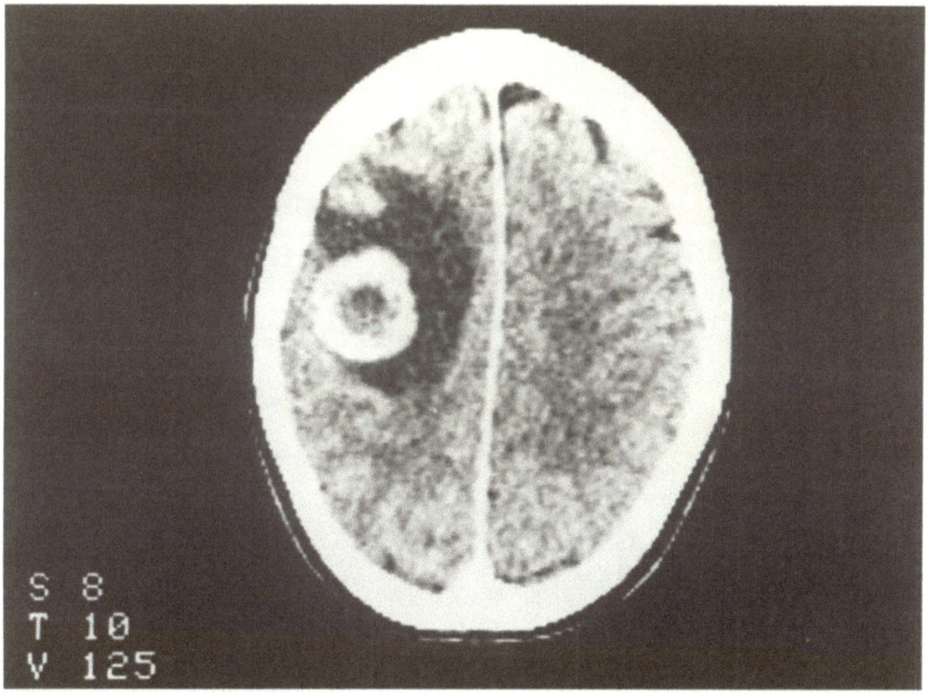

Fig. 1 CT-scan of a patient with a left fronto-parietal secondary.

tasis and perifocal oedema. Figure 2 shows the PET scans taken through the same plane. It can be seen that the rCBF, rOER and $rCMRO_2$ are lower in the region of the tumour and peritumour oedema than in the normal brain. It is evident from these PET scans that it is not easy to differentiate the region of the tumour from that of the surrounding oedema. This problem can be overcome by superimposing a conventional X-ray transmission CT scan taken through the same plane and defining the region of interest from the latter. From the quantitative data on patients with gliomas (grade III and IV) it can be seen that blood flow through tumour tissue is variable with a mean value lying close to that of contralateral white matter. The $rCMRO_2$ and rOER in every tumour studied was lower than that of corresponding normal brain. The rCBV was variable with considerable overlap with that of contralateral normal brain. These studies suggest that cerebral gliomas are overperfused in relation to their oxygen requirements. Studies involving the use of the glucose analogue ^{18}FDG have shown that in contrast to oxygen metabolism there appears to be no depression of the cerebral metabolic rate for glucose within tumour tissue [5]. In fact the values for the regional glucose extraction ratio were similar for both tumour and normal brain tissue. This metabolic uncoupling between $rCMRO_2$ and rCMRGlu is suggestive of a 'preferential' increase in glycolysis within cerebral tumours.

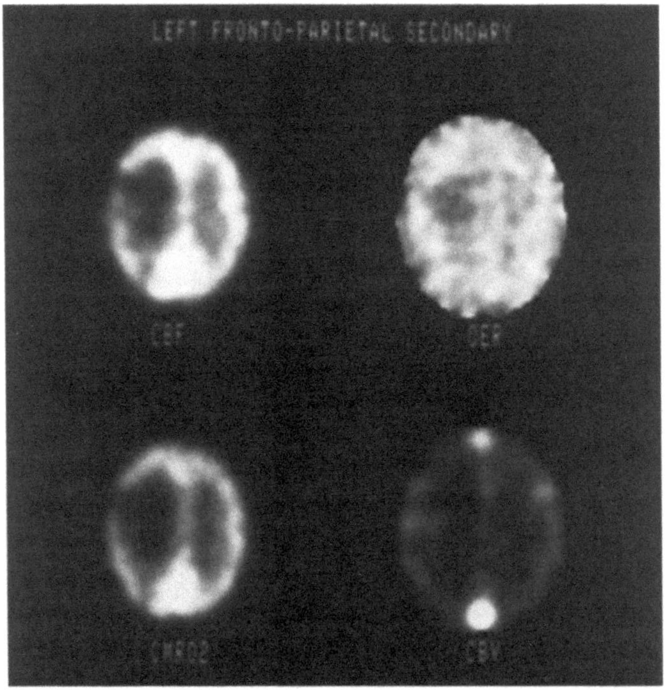

Fig. 2 PET scans of the same patient as in figure 1. The left side of the brain is on the left side of the image and the frontal lobe is at the top of the image. The CBF, OER and $CMRO_2$ are lower in the region of the tumour.

Effects of dexamethasone

Although dexamethasone is widely used for treating intracerebral oedema, its mode of action is not well understood. Apart from the local effects on oedema, more generalised effects have been reported on intracranial pressure and cerebral blood flow [12–16]. A direct action on the blood vessel wall has also been postulated [17, 18]. PET scans to measure rCBF (fig. 3), rOER, $rCMRO_2$ and rCBV (fig. 4) in patients with cerebral tumours both before and after treatment with dexamethasone have been carried out. Ten patients (seven secondaries, two astrocytomas and one lymphoma) were scanned twice. The interval between scans was 1–5 days and dexamethasone was given as a loading dose of 20 mg iv and thereafter 4 mg orally 4 times daily.

Subjectively all patients improved. No moderately or severely ill patients could be scanned because of technical limitations (the duration of one scanning procedure is about two hours).

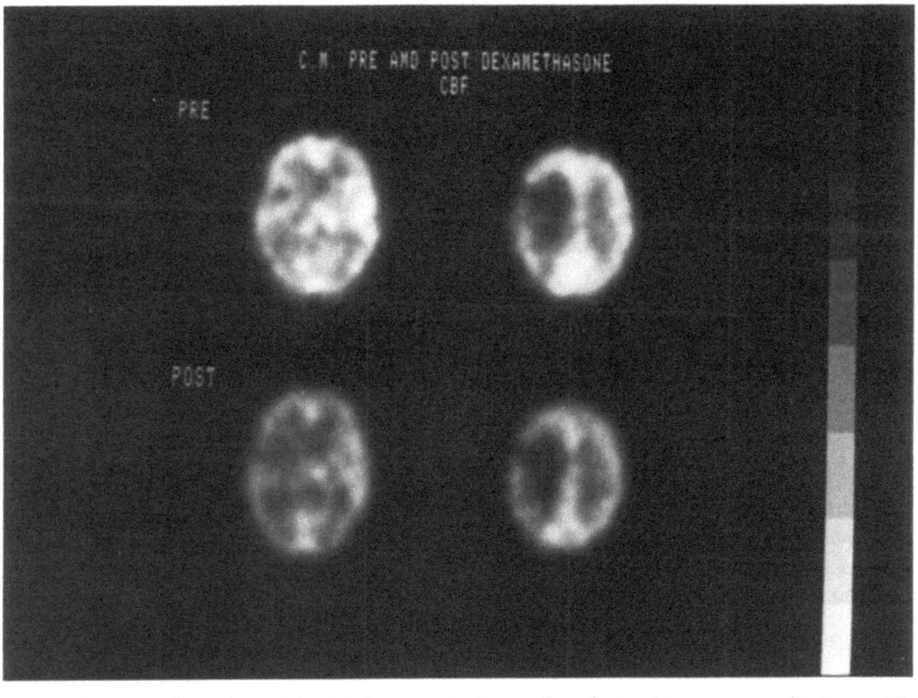

Fig. 3 The rCBF of a patient with a left frontoparietal secondary depicted in a tomographic image. The top of the image is the front of the brain. The left side of the brain is on the left side of the image. The image on the right side of the illustration is cutting through the tumour. The left hand side image is 2 cm lower. The grey scale is identical for all images. The higher the rCBF, the whiter the picture-element. After dexamethasone there is a diffuse decrease of rCBF.

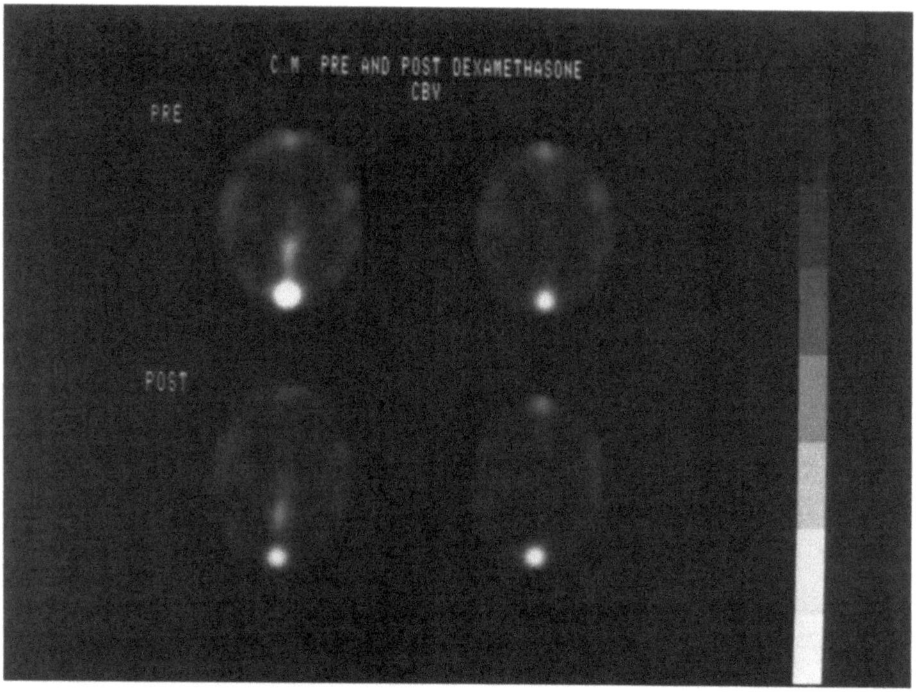

Fig. 4 The rCBV of the same patient as in figure 1. The blood volume decreases slightly in all regions after dexamethasone.

The scan results are summarised in table 1 and illustrated in the figures 1 and 2. Surprisingly the rCBF decreased after dexamethasone in all regions except in the oedematous territories. The $rCMRO_2$ generally decreased slightly or remained the same, accompanied by a regional slight increase in fractional oxygen extraction (rOER). There was a decrease in blood volume (rCBV) (fig. 4) in parallel with the decrease in rCBF (fig. 3) in the corresponding territories.

These results suggest that there is a direct diffuse influence of dexamethasone on the blood vessel wall resulting in both decreased blood flow and decreased rCBV. As the brain is a closed container of fluid, a reduction of rCBV may lead to decreased intracranial pressure with improvement of the clinical condition of the patient. The mechanisms by which dexamethasone acts on the blood vessel wall is thought to involve inhibition of the production of prostacyclin, a potent vasodilator, in the vascular endothelial cells [17].

A complicating factor in these measurements is the as yet unknown influence of dexamethasone on the extraction of water. Animal work has shown some decrease of permeability-surface (PS) product for water after administration of dexamethasone [19]. A big decrease of PS product in man would result in artefactually lower rCBF measurements. This has to be clarified before our data can be assessed properly.

Table 1 Effects of dexamethasone on brain. The values are the mean of 10 patients, without (pre) dexamethasone and after (post) 1–5 days of treatment. The samples of white matter and cortex are taken from the contralateral hemisphere. rCBF and $rCMRO_2$ are given as ml/100 ml tissue/min and rCBV as ml/100 ml tissue.

		Tumour	Edema	White	Cortex
rCBF	pre	20.8	14.5	20.1	38.5
	post	18.7	14.6	17.2	34.0
rOER	pre	30.6	43.7	39.5	43.8
	post	35.4	42.5	45.0	47.0
$rCMRO_2$	pre	1.12	1.11	1.60	3.03
	post	1.08	0.92	1.60	2.80
rCBV	pre	3.8	1.9	2.4	4.3
	post	3.0	1.6	2.1	3.8

Effects of craniotomy

Eight patients with brain tumours (six astrocytomas, one secondary and one meningioma) were scanned before craniotomy and again about one week afterwards. The mean values of the physiological data are summarised in table 2. Only samples from the cortex contralateral to the tumours are shown. The rCBF increased markedly after operations coupled with an increased rCBV. The oxygen utilisation improved after craniotomy, whereas the fractional oxygen extraction remained the same. The increase in oxygen utilisation did not correlate very well with the increase in rCBF. However, there was a tight correlation with the change in haemoglobin before and after craniotomy (fig. 5). The rCBF in these cases is therefore not only regulated by the demand for oxygen but also by the oxygen carrier capacity.

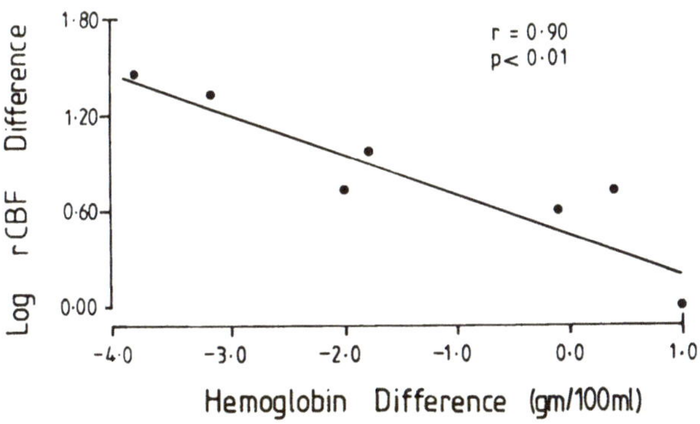

Fig. 5 The relationship between the differences of Hb and the log of the differences of rCBF before and after craniotomy.

Table 2 Effects of craniotomy on brain. The values are the mean of 8 patients before (pre) and after (post) craniotomy. The rCBF and $rCMRO_2$ are given as ml/100 ml tissue/min, rCBV ml/100 ml, and Hb as g/100 ml.

	pre	post
rCBF	27.8	37.6 ($p < 0.025$)
rOER	50.2	50.7
$rCMRO_2$	2.43	2.84 ($p < 0.025$)
rCBV	3.93	3.96
Hb	13.1	11.7 ($p < 0.05$)

Conclusions

These studies show that PET scanning is a useful method for investigating conditions such as cerebral tumours. Quantitative measurements can be made concerning the pathophysiology of brain tumours both before and after therapeutic intervention. In particular measurements of several different physiological values at one time can give increased insight into the metabolic state of brain tissue. Combining flow and oxygen utilization studies results in estimates of fractional oxygen extraction, an indicator of whether tissues are ischaemic or have a luxury perfusion. The combination of glucose and oxygen consumption gives an indication of whether aerobic or anaerobic metabolism is occuring. rCBF and rCBV measurement enables A-V shunting in tumours to be estimated. It is hoped that PET scanning will become a useful tool in assessing the effects of therapeutic intervention in cerebral tumours as well as leading to an increased insight into tumour metabolism.

References

[1] Frackowiak, R. J. S., G. L. Lenzi, T. Jones, et al.: Quantitative measurement of regional cerebral blood flow and oxygen metabolism in man using ^{15}O and positron emission tomograph: Theory, procedure, and normal values. J. Comput. Assist. Tomogr. **4** (1980) 727–736.

[2] Jones, T., D. A. Chesler, M. M. Ter-Pogossian: The continuous inhalation of oxygen-15 for assessing regional oxygen extraction in the brain of man. Brit. J. Radiol. **49** (1976) 339–343.

[3] Lammertsma, A. A., T. Jones, R. S. J. Frackowiak, et al.: A theoretical study of the steady-state model for measuring regional cerebral blood flow and oxygen utilisation using oxygen-15. J. Comput. Assist. Tomogr. **5** (1981) 544–550.

[4] Rhodes, C. G., R. J. S. Wise, J. M. Gibbs, et al.: *In vivo* disturbance of the oxidative metabolism of glucose in human cerebral gliomas. Annals of Neurology (in press).

[5] Ito, M., A. A. Lammertsma, R. J. S. Wise, et al.: Measurement of regional cerebral blood flow and oxygen utilisation in patients with cerebral tumours using ^{15}O and positron emission tomography: Analytical techniques and preliminary results. Neuroradiology **23** (1982) 63–74.

[6] Lammertsma, A. A., T. Jones: The correction for the presence of intravascular oxygen-15 in the steady state technique for measuring regional oxygen extraction ratio in the brain: 1. Description of the method. J. Cereb. Blood Flow. Metabol. **3** (1983 a) 416–424.

[7] Lammertsma, A. A., R. J. S. Wise, J. D. Heather, et al.: The correction for the presence of intravas-

cular oxygen-15 in the steady-state technique for measuring regional oxygen extraction ratio in the brain: 2. Results in normal subjects and brain tumour and stroke patients. J. Cereb, Blood Flow Metabol. **3** (1983 b) 425–431.

[8] Phelps, M. E., S.-C. Huang, E. J. Hoffman, et al.: Validation of tomographic measurement of cerebral blood volume with C-11 labeled carboxy-hemoglobin. J. Nucl. Med. **20** (1978) 328–334.

[9] Phelps, M. E., S.-C. Huang, E. J. Hoffman, et al.: Tomographic measurement of local cerebral glucose metabolic rate in humans with (F-18) 2-fluoro-2-deoxy-D-glucose: validation of method. Ann. Neurol. **6** (1979) 371–388.

[10] Huang, S.-C., M. E. Phelps, E. J. Hoffman, et al.: Noninvasive determination of local cerebral metabolic rate of glucose in man. Am. J. Physiol. **238** (1980) E69–E82.

[11] Crane, P. D., W. M. Pardridge, L. D. Braun, et al.: Kinetics of transport and phosphorylation of 2-Fluoro-2-Deoxy-D-Glucose in rat brain. J. Neurochem. **40** (1983) 160–176.

[12] Alberti, E., A. Hartmann, H.-D. Schirtz, et al.: The effect of large doses of dexamethasone on the cerebrospinal fluid pressure in patients with supratentorial tumours. J. Neurol. **217** (1978) 173–181.

[13] Brock, M., H. Wiegand, C. Zillig, et al.: The effect of dexamethasone on intracranial pressure in patients with supratentorial tumours. In: Dynamics of brain edema (H.M. Pappius, W. Feindel, eds.), pp. 330–336. Springer-Verlag, Berlin–Heidelberg–New York 1976.

[14] Buttinger, C., A. Hartmann, R. von Kummer, et al.: The effect of high doses of dexamethasone on cerebral blood flow in patients with cerebral tumours. In: Treatment of cerebral edema (A. Hartmann, M. Brock, eds.), pp. 132–138. Springer-Verlag, Berlin–Heidelberg 1982.

[15] Hossman, K.-A., M. Blöink: Blood flow and regulation of blood flow in experimental peritumoral edema. Stroke **12** (2) (1982) 211–217.

[16] Reulen, H.J., A. Hadjidimos, K. Schürmann: The effect of dexamethasone on water and electrolyte content and on rCBF in perifocal brain edema in man. In: Steroids and brain edema (H. J. Reulen, K. Schürmann, eds.), pp. 239–252. Springer-Verlag, Berlin–Heidelberg–New York 1972.

[17] Axelrod, L.: Inhibition of prostacyclin production mediates permissive effect of glucocortocoids on vascular tone. Lancet i (1983) 904–906.

[18] Altura, B. M.: Role of glucocorticoids on local regulation of blood flow. Am. J. Physiol. **211** (1966) 1393–1397.

[19] Reid, A. C., G. M. Teasdale, J. McCulloch: The effects of dexamethasone administration and withdrawal on water permeability across the Blood-Brain-Barrier. Ann. Neurol. **13** (1983) 28–31.

Remarks on the follow-up of cerebellar astrocytomas (Brief communication)

A. Ferbert, F. Gullotta

The so-called astrocytoma of the cerebellum is a benign tumour and essentially different in its biology from the astrocytoma of the cerebral hemispheres. To operate is the method of choice. However, it is controversial whether a further treatment by irradiation or chemotherapy could improve the outcome.

To analyse this problem more fully a retrograde study in 105 patients operated on between 1950–1972 for a cerebellar astrocytoma has been made. No data were available for nine patients, incomplete data for the periods between 5 months and 12 years for 7 patients. For 89 patients complete histories were available. 45 patients died within the first three months p.o. 32 patients were still alive of whom 14 patients were operated on 20–30 years ago and 18 patients 10–19 years ago. In 12 patients having succumbed 3 months after operation, six died of recurrence of tumour. Irradiated p.o. were only 7 patients of whom 5 died. In 26 cases the tumour had infiltrated the brain stem and only 7 patients survived the operation. However, two patients are still alive after 25 resp. 10 years.

Conclusions

1. Patients operated for a localized cerebellar astrocytoma can be considered to be cured and irradiation and chemotherapy are not indicated.
2. In case the tumour has transgressed the border of the cerebellum and has infiltrated the brain stem, a survival period of over 20 years after partial resection seems possible.
3. 'Successes' of radio- and chemotherapy have to be evaluated against this background.

Cerebral cysticercosis – a contribution to the differential diagnosis of supratentorial and infratentorial gliomas

D. Voth, E. Polar Salinas, J. Bohl

Introduction

In this interesting form of cysticercosis with its cerebral manifestations man serves as the intermediate host. The infestation results from the ingestion of eggs of the pork tape-worm with unwashed or insufficiently washed vegetables, by transmission with the hands as a result of inadequate personal hygiene, by consumption of contaminated water or other foodstuffs. The living embryo is released after digestion of its covering by the gastric juices, penetrates the gastro-intestinal mucosa and is conveyed by the blood stream to the various tissues and organs of the host, where it becomes quiescent and transformed into a cyst. It reaches its full size as a larva in 2–3 months. In man these larvae (cysticercus cellulosae) are found mainly in the central nervous system (CNS), in the eyes and in the muscles [9, 17, 19, 21].

Even though cysticercosis has largely disappeared from Europe at the present time, there is a very considerable, but nevertheless falling, morbidity in India, Africa, in the Far East and above all in the Latin-American countries. Having regard to the slightly less typical clinical picture [24, 29] and especially as we have the impression that there is a definite change in the form of the malady, it seemed worth while to present a communication on this topic, especially as the clinical picture of cysticercosis is able to imitate absolutely the symptoms of a space-occupying lesion produced by a tumour [30, 40].

Pathology of cysticercosis

Even with the falling morbidity, the incidence of the cerebral form among tumour patients in the neurosurgical clinics in Peru, Chile or Mexico, still shows a figure of between 1.3% and a maximum of up to 25% in Mexico, for instance. If infestation occurs in man as the intermediate host, the CNS will be involved in up to 82% of the cases.

Whereas in the past the size of the parasite in the CNS was usually given as 6–14 mm (cyst diameter), with the size occasionally up to 50 mm, the occurrence of a giant form [8, 33] (giant cystic parasitosis) has been observed in Peru particularly, but also to an increasing extent in Chile and Bolivia, with a diameter up to 8 cm and a maximum volume of 268 ml (fig. 1). The occurrence of this form has been described in Peru since 1975. The reasons for this change in the pattern of the disease are not, as yet, definitely known.

The following forms of cysticercosis are distinguished (tab. 1):
1. The cystic form with multiple cysts, whitish in appearance and about the size of a pea, situated in the pia and the white matter (parenchymatous form with single or multiple cysts, fig. 2).
2. The racemose form, frequently found in the basal cisterns, with spread into the posterior fossa. There is a grape-like growth with development of multilocular, usually small, cysts (fig. 3).

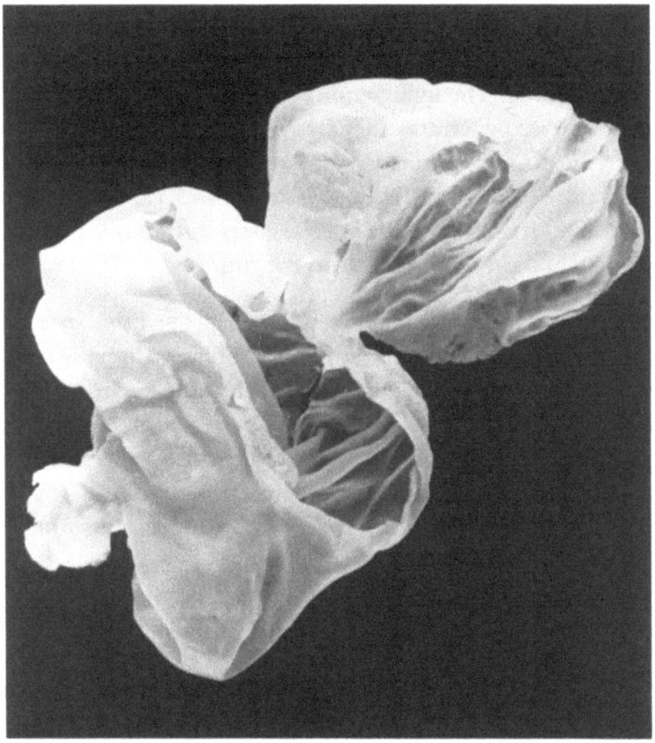

Fig. 1 Macroscopic view of a cerebral cysticercus cellulosae (Giant cystic cysticercosis) from the parietal lobe of a 34-year-old woman. The cyst wall has been opened transversely. Note the large cystic bladder with a thin irregulary folded wall and a firm small nodule at one side (left). Microscopically this nodule contains degenerated parts of the parasite with many calcifications. Operation specimen, fixed with formalin.

Table 1 Survey of the various forms of cysticercosis. The general distribution of the various manifestations present quite marked differences. Thus, in Poland, Mexico and South America one finds the meningeal type and the intraventricular forms, more frequently for instance, than in India, where the parenchymatous form is the most frequently described.

1. Meningeal, racemose form
2. Parenchymatous form, with single or multiple cysts in the white matter
3. Intraventricular form. Usually solitary
4. Mixed forms

3. "Giant cystic cysticercosis" with a preferential location in the cerebral white matter and subcortical region.
4. The intraventricular form, which occurs not only in the lateral ventricle but also in the fourth ventricle.

Whether the meningo-encephalitic form described by Chandy and Isaiah [5] represents a separate type is not certain.

All the same, numerous reactions to the parasitic infestation are found in the CNS, so that for instance in the brain tissue there are signs of ganglion cell damage and an astrocytic reaction. The vascular system reacts with perivascular infiltrates, sometimes with a panangiitis or endangiitis. Not uncommonly in the ependyma as well as in the meninges we find granulomatous inflammatory changes resembling a chronic leptomeningitis, often with eosinophilic infiltration (tab. 2).

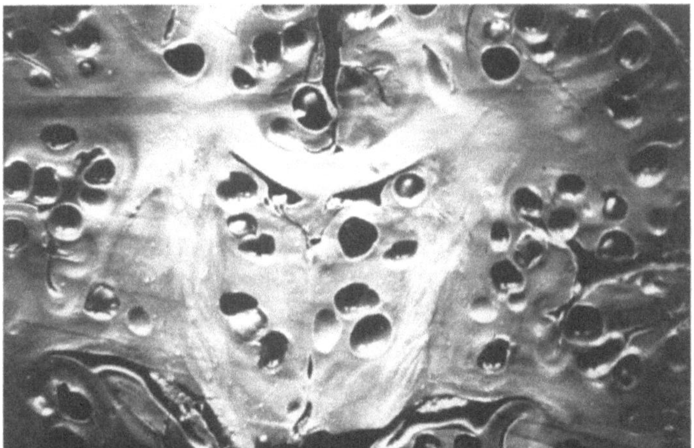

Fig. 2 Cerebral cysticercosis (parenchymatous form) with multiple, relatively small cysts, which are scattered in the white matter and the cortex. Operation has nothing to offer in these cases. (Autopsy specimen.)

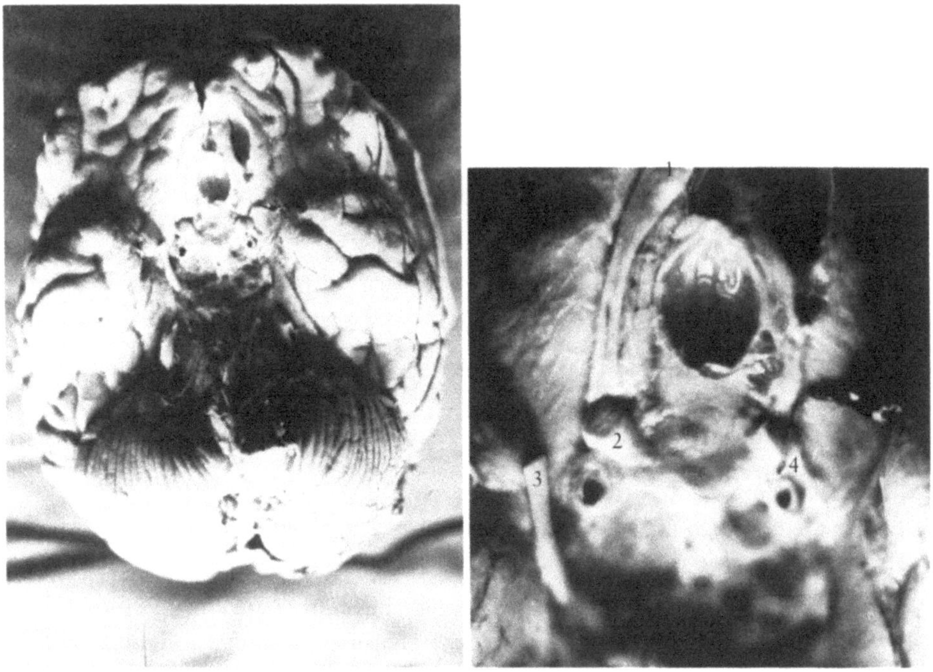

Fig. 3 a) The base of the brain with chiasmal cysticercosis. This was a pretty typical manifestation (meningeal racemose form) which is responsible for the visual disturbances.
b) Detail from Fig. 3a. The thikened and fibrosed leptomeninx can be seen with solitary cysticerci. 1 = Right olfactory nerve, 2 = Right optic nerve, 3 = Right oculomotor nerve, 4 = Left internal carotid artery.

Figures 4–6 demonstrate the histological appearance und the ultrastructure of the bladder wall (Cysticercus racemosus). Ref.: W. J. Brown, M. Voge: Neuropathology of parasitic infections. Oxford, New York, Toronto: Oxford University Press 1982.

Symptoms of cerebral cysticercosis

The clinical picture [3, 7, 10, 16, 25, 26, 28, 35, 38] has already been classically described, so that apart from headaches, which are often localised in the region of large cysts, there are unspecific manifestations such as giddiness, nausea and vomiting, which taken together convey the impression of raised intracranial pressure. Symptomatic epilepsy is very frequent, rarely with generalized convulsions, but more often with focal attacks [2, 6, 39, 41]. Neurological deficits with unilateral motor or sensory signs may not present for a long time and are often completely absent. Most conspicuous are the psychic changes, with depression, flight of ideas, suicidal remarks, which however are never actually realised, and in addition increased irritability and aggression.

Table 2 The morbid anatomical findings are very diverse and include all the variations described (after Tandon [38])

Morbid anatomical findings in cysticercosis
1. Meningoencephalitis
2. Granulomatous meningitis
3. Focal granuloma (aseptic abscess!)
4. Internal hydrocephalus, communicating or obstructive
5. Ependymitis
6. Arteritis

It must already be apparent that these symptoms can resemble completely the clinical picture of a supratentorial glioma. The "giant cystic cysticercosis" progresses for the most part with the pattern of an increasing space-occupation and shows the clinical picture of a unilateral circumscribed tumour with signs of cerebral compression.

With the intraventricular type the entire clinical picture is usually determined by the presence of an obstructive hydrocephalus and in this case a posterior fossa glioma may well be considered, but the absence of any cerebellar deficits can give a hint as to the true character of the illness. On the other hand, lesions of the ninth or tenth cranial nerves can develop in association with cysticercosis [10].

A fairly typical clinical picture is produced by involvement of the cisterna magna. This can include paresthesiae (formication), psychic changes, increased aggression, lesions of the lower cranial nerves, bilateral pyramidal signs, motor disturbances and impairment of vision as a result of obstructive hydrocephalus.

The course of the disease is rarely very acute. As a rule the patient has been complaining for several months before coming under medical treatment. Of course, the special features of the Latin-American countries certainly play an additional rôle here.

Diagnosis of cysticercosis

When confronted with such a pattern of complaints and neurological signs, it is rarely possible to distinguish cysticercosis from a space-occupying neoplasm [24, 29]. Radiographs of the skull may give the first hint with evidence of calcified parasites, although these are by no means always seen. Echo-encephalography may sometimes reveal large cysts, as well as marked internal hydrocephalus.

The electroencephalogram (EEG) is often pathological, more often with focal findings, but less often with generalized changes. Space-taking cysts may be indirectly apparent in the angiogram because of an avascular area.

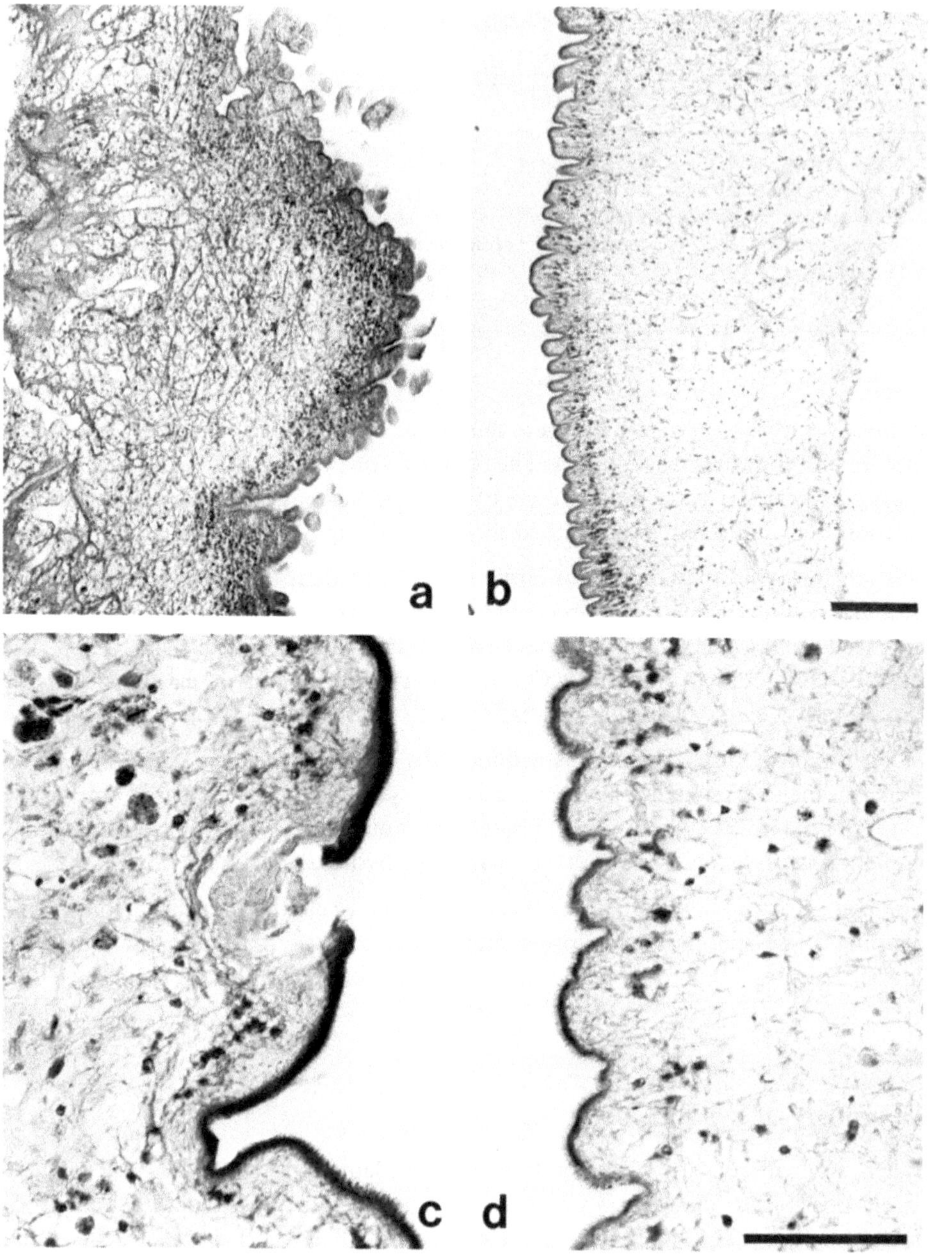

Fig. 4 Transverse sections through the bladder wall of racemose form of Cysticercus.
At a lower magnification (a, b) the wall shows three distinct layers: A markedly convoluted outer layer with a dense membrane, a small zone with many rounded dark bodies and a thick layer, consisting of loose connective tissue with a lot of fibrils. At a higher magnification (c, d) numerous microvilli can be detected at the surface. At some places the outer membrane is interrupted by an outlet of a special submembraneous organelle of the bladder wall. Paraffin embedding: a) van Gieson staining; b–d) HE staining. The scale bar represents in a) and b) 100 μm and 50 μm in c) + d).

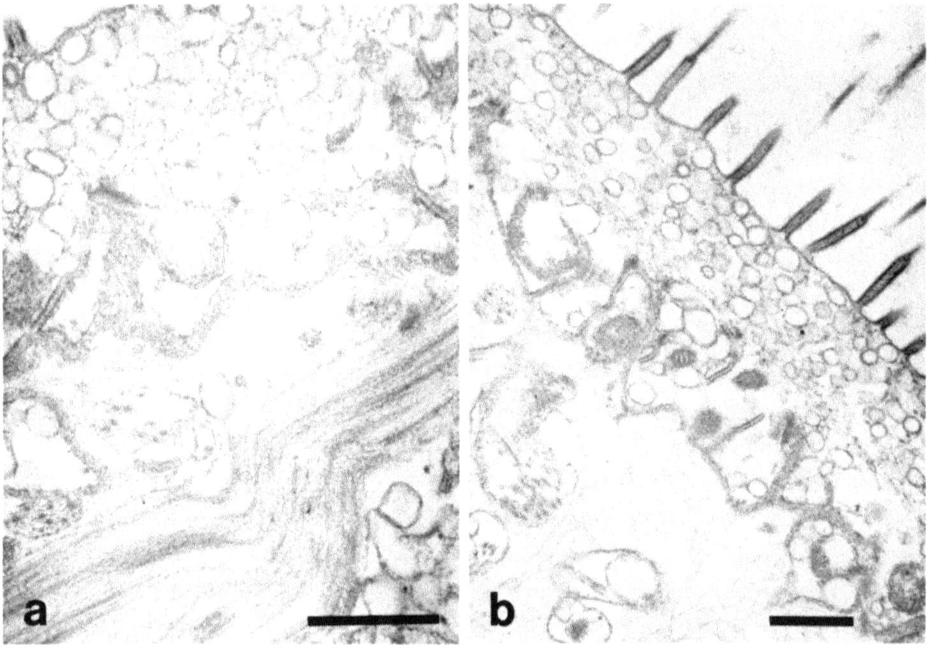

Fig. 5 Ultrastructure of the outer layer of the bladder wall of a Cysticercus racemosus. Note the microvilli-like processes at the surface and the vesicular structure of the dense superficial membrane. The tissue beneath often contains a lot of fibrils and fibres. Embedding in Epoxy resin; photographs were taken with a Philips EM 301. The scale bar in a. and b. represents 0,5 μm.

Pneumoencephalography is playing a diminishing rôle, even in Latin America and in view of its complications this is to be welcomed.

The introduction of computer tomography has produced real progress [13, 37] and in many instances it can confirm the diagnosis. It should be mentioned that isotope scintigraphy is, as a rule, of no value in the diagnosis of cysticercosis. Laboratory investigations can also give additional hints. The CSF shows a pleocytosis, in which case one often finds a few eosinophil cells, also an increase in the total protein and a positive complement fixation reaction to the specific antibody.

Distinguishing cysticercosis from the various sorts of glioma no longer causes any difficulties since the introduction of computer tomography, especially as the finest calcification from multiple parasites is very well shown. Anyway, the diagnosis of the distinctive large cysts from the solitary lesion of a tumour presents no problems. Superficial consideration of a "giant cystic cysticercosis" may mimic a cystic tumour, but the differential diagnosis should pose no difficulties to the experienced.

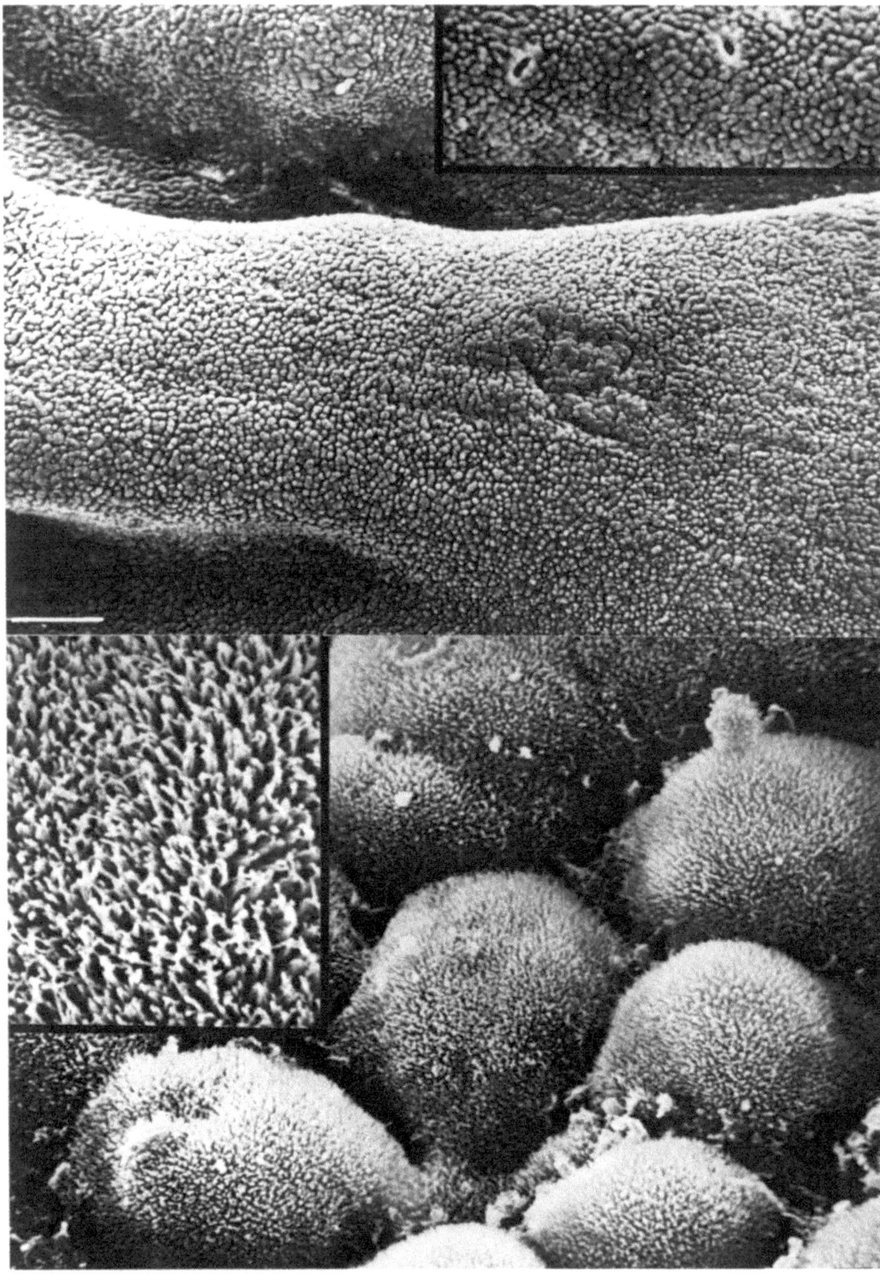

Fig. 6 Scanning electron microscopic view of the outer surface of a Cysticercus racemosus bladder in various magnifications.
The upper view shows big folds of the bladder wall with two openings in the outer layer (see inset!) for small outlets of special organelles. The view below shows small mountain-like protuberances at a higher magnification with many microvilli at the surface (see inset!). The scale bar in the upper figure represents 500 μm (white). The black scale bar below represents 5 μm.

The treatment of cerebral cysticercosis

It should be said that while *chemotherapy* with Praziquantel has shown some successes, it is not however adequate on its own for the treatment of cerebral cysticercosis. Apart from specific chemotherapy the administration of corticosteroids has proved of value. In many cases treatment with Prednisolone has been successful in avoiding an operation and definitely improving the patient's condition. According to our experience in the neurosurgical department at Santa Toribio de Mogrovejo in Lima (Peru) one should start with a daily dose of 40–80 mg intravenously. The subsequent treatment should proceed as follows – 0.5 mg Prednisolone/kg body weight, twice daily in the first two weeks, once daily in the third and fourth weeks, then in the fifth and sixth weeks two or three times weekly and finally once weekly for a further twelve weeks. Throughout the general condition shows a rapid and decisive improvement and even the specific signs and symptoms are favorably affected. Nevertheless relapses do occur.

Surgical treatment is indicated for racemose cysticercosis in the cisterna magna and the fourth ventricle, also in isolated "giant cysts", where sometimes two or more cysts can be successfully removed. Intraventricular cysts can be removed by a transventricular approach. Purely symptomatic treatment includes putting in a ventriculo-atrial shunt or a ventriculo-peritoneal shunt for obstructive hydrocephalus which cannot be dealt with immediately.

Discussion

The management of cysticercus has undergone such a transformation, that the morbidity figures are definitely falling. This has resulted from an improvement in hygiene and through education of the population even in the Latin-American countries, where it still occurs relatively frequently. In spite of this it is still necessary for every neurosurgeon in these regions to consider cysticercosis in the differential diagnosis of space-occupying lesions, as the clinical picture of cerebral cysticercosis and of an intrinsic brain tumour, is often identical [15, 38].

Treatment with praziquantel [4, 20, 37, 42] and corticosteroids [23, 38] can influence the condition of the patient very positively. It has become apparent over the years that surgical intervention is not necessary in many cases and in these circumstances may be even longer avoided. In the meantime, as a palliative measure, it is often enough to implant a shunt system to treat a possible developing obstructive hydrocephalus [14].

The basal form of cysticercosis with marked arachnoid thickening, especially in the chiasmal region with its consequent visual impairment, is still not surgically rewarding. The formerly quite rare, pure intracentricular cysticerci which arise mostly from the choroid plexus are easily accessible [24, 31, 32] by a transventricular approach. The same holds true for cysticercosis of the fourth ventricle and the cisterna magna which is easily through a suboccipital craniotomy [1, 11, 18, 22].

The "giant cystic cysticercosis" [8, 33] which apparently has become more frequent in recent years, are worth exploring, if the cysts are easily accessible and can be removed with their membranes, without causing further damage. As these cysts are sometimes found in the Sylvian fissure or the medial longitudinal fissure, removal is then possible without any problems.

It seems likely in the future that, by education of the population and a general improvement in hygienic conditions, cysticercosis will disappear, even in Latin America as it already has for a long time in Europe. Nevertheless at the present time the achievement of this possibility still poses many difficulties.

Summary

In spite of a general fall in the morbidity, cerebral cysticercosis in Latin America shows a certain change in its presentation, with the appearance of a "giant cystic cysticercosis" which previously occurred infrequently, or not at all.

While the clinical picture can completely mimic a space-occupying neoplasm, the differential diagnosis should now present no problems with the help of computer tomography.

Meanwhile, conservative treatment with Praziquantel and corticosteroids has produced some favourable results. Surgical intervention is necessary in the case of "giant cystic cysticercosis", the rare, purely intraventricular cysts, as well as those involving the cisterna magna and the fourth ventricle. Operation is less successful for the basal type in the chiasmal region, or with multiple small cysts which may be distributed over the whole brain. Palliative measures for treatment of an obstructive hydrocephalus are quite frequently necessary.

The results of treatment by these combined procedures are encouraging.

References

[1] Adelstein, L.J.: Cysticercus cyst of fourth ventricle with surgical removal. J. nerv. ment. Dis. **92** (1940) 623–629.

[2] Arseni, C., A. Cristensen: Epilepsy due to cerebral cysticercosis. Epilepsia **13** (1972) 253–258.

[3] Asenjo, A., E. Rocca: Compromiso de los lares craneanos en la cisticercosis cerebral. Rev. méd. Chile **74** (1946) 605–612.

[4] Botero, D., S. Castaño: Treatment of cysticercosis with praziquantel in Colombia. Am. J. Trop. Med. Hyg. **31** (1982) 811–821.

[5] Chandy, J., P. Isaiah: Clinical manifestation of cysticercosis of the brain. Indian J. Surg. **14** (1952) 53–56.
[6] Chopra, J. S., U. Kaur, R. C. Mahajan: Cysticercosis and epilepsy: a clinical and serological study. Trans. R. Soc. Trop. Med. Hyg. **75** (1981) 518–520.
[7] Flisser, A., I. Bulnes, M. L. Diaz, et al.: Estudio seroepidemiologico de la cysticercosis humana en poblociones predominantemeute indigenas y rurales del Estado de Chiapas. Arch. Invest. Med. **7** (1976) 107–133.
[8] Franco-Ponce, J., J. Urquiaga: Giant cystic parasitosis of the nervous system. Neurol. Surg., p. 30. Thieme, Stuttgart, New York 1981.
[9] Fuller, G. A., P. van Dellen, jur., J. C. Tyrell: Inadvertently self-induced cerebral cysticercosis. A. Afr. Med. J. **62** (1982) 591.
[10] Grisolia, J. S., W. C. Wiederholt: CNS cysticercosis. Arch. Neurol. **39** (1982) 540–544.
[11] Jankowski, R. et al.: Cysticercosis presenting as a mass lesion at the foramen of Monro. J. Comput. Assist. Tomogr. **3** (1979) 694–696.
[12] Kean, J. R.: Neuro-ophthalmologic signs and symptoms of cysticercosis. Arch. Ophthalmol. **100** (1982) 1445–1448.
[13] Lamas, E., J. Estevez, M. Sato, et al.: Computerized axial tomography for the diagnosis of cerebral cysticercosis. Acta neurochir. **44** (1978) 197–205.
[14] Lobato, R. D., E. Lamas, J. M. Portillo, et al.: Hydrocephalus in cerebral cysticercosis. Pathogenic and therapeutic considerations. J. Neurosurg. **55** (1981) 786–793.
[15] López, L. N., L. Rodriguez: Neurocysticercosis: Radiological and surgical aspects. Neurol. Surg., p. 30. Thieme, Stuttgart, New York 1981.
[16] López-Hernández, A., C. Garaizar: Childhood cerebral cysticercosis: clinical features and computed tomographic findings in 89 Mexican children. Can. J. Neurol. Sci. **9** (1982) 401–407.
[17] Lorentz, I. T.: A case of spinal cysticercosis. Clin. exp. Neurol. **15** (1978) 85–91.
[18] Madrazo, I., J. A. Carcia Renteria, J.A. Maldonado, et al.: Intraventricular cysticercosis. Neurol. Surg., p. 29. Thieme, Stuttgart, New York 1981.
[19] Mann, I.: Integrated multidisciplinary environmental approach to the study of taeniasis and echinococcosis. Ann. Ist. Super. Sanita. **14** (1978) 235–244.
[20] Markus, M. B.: Treatment of cerebral cysticercosis. Arch. Neurol. **40** (1983) 392.
[21] Mattos-Pimenta, A., P. Brandt-Martinez: Die tierischen Parasiten und Pilzinfektionen im zentralen Nervensystem. In: Hdb. Neurochir. Vol. IV/1, pp. 673–773. Springer-Verlag, Berlin–Göttingen–Heidelberg 1960.
[22] Milenković, Z., G. Penev, P. Stojanovic, et al.: Cysticercosis cerebri involving the lateral ventricle. Surg. Neurol. **18** (1982) 94–96.
[23] Minguetti, G., M. V. Ferreira: Acao de corticóides na fase aguda da neurosisticercose: nota preliminar. Arg. Neuropsiquiatr. **40** (1982) 77–85.
[24] Misra, R. C., M. P. Shrivastava, V. Saxena: Cerebral cysticercosis (A profile of two cases). J. Assoc. Physicians India. **30** (1982) 163–164.
[25] Obrador Alcalde, S.: Clinical aspects of cysticercosis. Arch. Neurol. Psychiat. **59** (1948) 457–468.
[26] Obrador Alcalde, S.: Parasitosis del encéfalo (revisioń clinica de 41 casos de cisticercosis e hidatidosis). Acta neurol. lat.-amer. **1** (1955) 35–45.
[27] Oscar Colli, B.: Surgical treatment of neurocysticercosis. Gac. Med. Max. **117** (1981) 251–257.
[28] Percy, A. K., S. E. Nyrd, G.E. Locke: Cerebral cysticercosis. Paediat. **66** (1980) 967–971.
[29] Pinto Pupo, P., J. B. Dol Reis: Evolucão favoravel de um caso de cisticercose cerebral observado durante 10 anos. Arch. Neuro-psiquiat. (São Paulo) **12** (1954) 267–271.
[30] Popper, H., G. Bertha, G. F. Walter, et al.: CNS cysticercosis – a problem of differential diagnosis. Arch. Psychiat. Nervenkr. **23** (1982) 369–374.
[31] Rocca, E., E. Monteagudo: Tratamiento quirúrgico en la neurocisticercosis racemosa Bol. Acad. Perú Cir. **6** (1953) 34–38.
[32] Rocca, E., E. Monteagudo: Neurocisticercosis racemosa y su conducta quirúrgica. Rev. méd. Hosp. Obrero (Lima) **3** (1954) 141–146.
[33] Rocca, E. D., U. F. Rocca: Unusual forms of cerebral cysticercosis, clinical and angiographic. Presentation of two cases. Neurol. Surg., p. 30. Thieme, Stuttgart–New York 1981.
[34] Rodriguez, J. C., R. A. Gutierrez, O. D. Valdies, et al.: The role of computed axial tomography in

the diagnosis and treatment of brain imflammatory and parasitic lesions. Our experience in Mexico. Neuroradiology **16** (1978) 458–461.
[35] Shanley, J. D., M. C. Jordan: Clinical aspects of CNS cysticercosis. Arch. Intern. Med. **14** (1980) 1309–1313.
[36] Skromme-Kadlubik, G., C. Celis, A. Ferez: Cysticercosis of the nervous system: Treatment by means of specific internal radiation. Arch. Neurol. **38** (1981) 288.
[37] Spina-Franca, A., J. P. Nobrega, J. A. Livramento, et al.: Administration of praziquantel in neurocysticercosis. Tropenmed. Parasitol. **33** (1982) 1–4.
[38] Tandon, P. N.: Cerebral cysticercosis. Neurosurg. Rev. **6** (1983) 119–127.
[39] Tolosa, E., P. Fuenmayor: Experiencia neuroquirurgica sobre la epilepsia por cisticercosis cerebral. Rev. clin. esp. **66** (1957) 21–30.
[40] Vijayan, G. P., S. Venkataraman: The syndrome of raised intracranial pressure without localising neurological signs: an analysis of 68 cases. J. Assoc. Physicians India. **30** (1982) 521–526.
[41] de Villiers, J. C.: Cysticercosis of the nervous system. S. Afr. Med. J. **63** (1983) 769–772.
[42] Zhu, D. Y., H. L. Sun, W. C. Xu, et al.: Clinical evaluation of Biltricide (Praziquantel) in cysticercosis cellulosae. Chung Kuo I Hsueh Ko Hsueh Yuan Hsueh Pao **4** (1982) 220–223.
[43] Zülch, K. J.: In: Handbuch Neurochirurgie, Vol. III., pp. 590–594, "Zystizerken" (Cysticercus cellulosae). Springer-Verlag, Berlin–Göttingen–Heidelberg 1956.

Acknowledgements

I would like here to express my thanks for the kind hospitality of my Peruvian collegues, whom I was pleased to meet in Lima in 1982!

D. V.

We are indebted to Prof. Dr. R. Wagner, Department of Pathology, J. Gutenberg-University Mainz, for his scanning electron microscopic investigation of the bladder wall of a Cysticercus racemosus.

Measurement of intracranial pressure. Technique and indications

M. Schwarz, G. Keßel, E. Mahlmann, D. Voth

Introduction

The anatomical position of the soft tissues of the brain within the skull is important in relation to its pathophysiology, particularly when one considers that after the closure of the sutures it is virtually enclosed in a rigid, unyielding box. As the skull cavity contains incompressible fluid, it follows that any fluctuation in the intracranial volume, which can no longer be adjusted by compensatory movements of the fluid contents, must lead to changes in the intracranial pressure. In primary diseases of the central nervous system such effects on the intracranial volume relationships are, of course, the rule.

With intracranial space-occupying lesions caused by tumours, the patient is not endangered so much by the primary disturbances of neurological function as by the slowly developing rise of intracranial pressure. In comparison a disturbance of the CSF pathways produced by a tumour leads to a generalised increase in intracranial volume, as is so frequently found with tumours in the midline, the posterior fossa and the ventricular cavities.

The intracranial pressure in living patients was measured in the cerebrospinal cavity for the first time by Quinke and von Bergmann [13] by lumbar puncture. In a patient with communicating hydrocephalus they recorded a pressure of 37 mm Hg through a lumbar needle. In 1951 the continuous pressure recording used by Guillaume and Janny [9] finally standardized the method of Lundberg [11] for clinical use.

At the present time we have basically two different methods available for the measurement of pressure, or tension [3, 4, 7, 10, 14, 15, 18]. Firstly, external measurement of the fluid pressure which is conducted through suitable tubing from the cerebrospinal space to an external pressure recorder, or secondly the direct measurement of pressure by means of a pressure transducer implanted in the intracranial cavity.

Methods

The measurement of the intraventricular fluid pressure.

A burr-hole is made at the level of the coronal suture about 2.5–3 cm from the midline on the side of the non-dominant hemisphere and a plastic catheter is introduced into the frontal horn of the lateral ventricle. After fixation of the catheter it is connected through a three-way tap to a Statham-element and a drainage reservoir in the by-pass. The transducer conducts the analogue of the recorded pressure to the display, through a connector. This connector can then be plugged in to a two-channel writer which displays the pressure with a predetermined paper speed (fig. 1).

Alternatively the pressure can be measured by using an epidural pressure recorder. In present day clinical practice the gaeltec* miniature recorder [6, 7, 8] is generally used (Fig. 2). The actual recorder, with a membrane on one side is 6 mm long, 4 mm wide and 1.5 mm thick. This flattened piriform design discourages any rotation in the long axis. The membrane lies on the dura. The attached lead is flexible, electronically screened and tension proof. It can be inserted through a burr-hole or it can be put in after a craniotomy in the same way that one would insert a drain. The lead can then be brought out to the manometer through the wound or else through a laterally placed stab wound. At the conclusion of the recordings the instrument is pulled out just like a drain.

Continuous recording by either of these methods not only provides reliable values for the basal and mean pressures, but can also show a series of so-called pressure waves of typical pattern. According to their amplitude and frequency these are classified as 'A'-plateau waves, and 'B' waves or 'R' waves. The appearance of these waves is important in postoperative monitoring and control of treatment [1, 2, 6, 16, 18].

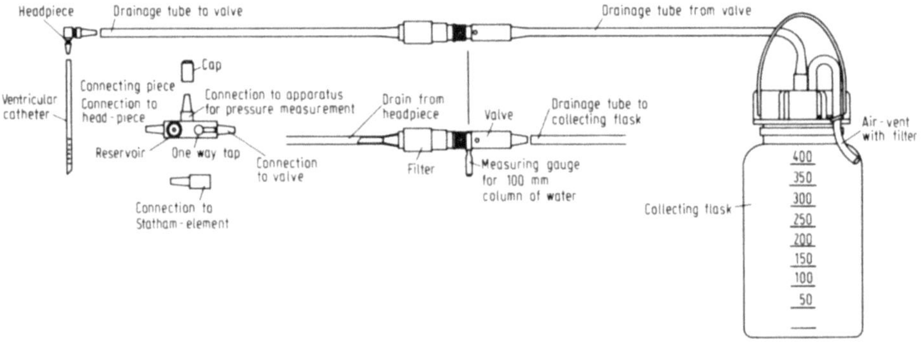

Fig. 1 Diagrammatic representation of a system for the measurement of ventricular pressure.

* Gaeltec, produced by Gaeltec and Co., Dunvegan, Isle of Skye, Scotland.

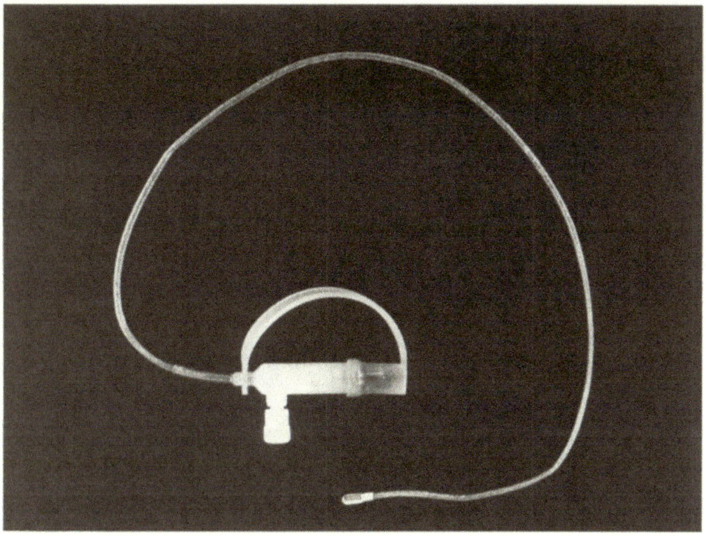

Fig. 2 Gaeltec miniature pressure recorder for epidural measurements.

Indications and complications

The development of increased intracranial pressure with tumours, depends first of all on their speed of growth and/or the development of perifocal edema. Even quite large tumours with marked midline shifts but minimal edema and no obstruction of the CSF pathways show only a slightly raised average pressure, whereas tumours with massive perifocal edema or disturbance of the fluid circulation can quickly cause decompensation. Hence, there is very rarely any definite or absolute indication pre-operatively for measurement of intracranial pressure. However, an exception does exist if the tumour is causing disturbance of the CSF pathways. With obstructive hydrocephalus produced by a tumour, measurement of ventricular pressure with simultaneous drainage is always indicated pre-operatively [15]. This is particularly the case with tumours of the posterior fossa (fig. 3) or midline tumours (fig. 4). As the measurement of the intraventricular pressure involves an invasive method, one must be aware of possible complications:

1. The necessity of opening the dura and penetrating the brain parenchyma in order to reach the ventricular system.
2. The danger of infection as a result of opening the dura.
3. The danger of undesirable loss of fluid as a result of the drainage tubing becoming detached.

A further definite disadvantage is that, because of the fear of a possible separation of the drain, the mobility of the patient and possibly also nursing measures are made more difficult. The risk of infection is quoted in the literature as 2%–19.6% [6, 10,

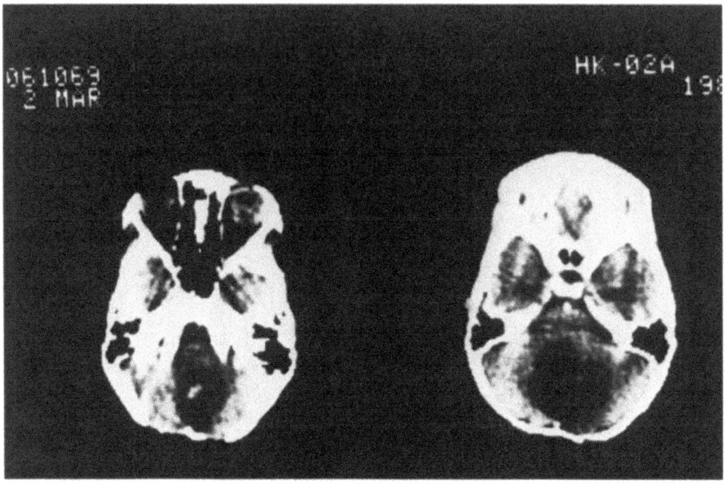

Fig. 3a Pre-operative CT of a recurred spongioblastoma (pilocytic astrocytoma of the posterior cranial fossa). A ten-year-old girl.

11, 12]. In 150 ventricular pressure measurements we have seen altogether four confirmed cases of meningitis i. e. with positive cultures, and also two local disturbances of wound healing. In our experience if an infection is to be avoided, the technique must be most scrupulous during the implantation of the catheter. We recommend a long, subgaleal course, and the care of the catheter at its place of exit by means of a regular renewal of the sterile dressings. A second factor is the duration of the implantation. In all confirmed cases of meningitis the catheter had remained *in situ* for more than 96 hours.

On the other hand complications with epidural pressure measurements are few as this procedure is, in comparison with ventricular pressure measurements definitely less invasive. The nursing care and the mobility of the patient are not restricted, as

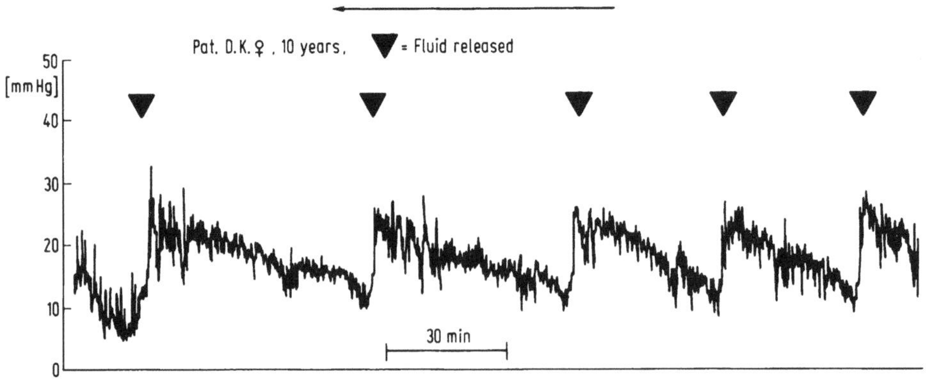

Fig. 3b Corresponding intraventricular pressure measurement in obstructive hydrocephalus resulting from obstruction of the lower end of the aqueduct. Typical pattern resembling plateau waves.

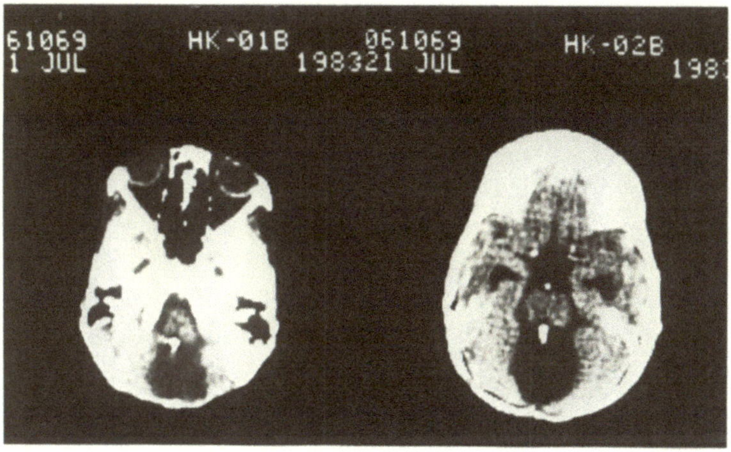

Fig. 3c Postoperative CT with Leksell drain in the operative defect.

these activities do not produce any artifacts in the measurements. Conscious patients can themselves detach the pressure recorder from the connecting cable and re-attach it, so that any recalibration is unnecessary. The high frequency resolution of the measurement by a direct pressure transducer allows one to distinguish easily on the pressure tracing the artificial variations in pressure produced by coughing, suction and changes of position, from pressure waves which are important for diagnosis and treatment. Further advantages of the implanted miniature pressure recorder are:

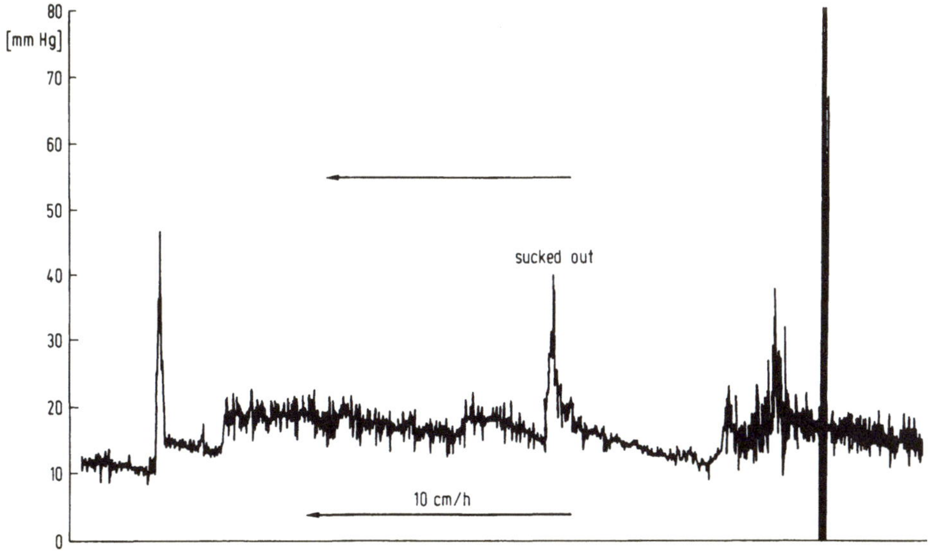

Fig. 3d Postoperative ventricular pressure measurements. The intraventricular pressure has returned to normal.

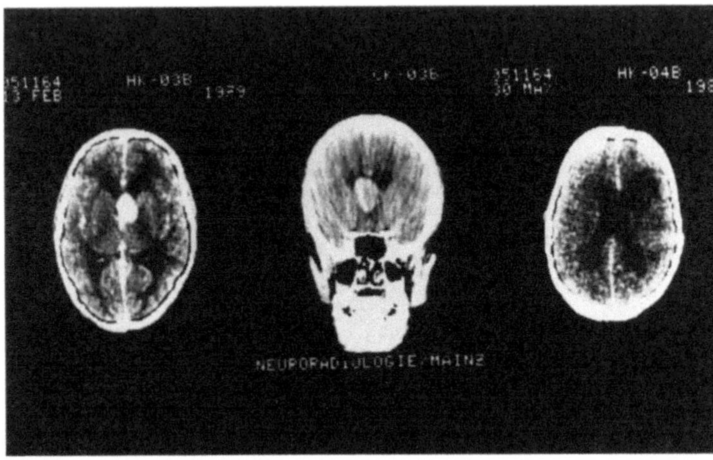

Fig. 4a Pre- and post-operative CT of a ventricular tumour (astroblastoma) with incomplete block of the foramen of Monro.
Thirteen-year-old girl.

1. No injury to the brain.
2. No operative problems with its use (with ventricular pressure measurements frequent ventricle punctures are sometimes necessary).
3. Less risk of infection.
4. No problems of blockage of the catheter with the consequent loss of useful measurements.
5. No danger at all of provoking herniation (as for example in space-occupying lesions of the posterior fossa and unwanted/unnoticed disconnection of the drainage system).

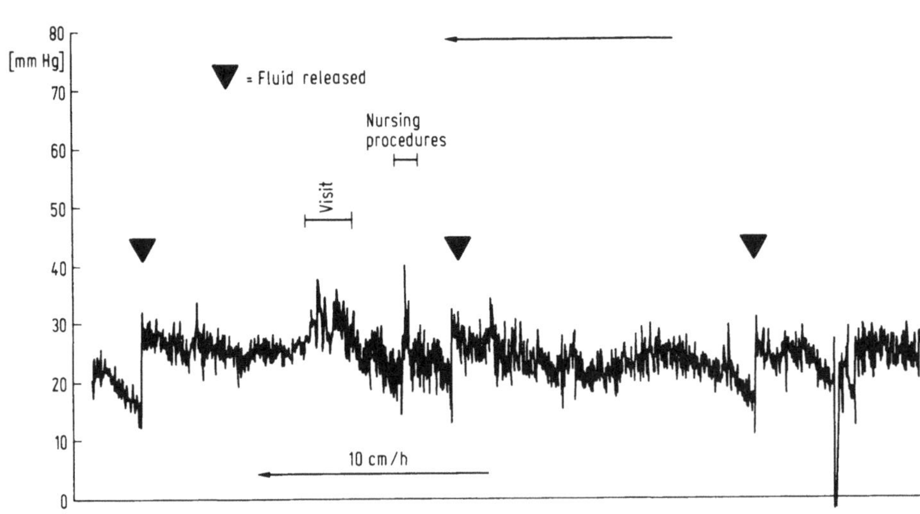

Fig. 4b Pre-operative pattern of pressure with basal pressure between 25 and 30 mm Hg.

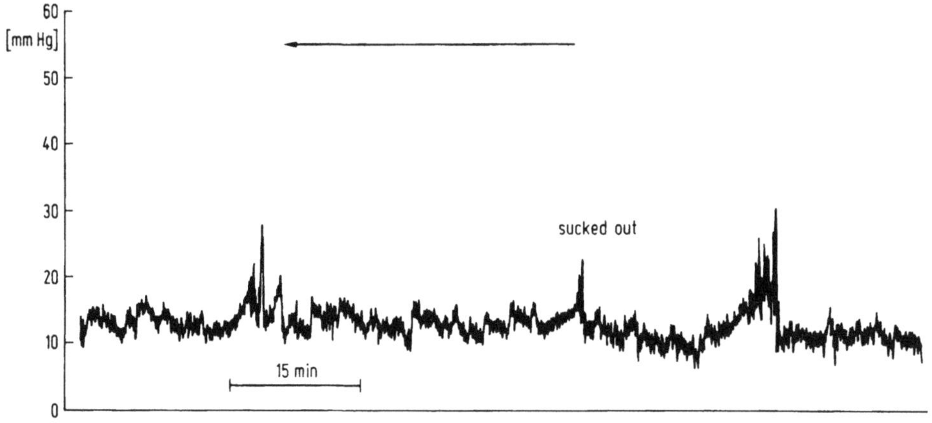

Fig. 4c Postoperative recording with return of ventricular pressure to normal.

Summary

The only indication for pre-operative intraventricular pressure measurement in space-occupying lesions is when the actual lesion is causing a disturbance of the CSF circulation, which can lead to a sudden decompensation. On account of the possibility of simultaneous fluid drainage deliberate and controlled lowering of the pressure is guaranteed. The postoperative measuring of ventricular pressure proves that there is free fluid drainage. This is of particular significance after interventions in the posterior fossa, and also with tumours of the third ventricle.

Continuous postoperative epidural pressure monitoring is suitable as a minimally invasive procedure, to record promptly any possible complications such as haemorrhages and brain swelling and to enable one to initiate further diagnostic and therapeutic measures.

References

[1] Arnold, H., R. Laas: Die Ursache der Plateauwellen: Kompression der sinusnahen Brückenvenenabschnitte. XXXI. Jahrestagung Dtsch. Ges. Neurochir. Erlangen Mai 1980. Adv. Neurosurg. **9** (1980) 351–354.

[2] Brawanski, A., M. Gaab: Intracraniel pressure gradients in the presence of various intracraniel space-occupying lesions. Adv. Neurosurg. **9** (1980) 355–362.

[3] Dorsch, N. W. C., L. Syman: A practical technique for monitoring extradural pressure. J. Neurosurg. **42** (1975) 249–257.

[4] Espaza, J., A. Manrique, R.D. Lobato, et al.: Simultaneus epidural and intraventricular pressure measurement during the occurence of supratentorial expanding lesions. In: Intracranial Pressure IV (K. Staubman, A. Marmarou, J. D. Mitter et al., eds.), pp. 377–380. Springer-Verlag, Berlin–Heidelberg–New York 1980.

[5] Fuchs, E. L.: Quantitative CSF drainage in cases of posterior fossa tumor. Adv. Neurosurg. 5 (1978) 211–215.

[6] Gaab, M.: Die Registrierung des intrakraniellen Druckes. Grundlagen, Techniken, Ergebnisse und Möglichkeiten. Habil. Schr., Med. Fak. Würzburg 1980.

[7] Gaab, M., O. E. Knoblich, K. Dietrich: Miniaturisierte Methoden zur Überwachung des intrakraniellen Druckes. Techniken und klinische Ergebnisse. Langenbecks Arch. Chir. **350** (1979) 13–31.

[8] Gaab, M., N. Sörensen: Extradurale Langzeitmessung des intrakraniellen Druckes in der Pädiatrie. Methodik und klinische Anwendung. Kinderarzt **11** (1980) 11–20.

[9] Guillaume, J., P. Janny: Manométrie intracranieme continue. Intérêt de la méthode et premiers résultats. Rev. neurol. (Paris) **84** (1951) 131–142.

[10] Hase, U.: Intracranielle Drucksteigerung. Meßmethoden, Pathophysiologie, Therapie. Neurochirurgia **21** (1978) 145–157.

[11] Lundberg, N.: Continous recording and control of fluid pressure in neurosurgical practice. Acta Psych. Neurol. Scand. **36** (1960) Suppl. 149.

[12] Pöll, W., W. v. Waldthausen, M. Brock: Infection rate of continous monitoring of ventricular fluid pressure with and without open cerebro-spinal fluid drainage. Adv. Neurosurg. **9** (1980) 363–366.

[13] Quincke, H.: Über Hydrocephalus. Verhandl. d. Cong. für Inn. Med. **10** (1891) 321–340.

[14] Schwarz, M., D. Voth: Palliative operations: internal shunt, ventricular fluid drainage, ventriculocisternostomy (Torkildsen) and interventriculostomy (Leksell). In: Tumours of the Central Nervous System (D. Voth, P. Gutjahr, C. Langmaid, eds.), pp. 214–217. Springer-Verlag, Berlin–Heidelberg–New York 1982.

[15] Schwarz, M., G. Keßel, D. Voth: Über die Bedeutung der intraventrikulären Druckmessung im Rahmen der Diagnostik des Hydrocephalus internus. In: Hydrocephalus im frühen Kindesalter (D. Voth, P. Gutjahr, P. Glees, eds.), pp. 105–111. Enke-Verlag, Stuttgart 1983.

[16] Tsementzis, S. A.: Significance of the ventricular-fluid pressure wave form. Acta Neurochirurg. **40** (1978) 191–202.

[17] Voth, D., N. Nakayama: Ein neues ventilgesteuertes System für die präliminare Ventrikeldrainage (Technische Beschreibung und klinische Erfahrung). Neurochirurgia **19** (1976) 196–201.

[18] Voth, D., O. Hey, N. Nakayama, P. Emmrich: Die kontinuierliche Registrierung des intrakraniellen Druckes (Intraventrikuläre Messung) im Rahmen der pädiatrischen Intensivmedizin. In: Pädiatrische Intensivmedizin (P. Emmrich, ed.), pp. 104–109. Thieme-Verlag, Stuttgart 1977.

Intracranial pressure monitoring in postoperative treatment of supratentorial and infratentorial gliomas
(Brief communication)

K. E. Richard, K. Radebold

This investigation deals with the significance, indication and technique of measurement of intracranial pressure in the postoperative intensive care unit after operation for a supra- (fig. 1) or infratentorial glioma.

During the period of 1973–1982 166 patients suffering from a glioma – supratentorially (No. 78) – infra-tentorially (No. 88) had their intra-cranial pressure recorded for an average of five days.

The normal p.o. course was characterised by a quick normalization of ICP (fig. 2) within the first three days, parallel to the recovery of neurological and mental functions.

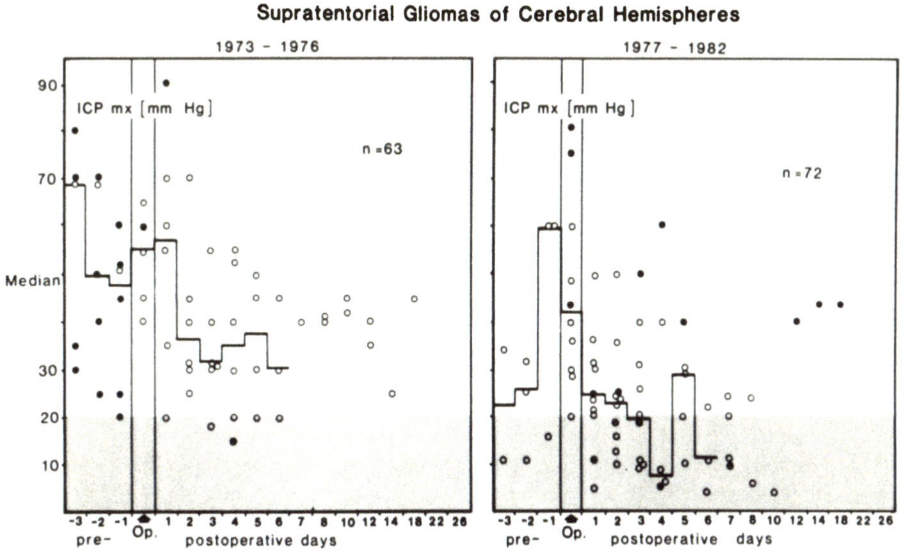

Fig. 1 Maximum ICP-values in the pre-and postoperative course of patients with *cerebral gliomas*, divided into two different periods of treatment:
(Open circles: ICP-peaks of patients with favorable outcome; closed circles: ICP-peaks of patients with fatal outcome).

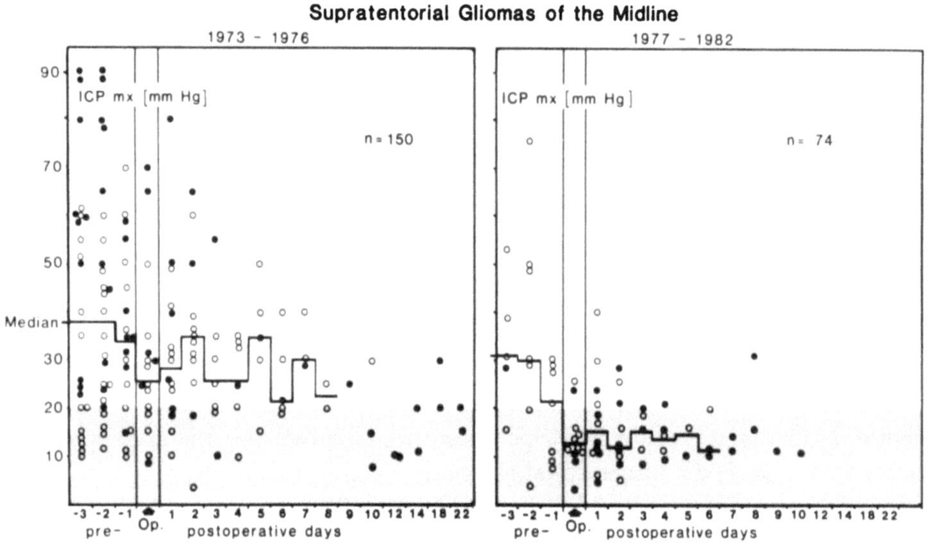

Fig. 2 Maximum ICP-values in the pre-and postoperative course of patients with *supratentorial midline gliomas*.

Acute rise of ICP were recorded after subtotal resection of the glioma, which had infiltrated peri-central cortical regions, basal ganglia, thalamus or hypothalamus, midbrain, pons or medulla. Reactive brain oedema, brain swelling following pressure by spatula, or interruption of venous drainage, haemorrhagic softening in the tumour border and impairment of CSF circulation were sources for acute rise of ICP in the post-operative course.

A continuous surveillance of ICP is the precondition for early assessment of an acute pressure crisis. Disturbance of the CSF circulation after glioma operation with suspected ventricular infiltration are reliably realized with a ventricular catheter. Pressure rises following brain oedema or brain swelling after resection of supratentorial gliomas of the hemispheres are both recorded via an epi-dural transducer.

To Professor Dr. R. A. Frowein on the occasion of his 60th birthday

EEG, SEP and VEP examinations during the treatment of malignant gliomas

A. Pobloth, J. Jörg, W. Kass

During the last four years we have investigated the clinical, psychological and neurophysiological findings in 52 patients with intracranial gliomas. In most of the cases a more or less total operation had been performed with the aim of reducing the bulk of the tumour as far as possible. They had all been given radiation with 40 Gy to the brain and also 20 Gy directly to the tumour residue. They were subsequently given chemotherapy with six courses of CCNU over a year. The neurophysiological investigations included the EEG and recordings of SEP and VEP in all cases. It was felt that these investigations might help in findings answers to the following questions:

1. Do the clinical and psychological results correlate with the results of the neurophysiological tests?
2. Can the side-effects of radiation and chemotherapy be assessed by neurophysiological methods?
3. How far do the site and histology of the tumour correspond with the results of the EEG, SEP and VEP?

Material

Fifty-two patients with brain tumours which have been treated during the last four years were available for assessment. Among the pathological types encountered were astrocytoma, glioblastoma multiforme, undifferentiated oligodendroglioma and four glioblastomas arising in the corpus callosum (butterfly glioma). They were examined before treatment, after operation, after the radiotherapy and before the courses of treatment with CCNU. Complete data were only available in 26 patients. This difference in the numbers was the result of loss of patients agreement, unfavourable prognosis and a failure to attend for follow-up examinations.

Methods

The EEG was recorded using the usual standard electrode placements. The VEP was obtained with central fixation by full-field and half field stimulation from a checkerboard. It was recorded from each eye separately from Oz-Fz by full-field stimulation, 01-Fz and 02-Fz by half-field stimulation. The median nerve was stimulated at both wrists and the SEP was obtained contralaterally and ipsilaterally from the mastoid versus C/P and the scalp C/P-F, as well as a recording from Erb's point from ipsilateral stimulation only.

Results

If we now compare the results in relationship to the site of the tumour and the clinical symptoms, it may be noted that localisation of the tumour cannot be bettered by EEG, SEP and VEP acting as a confirmation of the results of the cranial CT, even considering that the P15 of the median scalp SEP is a secured peak generated in the brain stem. The results of VEP and SEP correlate very well with the clinical findings of vision and sensation at the initial stage and during subsequent progress. In contrast to some publications, in only a few cases did the half-field stimulated VEP prove to be a more sensitive method than the perimetric examination as evidence of a visual field loss.

In most of the cases the P15 peak could not be obtained after the operation and radiation treatment, even in the absence of any clinical brain stem involvement. It was in checking the patients postoperatively, that we obtained the most pathological clinical and neurophysiological results.

Because of the administration of a minimum of 40 Gy to the healthy hemisphere, the side-effects of radiation had to be studied. We were able to identify not a slowing but an acceleration of the basic rhythm in the EEG. The contralateral scalp SEP showed an increase in latency when recorded from the healthy hemisphere. This increase was not of statistical significance, with a mean of 1.53 ± 1.06 ms for N1. We found no disturbance of visual function, i.e. there were no lesions of the optic nerve which could be attributed to the radiation.

During treatment with CCNU we found no changes in the clinical findings, neither were there any changes in the neurophysiological results which could be attributed to the treatment with nitroso-urea. The radiosensitizer misonidazole was given to five patients. We measured the nerve conduction velocity (CV) from the wrist to Erb's point. The velocity of nerve conduction slowed down from 77 to 66.9 m/s during the six weeks when it was being recorded. In comparison with a group of patients, operated on and also radiated with a change in CV from 72.9 to 69.6 m/s no significant decrease could be established during the administration of misonidazole. This result would suggest a subclinical neuropathy as described by Mamoli et al. [1, 8, 10]. It would be interesting to check these findings in a larger group of patients.

Summary

1. Compared with the cranial CT the EEG, SEP and VEP do not have any additional value in the localisation of cerebral gliomas.
2. The clinical results as regards sensation and visual function show a good correlation with the EEG, SEP and VEP.
3. Significant adverse effects can be demonstrated by SEP and VEP [4–6] either after X-ray [3, 7] therapy or during CCNU [2, 9] medication. The slight increase in latency may be caused by oedema.
4. In the absence of PM findings and other evidence it cannot be stated whether SEP and VEP in association with the CT are suitable for distinguishing between a recurrence and radiation necrosis.
5. Misonidazole is able to decrease the nerve conduction velocity. This is possible evidence of a subclinical neuropathy.

References

[1] Budka, H.: Neuropathologie der Therapieschäden durch intensive Strahlen- und Chemotherapie von Tumoren im Bereich des ZNS. In: Haemoblastosen, Zentrale Motorik, Iatrogene Schäden, Myositiden (D. Seitz, P. Vogel, eds.). Springer-Verlag, Berlin–Heidelberg, New York 1983.

[2] Crafts, D. C., C. B. Wilson: Basis and results of chemotherapeutic treatment of gliomas. Bull. Cancer **64** (1977) 101–114.

[3] Holdorff, B.: Strahlenschäden des Gehirn und Rückenmark. In: Haemoblastosen, Zentrale Motorik, Iatrogene Schäden, Myositiden (D. Seitz, P. Vogel, eds.). Springer-Verlag, Berlin–Heidelberg–New York 1983.

[4] Jörg, J.: Praktische SEP-Diagnostik. Enke-Verlag, Stuttgart 1983.

[5] Jonkman, E. J.: EEG, Computertomographie und Echoenzephalographie bei Patienten mit Astrozytom Grad III–IV. Ztschr. EEG–EMG **11** (1980) 89–96.

[6] Kuroiwa, Y., G. G. Celesia: Visual evoked potentials with hemifield pattern stimulation. Their use in the diagnostic of retrochiasmatic lesions. Arch. Neurol. **38** (1981) 86–90.

[7] Krauseneck, P., H. G. Mertens: Therapie maligner Neoplasien des Gehirns. Perimed Verlag, Erlangen 1983.

[8] Mamoli, B., P. Wessely, H. D. Kogelnik, et al.: Electroneurographic investigations of misonidazole polyneuropathy. Eur. Neurol. **18** (1979) 405–414.

[9] Neundörfer, B.: Neurotoxische Nebenwirkungen der Zytostatika-Therapie. In: Haemoblastosen, Zentrale Motorik, Iatrogene Schäden, Myositiden (D. Seitz, P. Vogel, eds.). Springer-Verlag, Berlin–Heidelberg–New York 1983.

[10] Strian, F., R. Maurach: Neurotoxische Nebenwirkungen der zytostatischen Therapie. Fortschr. Neurol. Psychiat. **49** (1981) 152–163.

CEA and TPA in plasma and cerebrospinal fluid of patients with intracranial tumours

D.-K. Böker, P. Oehr, J. Kirsch

Introduction

Diagnosis of intracranial tumours is dominated by computed tomography, but there is still a need for some other standards by which the completeness of tumour removal can be controlled. Such a one exists in the treatment of gastrointestinal tumours, by controlling plasma levels of carcino-embryonic antigen (CEA) which was described by Gold and Freedman [4]. As regards intracranial tumours there are some communications that mostly stress the value of determinations of CSF-CEA for reasons of differential diagnosis [6, 9, 10], but there is still a need for further investigation.

Another antigen which seems to be related to proliferative disease without exhibiting any organ specificity [7, 8] is TPA (tissue polypeptide antigen), first described by Björklund [1]. The value of this antigen in controlling the management of intracranial tumours remains still to be established. To our knowledge there are still no other communications on this subject.

Materials and methods

Fifty patients with various intracranial tumours were investigated: glioblastomas (n = 8), astrocytomas grade I–III (n = 16, including pilocytic astrocytomas), oligodendrogliomas (n = 3), ependymomas (n = 2), meningiomas (n = 13), neurinomas (n = 2), craniopharyngiomas (n = 2), metastases (n = 3), echinococcus (n = 1).

In 14 of the patients the levels of TPA and CEA were determined in tumour extract. In 18 patients plasma levels of both antigens could be determined, and in 47 patients the CSF concentrations of both antigens were controlled. For antigen determination blood and CSF samples were collected at the time of operation.

For normal values of TPA we investigated the cerebrospinal fluids of 20 patients with lumbar disc herniation. The CSF concentration of CEA was not determined in the control group because this antigen is not usually found in healthy persons [2, 3, 5, 9].

Specimens of normal brain were obtained from one patient with brain injury and two with spontaneous intracerebral haematomas to determine the concentrations of CEA and TPA in non-tumorous brain.

Determinations of the antigen levels were performed by radioimmuno-essays (CEA: Abbott, Wiesbaden-Delkesheim, FRG; TPA: Sangtec Medical, Bromma, Sweden).

Results

CEA concentrations in non-tumorous brain were 0.3, 0.4 and 0.5 μ/l. TPA showed figures of 99, 160 and 471 U/l, thus indicating a much greater variability. In the group of patients with lumbar disc herniation CSF concentrations of TPA were below 30 U/l.

In two glioblastomas, one astrocytoma, two craniopharyngiomas and one meningioma we found markedly raised CEA-levels (> 6μg/l). Values higher than 2.5 μ/l were found in two additional astrocytomas and two meningiomas. Plasma levels for CEA were below 3.0 μg/l in all patients.

TPA values in tumour extracts ranged between 20 U/l and 3000 U/l, the highest levels being found in an astrocytoma (1838 U/l) and in a craniopharyngioma (3000 U/l). Plasma levels which are to be regarded as normal up to 70 U/l [7, 8] were found in all cases but one below this value. We found a plasma TPA of 80 U/l only in one craniopharyngioma (see fig. 1).

CSF values for CEA were found to be 0.0 (n = 12) or less than 0.4 μg/l (n = 25) in most of the patients. In one meningioma we found a value of 1.3 μg/l. The only markedly raised CSF-CEA level was 3.2 μg/l in a patient with an intracranial echinococcus (see fig. 2).

TPA levels in the CSF of tumour patients were found to be below 70 U/l in all patients but one. The only markedly raised value was found in a patient with recurrent ependymoma. Values between 30 and 70 U/l were found in ten cases (one glioblastoma, two astrocytomas, four meningiomas, one neurinoma, one metastasis, and the echinococcus case), (see fig. 2).

Discussion

Both antigens are expressed by a number of intracranial tumours. But there is no correlation between the levels of CSF and TPA in plasma, CSF, and tumour extract, which is an accordance with the findings of Hill [5]. CEA is known not to pass the blood-brain-barrier, nor from blood to CSF [2]. This also seems to be true for TPA.

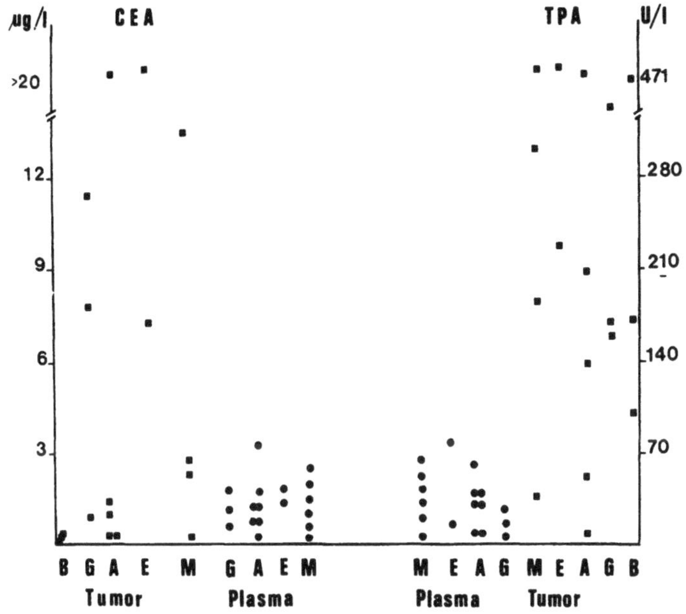

Fig. 1 CEA and TPA values in plasma and tumour extracts. B = normal brain, G = glioblastoma, A = astrocytoma, spongioblastoma, oligodendroglioma; E = ependymoma, neurinoma, craniopharyngoma; M = meningioma. See text for further explanation.

Plasma levels for CEA can be regarded as normal up to 2.8 µg/l, and up to 70 U/l for TPA. Als we found it slightly elevated in only one case of astrocytoma, plasma level determinations of CEA are not a very useful tool in managing intracranial tumours.

Plasma TPA was also normal in all cases but one. The value of 80 U/l in a craniopharyngioma patient is not very high. Thus controlling plasma levels in brain tumour patients does not seem to be very useful.

CSF levels of CEA were normally low, between 0.0 and 0.4 µg/l in 37 of the 47 cases in which we checked CSF levels. In the meningioma group CEA levels seem to be somewhat higher than in the other tumour groups, but they are not clearly raised. Furthermore with meningiomas completeness of tumours removal is more easy to determine during the operation. The only markedly raised level of CSF-TPA was found in a case of recurrent ependymoma. Possibly, alterations of the blood-CSF barrier are responsible for this finding, whereas we had some other cases of recurring tumour in this series (two astrocytomas, one oligodendroglioma) in whom we did not find elevated CEA or TPA levels. Still a little more pronounced than for CEA TPA levels are slightly raised in meningiomas, but quite naturally here the same reservations regarding its usefulness have to be made.

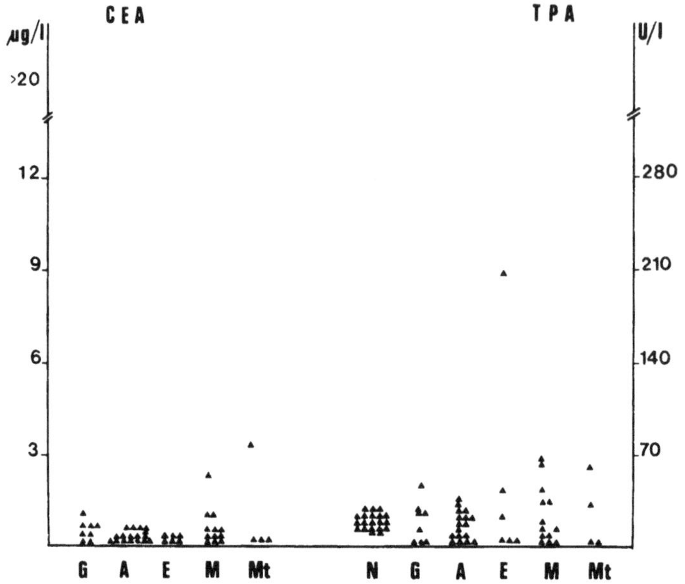

Fig. 2 CEA and TPA values in CSF. N = CSF from patients with lumbar disc herniation; Mt = metastases of various primary tumours. (The highest value of CEA as well as of TPA is from one patient with an intracranial echinococcus.)

As neither the CSF values nor the plasma values of CEA and TPA were found to be elevated in our material – even the three cases of brain metastases showed normal values – determination of these antigens does not seem to be a useful tool in controlling treatment or in recognizing a tumour recurrence. However, further investigations are necessary to confirm this, especially for TPA.

Summary

CEA and TPA levels have been determined in extracts of 14 intracranial tumours, plasma from 18 patients with intracranial tumours, and in CSF from 47 patients with intracranial tumours. Both antigens are expressed by some tumours, but they do not seem to pass the blood-brain-barrier, into the cerebrospinal fluid. Plasma levels as well as CSF levels were found to be raised only in one case each. Therefore estimating the CEA and TPA in plasma or CSF does not appear to be a useful tool in the management of intracranial tumours.

References

[1] Björklund, B., V. Björklund: Antigenicity of pooled human malignant and normal tissues by cytoimmunological technique: Presence of an insoluble, heatlabile tumour antigen. Int. Arch. Allergy *10*, (1957) 153–184.

[2] Corman, G., K. Felgenhauer, G. Uhlenbruck, et al.: CEA im Liquor Cerebrospinalis: Ein diagnostischer Parameter bei Metastasen des Zentralnervensystems? In: CEA und andere Tumormarker (G. Uhlenbruck, ed.), pp. 194–197. Verlag Tumor Diagnostik, Leonberg 1982.

[3] Dearnaley, D. P., P. Patel, T. J. Powles, et al.: Carcinoembryonic antigen estimation in cerebrospinal fluid in patients with metastatic breast cancer. Oncodev. Biol. Med. *2* (1981) 305–311.

[4] Gold, P., S. O. Freedman: Specific carcinoembryonic antigens of the human digestive system. J. Exp. Med. *122* (1965) 467–481.

[5] Hill, S., E. Martin, E. C. Ellison, et al.: Carcinoembryonic antigen in cerebrospinal fluid of adult braintumor patients. J. Neurosurg. *53* (1980) 627–632.

[6] Mikaye, E., M. Yamashita, K. Kitamura, et al.: Carcinoembryonic antigen (CEA) levels in patients with brain tumors. Acta Neurochir. *46* (1979) 53–57.

[7] Oehr, P., O. Bellmann, D. Hamann: Measurement of Tennessee antigen, carcinoembryonic antigen, tissue polypeptide antigen and alpha-feto-protein in body fluids associated with pregnancy. Clin. Biochem. *15* (1982) 13–16.

[8] Oehr, P., G. Derigs, R. Altmann: Evaluation and characterization of tumor-associated antigens of inverse distribution function values into specificity-sensitivity diagrams. Tumor Diagnostik 6 (1981) 283–290.

[9] Schold, C., W. R. Wasserstrom, M. Fleisher, et al.: Cerebrospinal fluid biochemical markers of central nervous system metastases. Ann. Neurol. *8* (1980) 597–604.

[10] Suzuki, Y., R. Tanaka: Carcinoembryonic antigen in patients with intracranial tumors. J. Neurosurg. *53* (1980) 355–360.

Sensitivity of human malignant brain tumours to chemotherapeutic agents as detected by the pro-assay: preliminary results of an in vivo/in vitro correlation*

U. Bogdahn, W. Kargl

Introduction

As the results of combined forms of treatment in highly malignant human brain tumours are still very disappointing – mean survival times of 58 weeks may be achieved with a combination of operation, radiation and chemotherapy in glioblastoma patients [5] – an *in vitro* system intending to predict the response of individual tumours to chemotherapeutic agents may provide an improvement in the results of treatment. Since Hamburger and Salmon's original [7] description of the human tumour stem cell assay a number of authors have tried to focus their attention on predictive *in vitro* systems. The application of the tumour stem cell assay to neurooncology with respect to predictive therapeutic capabilities has so far been disappointing [6], as *in vivo*/*in vitro* correlations for tumour sensitivity have merely matched 42% correct prediction. Among alternative non-stem cell based test systems [8] we have been able to develop a proliferation microassay (PRO) [3] that intended to predict equally accurately resistance and sensitivity of human malignant brain tumours to a number of chemotherapeutic agents.

Method

Patients: Tests were carried out on 17 patients harboring malignant brain tumours (seven glioblastomas, five anaplastic astrocytomas, three malignant ependymomas, one medulloblastoma, one angiosarcoma). All patients received a standard treatment including operation, radiation (55–62 Gy) and either BCNU (N = 12) or CCNU (N = 5) chemotherapy, plus optimal standard care. The clinical response of these patients was defined as the duration of recurrence free interval.

* This work is currently supported by the Deutsche Forschungsgemeinschaft.

Assay-system: The assay has been described in detail elsewhere [3]. Briefly fresh biopsy material was obtained from the Neurosurgical department, washed thoroughly and separated from debris. A tumour cell suspension was prepared by mechanical and enzymatic disaggregation (collagenase, neuraminidase, heparin). Cells were washed three times and then finally plated into 96-well microculture plates, employing BME with 20% fetal calf serum and 0.1% penicillin and streptomycin. Tumour cells were also grown in Labtek® tissue culture slides under identical conditions (37° C, 5% CO_2,H_2O-saturated atmo.) for further characterization. After 24 hours cells were treated with a range of chemotherapeutic agents according to their *in vivo* pharmacokinetic data; an incubation period of 72 hours was employed. Afterwards cells were washed and allowed to grow in fresh culture medium for another nine days (this has been recently changed to 8 cell doublings). Finally, ^{3}H-uridine uptake (5.6-^{3}H-uridine, spec. activity 40 Ci/mmol) as an indicator of RNA-synthesis and cell proliferation was measured after a 9-hour incubation period by a liquid scintillation counting protocol. The effect of different drugs on cell proliferation was expressed as per cent inhibition of RNA-synthesis compared to untreated controls. An inhibition of more than 50% at the concentration comparable to the maximum *in vivo* attainable plasma concentration was regarded as an indication of the tumour being sensitive to the corresponding drug. More recently this has been changed to achieve improved comparability of *in vitro* and *in vivo* data by employing the area-ratio method [2]. Tumour cells were characterized by morphological and cytochemical characteristics, and in addition, more recently, by immunological properties.

Results

In vitro results for BCNU: As BCNU is the most frequently used single agent in brain tumour therapy, we want to focus on the results for this drug. Although all our patients were treated either with BCNU or CCNU, in these experiments only BCNU was tested *in vitro*. However, patients treated with CCNU will be included in our correlation, as the mode of action and the pharmacokinetics of both drugs are more or less similar. *In vitro* chemosensitivity to BCNU was evaluated at a concentration of 1 µg/ml, being equal to 4.5 uM. The maximal pharmacological achievable concentration is 2 µg/ml [1], the concentration-time product achievable is 1.02 µghr or 4.58 µMhr. Taking an *in vitro* $T_{1/2}$ of 21 min and the incubation period of 72 hrs into account [4], the comparable maximum *in vitro* concentration was calculated as 8.8 µM. The concentration of 4.5 µM corresponding 2.5 µMhr is thus well below the maximal achievable dose, assuming that tumour tissue concentrations are also below peak plasma concentrations. At this concentration 7 out of 17 tumours showed sensitivity to BCNU *in vitro* (fig. 1).

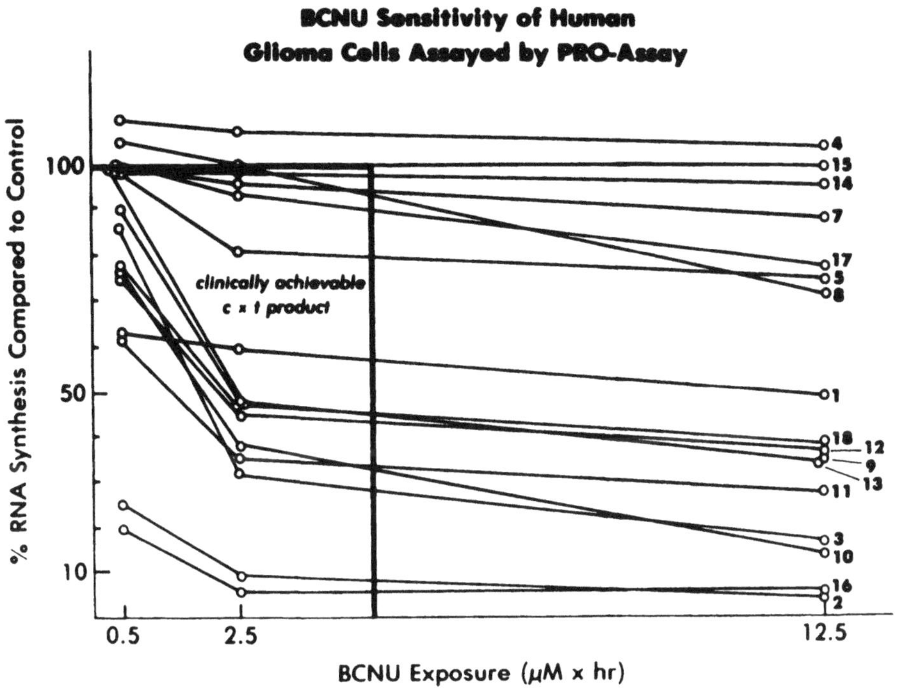

Fig. 1 Sensitivity of human brain tumour cells to BCNU, assayed by PRO-assay. Numbers on the right relate to the original tumour biopsy.

In vivo/in vitro correlation: as mentioned above, patients (N = 5) treated with CCNU are included in the correlation. The median postoperative recurrence free interval for *in vitro* BCNU-sensitive patients was 17 months (mean 15.1 months, σ = 4.42), for *in vitro* resistant patients 5 months (mean 6.38 months, σ = 2.96, difference statistically significant at $p<0.001$) (fig. 2).

Radiation therapy results in a mean postoperative survival time of about 46 weeks and on this basis we took an arbitrary clinical cut-off for patients who were clinically BCNU-sensitive or -resistant, as one year. The individual *in vitro* prediction of our assay for *in vivo* resistance was correct in all cases (10/10), for *in vivo* tumour sensitivity it was incorrect in one case with a borderline *in vitro* BCNU sensitivity of 48% and a postoperative recurrence-free interval of 11 months. This amounts to a predictive capacity for *in vivo* tumour sensitivity of 85.8% for the assay.

Tumour-sensitivity to alternative drugs. As space is limited, only a brief summary of results with alternative drugs may be given here – for further detail see [3]. All drugs have been tested in at least 4 doses, for each the dose of evaluation will be given. VM 26 was effective in 5/12 tumours at a concentration of 0.4 μg/ml and in one tumour enhancement of 150% was observed. Procarbazine-sensitivity was estimated at 2.5 μg/ml; although it has doubtful *in vitro* activation, 4/15 tumours were sensitive

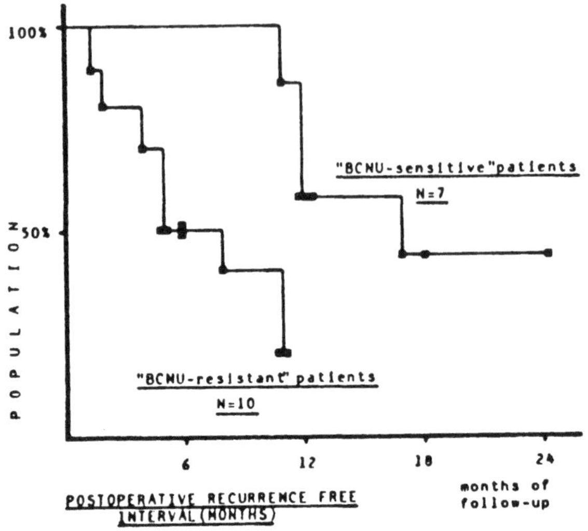

Fig. 2 Correlation of *in vivo* and *in vitro* BCNU-sensitivity of patients and their tumours. Patients with *in vitro* sensitive tumours had a significantly longer median survival time (17 months) than patients with in vitro BCNU-resistant tumours (5 months).

to the drug, enhancement was observed in three tumours. At 10 mU/ml 7/15 tumours showed sensitivity to Bleomycin. Methotrexate (penetrating the Blood-Brain-Barrier only in high-dose-regimen) was effective in 6/13 tumours at 5 μg/ml (2×10^{-5}M). For Cisplatin (only doubtful penetration of BBB) 7/16 tumours displayed sensitivity at 2.5 μg/ml. Cytosine-Arabinoside (ARA-C) was effective in 10/15 tumours tested at 10 μg/ml. Adenine-Arabinoside (ARA-A) showed an effect in 4/14 tumours at a concentration of 1μg/ml, and in 5/14 at 10 μg/ml. For ARA-C and ARA-A no inhibitor of deaminase-activity was employed, so activity for these drugs might be even better. Human Fibroblast interferon (kindly provided by Behringwerke, Marburg) was effective in 5/14 tumours at 100 IU/ml. Namalwa lymphoblastoid interferon (kindly provided by Behringwerke, Marburg and by Deutsche Wellcome, Burgwedel) was effective in 6/11 tumours, again at 100 IU/ml.

Discussion

Apart from clinical trials, *in vitro* and maybe *in vivo* drug sensitivity assays intending to predict the response of individual tumours to chemotherapeutic agents may finally improve the results of treatment in brain tumour patients. The results presented here are preliminary (as the number of patients is still small and some patients still have not yet had documented recurrences, and as the assay has been modified slightly in the recent past) and the *in vitro*/*in vivo* correlations presented are retrospective. Still it may be clearly seen that there seem to be chances to improve therapeutic efficiency by applying the assay in the future. As *in vitro/in vivo* correlations for brain tumour patients are better than with any other assay so far – the predictive capacity for *in vivo* sensitivity assayed by the tumour stemm cell assay [6] is only about 42% – there may be immediate benefits from employing the PRO-assay to two aspects of brain tumour therapy: 1. selection of the optimal drug for therapy of recurrent gliomas and 2. screening of new agents available and suitable for brain tumour chemotherapy. As for tumour biology the tumour stem cell assay is of irreplacable importance, efforts should be undertaken to compare the results obtained with different systems and to improve upon both in preparing for a future individualized chemotherapy.

Summary

The sensitivity of human malignant brain tumour cells to a number of cytotoxic drugs (BCNU, Cisplatin, VM 26, Methotrexate, Bleomycin, Procarbazine) and antiproliferative/antiviral agents (Adenine-arabinoside, Cytosine-arabinoside, alpha- and beta-interferon) was investigated in a micro-proliferation assay (PRO). Single cell suspensions from brain tumour biopsies were plated into 96-well micro-tissue-culture plates, and treated with drugs at pharmacologically achievable doses. Cells were then grown in fresh culture medium for approximately 8 population doublings. Cell proliferation was estimated subsequently by incorporation of (5.6-^{3}H)-uridine into tumour-cell RNA using a liquid scintillation counter. *In vitro* BCNU sensitivity was determined for a group of 17 brain tumour patients. Subsequent to surgery, all patients received radiotherapy (55–62 Gy) and chemotherapy consisting of either BCNU or CCNU. Patients whose tumours were sensitive to BCNU *in vitro* had a median postoperative recurrence free interval of 17 months (mean = 15.1 months), whereas patients with *in vitro* BCNU resistant tumours had a median recurrence free interval of 5 months (mean = 6.38 months, $p < 0.001$). All ten patients with *in vitro* BCNU-resistant tumours showed clinical resistance to either BCNU or CCNU. 6/7 patients with *in vitro* BCNU-sensitive tumours showed clearcut clinical sensitivity (postoperative recurrence free interval longer than 12 months) – the remaining patient with very borderline *in vitro* BCNU-sensitivity recurred after 11 months. The PRO-assay may be suitable for future selection of drugs to employ in recurrent gliomas and for screening new agents *in vitro* in respect to their activity in brain tumours.

References

[1] Alberts, D. S., et L.: Tabular summary of pharmacokinetic parameters relevant to *in vitro* drug assays. In: Cloning of human tumor stem cells S. Salmon, ed.), p. 351. Alan R. Liss, New York 1980.

[2] Ali-Osman, F., et al.: In vitro cytostatic drug testing in the human stem cell assay: a modified method for the determination of the sensitivity-index. Tum. Diag. Ther. *4* (1983) 1.
[3] Bogdahn, U.: Chemosensitivity of malignant human brain tumors. Preliminary results. J. Neuro-Oncol. *1* (1983) 149.
[4] Genini, D., et al.: Determination of in vitro pharmacokinetics of different nitrosoureas. Unpublished results. BTRC, UCSF, S.F., Ca., USA.
[5] Jellinger, K., et al.: Combination chemotherapy (COMP protocol) and radiotherapy in anaplastic supratentorial gliomas. Acta Neurochir. *51* (1979) 1–13.
[6] Rosenblum, M., et al.: Stem cell studies of human malignant brain tumors. J. Neurosurg. *58* (1983) 170–176.
[7] Salmon, S., et al.: Clinical correlation of in vitro drug sensitivity. In: Cloning of human tumor stem cells (S. Salmon, ed.). Alan R. Liss, New York 1980.
[8] Thomas, D. G. T., et al.: In vitro chemosensitivity assay of human glioma by scintillation autofluorography. In: Multidisciplinary aspects of brain tumor therapy (P. Paoletti, e.a., eds.), p. 19. Elsevier, North Holland 1979.

Acknowledgement

The authors are very grateful to Mrs. D. Zenglein for technical assistance and especially to the nurses of our neurooncological ward. Thanks is also given for the continuous support of H. G. Mertens. In addition, the authors are indebted to K. A. Bushe and the Neurosurgical Department for generously supplying tumour biopsy material.

III Principles of operative treatment and radiation therapy

Changes induced in anaplastic gliomas and brain tissue as a result of treatment

K. Jellinger

Introduction

Aggressive antineoplastic treatment has improved the prognosis of brain tumour patients, but has also increased the risk of therapy-induced adverse reactions of the CNS. However, the distinction between spontaneous tumour progression, tumour regrowth, and iatrogenic lesions of the CNS, all impairing the quality and duration of survival, can be difficult. By reviewing data on the morphological response to antineoplastic treatment of human glioma tissue and its proliferation zone, of the surrounding damaged, and intact CNS tissue, this paper should contribute to the understanding of therapy-induced changes which, it is hoped, will provide a basis for the design of more effective and less harmful therapeutic strategies.

Therapy-induced changes in tumour tissue

The morphological response of malignant gliomas to radiation and chemotherapy, studied both experimentally in animal, in tissue cultures [38, 46] and in humans [7, 12, 21, 43, 45, 53], is generally characterized by an increase in degenerative and regressive changes accompanied by loss of cells, development of extensive necroses, and a variety of cell and tissue alterations which, however, may also occur spontaneously in the natural course of anaplastic gliomas [39, 79]. The heterogeneity of human gliomas limits the evaluation of the morphologic effects of antitumour treatment due to

a) the great variability in cell and tissue morphology;

b) the possibility of spontaneous occurrence of morphological changes similar or identical to those induced by therapy, and

c) the variable intervals between treatment and morphological examination at biopsy and/or autopsy.

This is demonstrated in a personal series of 218 consecutive autopsy cases of anaplastic supratentorial gliomas, 100 of which had received aggressive adjuvant radiation and/or chemotherapy (tab. 1). While the incidence of spontaneous, non-surgical haemorrhages did not show essential differences, cerebral cyst resulting

Table 1 Autopsy series of anaplastic supratentorial gliomas (1976–1982)

Treatment Tumour type	Astrocytoma anapl. III	Oligo-Astro-cytoma III	Glioblastoma IV	Ependymoma anapl. III	Total
No operation	20	–	61	–	81
Operation	9	3	25	–	37
P. o. Radiother.	19	4	15	–	38
P. o. Chemother.	5	1	6	–	12
P. o. Radio + Chemother.	13	2	32	3	50
No operation No p. o. therapy	29	3	66	–	118
Postop. therapy	37	7	53	3	100
Total	66	10	119	3	218

from tumour necrosis were significantly more frequent after radiation and chemotherapy (14–22%) than in the natural course of gliomas (3–4%). In addition, there was a series of adverse CNS reactions, including radiation necrosis, internal hydrocephalus, etc. (tab. 2).

The *gross changes* of gliomas following antitumour treatment range from compact tumour to total or partial tumour destruction with solid necrosis, cysts and scar formation to progressive or secondary tumour regrowth. The essential effects of radiotherapy are large coagulative necroses with sharp demarcation of the tumour from the surrounding tissue. While complete eradication has been noted in some brain tumours, e.g. malignant lymphomas, germinomas, medulloblastomas and metastases, total destruction of malignant gliomas is very rare [18, 33], although radiation doses of 70 to 80 Gy and fast neutrons may induce total or almost complete tumour sterilization [1, 8, 41, 48]. In one autopsy series of neutron-irradiated glioblastomas, replacement of the tumour by solid necroses in all cases was associated with severe damage to adjacent and remote brain [1, 48]. In another neutron-treated group, at post-mortem examination no or only minimal tumour was found in 69% as compared to 14% after treatment with 50–60 Gy photons [8]. In most other series [7] including our own, complete eradication of malignant gliomas was not achieved in any case by irradiation, chemotherapy of multimodal treatment, although serial CT studies show transient reduction in tumour volume by 25–70% within 3–12 months after treatment with later increase in volume and density due to cell and vascular proliferation [23].

Lack of tumour progression after radiation and chemotherapy was seen in two of 21 autopsy cases [43, 44], and in some cases only a scant quantity of residual tumour is present at autopsy [7, 48]. In our autopsy series, lack of tumour progression was

Table 2 Major morphological changes in anaplastic gliomas and brains of glioma patients

Treatment	No Surgery		Surgery		P. o. Radioth.		P. o. Chemoth.		P. o. Radio + Chemother.		Total	
Type of	(N = 81)		(N = 37)		(N = 38)[a)]		(N = 12)		(N = 50)[b)]		(N = 218)	
Lesion	N	%	N	%	N	%	N	%	N	%	N	%
Enhancement (?) of anaplasia	–	0	–	0	–	0	1	8	3	6	4	2
Haemorrhage	9	11	3[c)]	8	1	2	2	16	3	6	18	9
Space-occup. cer. cysts	3	4	1	3	6	15	2	16	11	22	23	11
Radionecrosis	–	0	–	0	5	13	–	0	3	6	8	3
Int. hydroceph.	2	2,5	1	3	2	5	1	8	11	22	17	8
Transliquor. tumour seeding	14	17	12	32	10	26	5	42	17	34	65	26
Extracranial metastases	–	0	1	3	–	0	–	0	4	8	5	2

a) 40–67 Gy; 5 pat. 66,5 Gy photons + misonidazole
b) 40–66 Gy; 3 pat. 66,5 Gy photons + misonidazole
c) after operation

observed in one out of 12 cases after adjuvant polychemotherapy (survival 3 months), and in 4 among 50 cases with multimodal treatment (8%), death from secondary diseases or complications occurring 6–33 months (mean 15 months) after operation. The brains of these and four other patients undergoing a repeat operation (total survival 9–16 months) revealed large surgical defects with only small marginal rims or up to walnut sized areas of residual or recurrent tumour [12, 13]. The majority of malignant gliomas, however, despite aggressive treatment, show progressive tumour proliferation and regrowth with diffuse infiltration, pronounced mass effects, signs of increased intracranial pressure, and frequent dissemination via the CSF spaces.

Histologically, anaplastic gliomas are characterized by high cellularity, cellular and nuclear pleomorphism, frequent mitotic figures, extensive necroses and severe vascular and mesenchymal response [19, 39, 55]. Untreated anaplastic gliomas usually show three concentric zones:

a) a central necrosis of variable corresponding to the low-density centre seen on CT scan;
b) a dense proliferation area containing high cellularity, circumscribed necroses,

blood vessel proliferation with "pseudo-palisading" of tumour cells, and giant cells with monstrous nuclei;

c) the brain adjacent to tumour (BAT) with
   1. a peripheral region of infiltration and of diffuse astroglial proliferation, small necroses, vascular proliferation with glomeruloid endothelial hyperplasia, and occasional perivascular monocytic infiltration, corresponding to the hypervascularized marginal zone seen in angiography and to the ring-like enhancement in CT scan;
   2. the surrounding nervous tissue with oedema, myelin damage and astroglial hyperplasia with occasional giant nuclei.

After radiation and chemotherapy, the general histologic features are not much changed, but there is increased cell kill and tissue necrosis with more extensive hypocellular areas, decreased mitotic rate, nuclear and cytoplasmic changes, increase of cell and nuclear monstrosities, and enhanced vascular and mesenchymal reaction with endothel hyperplasia [7, 12, 21, 43–45]. Some of these changes that may also occur spontaneously in untreated gliomas appear to be unrelated to the time interval between treatment and morphological examination, while in general, there is a good correlation between the intensity of most histological changes and the total tumour duration, survival time, and the interval to treatment (tab. 3).

Schiffer et al. [43] have shown that the extent of large central necroses, of perifocal oedema, and mitotic rate is less after short survival than in patients who survive treatment for more than six months, where small necroses, vascular proliferation, nuclear polymorphism, and macrophage areas increase, while the mitotic rate which is significantly reduced immediately after treatment, later increases due to the regrowth of the tumour (tab. 3).

The *morphologic changes* in gliomas following treatment are induced by disturbances of the cell cycle which depend on the mechanisms and phase-specifity of the

Table 3 Correlation between time after treatment and post mortem histology in malignant gliomas [43]

Histological Features (Percent)	Autopsy within 2 mos of radiation and 1–2 chemother. cycles (n = 10)	Autopsy over 4 mos after radiation and more than 2 cycles (n = 15)
Cent. necrosis	90	87
Prolif. zone	90	93
Nuclear polymorphism	60	87
Monstrous cells	50	40
Mitoses	30	73
Small necroses	60	73
Vasc. proliferat.	60	80
Macrophage area	70	20
Oedema	60	60

lesions. As in other solid tumours, gliomas are composed of three populations of cells in terms of their kinetic behavior [16]: the proliferating pool A which, in anaplastic gliomas accounts for about 30%; i.e. one-third of the viable cells are in active division with a comparatively short cell cycle time of 2–3 days. The labelling index, i.e. the percentage of actively proliferating cells, in glioblastoma, as in metastases, is 5–15%, in anaplastic gliomas less than 5%, and in isomorphic gliomas 1%. The majority of glioma cells are in the G_0 state, i.e. in the "resting", non-proliferating compartement B retaining their potential for cell division, while in pool C, non-proliferating, sterile and dead cells accumulate (fig. 1). A reduction of the tumour mass due to spontaneous necrosis or treatment will influence the balance between these cell pools, with increased moving of cells from the G_0 state in the quiescent pool B into the proliferating pool A [16]. The amount of time required for cell transition to repopulate the decimated pool A is unknown in gliomas, but the doubling time of solid tumours is prolonged after radiation and/or chemotherapy.

Since a large proportion of cells in malignant gliomas *in vitro* and *in vivo* are in the postmitotic G_1 phase, inhibition in this phase will cause rapid cell kill and necrosis. Inhibition in the S-phase (DNA synthesis) caused by alkylating and other, non cycle-stage specific compounds, induce nuclear enlargement, degeneration of the nuclear envelope, with margination of chromatin, variation in the nuclear size or pyknosis, increased cytoplasmic density or vacuolation, with loss of cytoplasmic details. Radiation which, similar to podophyllotoxin, mainly acts on the post-DNA-synthesis phase G_2 and early mitosis, can induce the formation of multinucleated giant cells which is also caused by inhibition of the late mitosis M-phase, e.g. by vincristine, but also may occur spontaneously by polyploidy. Postmitotic unification of karyomeres results in the formation of intranuclear "inclusions" due to cytoplasmic invagination [21].

Studies in animal glioma models and tissue culture indicate that characteristic, although not specific *cytologic features* are likely to results from radiation and

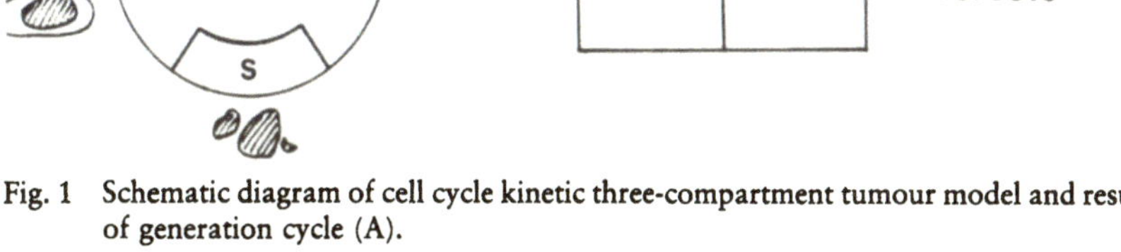

Fig. 1 Schematic diagram of cell cycle kinetic three-compartment tumour model and results of disorders of generation cycle (A).

chemotherapy, but the evaluation of these effects in human brain tumours is difficult because of their pleomorphic appearance. While some authors observed an increase of giant cells and bizarre nuclei after both radiation and chemotherapy [12, 20, 21, 53], others [43] failed to confirm alterations attributable to antitumor therapy, although in addition to increased necrosis and cell polymorphism, there was a tendency for a decrease in the number of mitoses and an increase of monstrous cells related to survival. Comparative evaluation of some cytologic and histologic features of gliomas in consecutive biopsies and autopsies using both the smear technique and paraffin preparations demonstrated a quantitative relationship of some changes to the type of treatment and to the time interval between treatment and microscopic examination (tab. 4):

a) The cytology of *untreated* anaplastic gliomas shows high cellularity with strong cellular and nuclear pleomorphism, marked variation in nuclear structure with one or several nuclei and many mitotic figures. Giant cells with large hyperchromatic or multiple nuclei, poor margination of nuclei or with nuclear fragmentation are frequent: cytoplasmic invagination is rare. During the spontaneous progression of tumour no appreciable changes are seen except for increased necrosis, vascular changes and meningeal invasion, apparently related to the time of tumour duration.

b) After *radiation* in addition to increased necrosis and vascular reaction, there is an increase of giant cells with abundant, bizarre cytoplasm, nuclear monstrosities with frequent pyknosis, irregular fragmentation and uneven distribution of nuclear fragments within the cytoplasm often showing basophilia or vacuolation (fig. 4). There is an increase of atypical mitoses with disappearance of typical mitoses. These changes are considered as effects of radiation and suggest a slowing of the tumour growth which is supported by the disappearance of circumscribed necroses with pseudopalisading being an expression of rapid growth [43].

c) After *chemotherapy* and radio-chemotherapy, in addition to the above changes, there is frequent formation of multinucleated giant and monstrous cells (fig. 3) reticular or vacuolar degeneration of the cytoplasm with loss of structural details and degeneration of nuclear and cellular membranes. The large, hyperchromatic nuclei often show budding and herniation, dissemination of fragments within the cytoplasm, large cytoplasmic inclusions, intranuclear cytoplasmic invaginations, and isolated giant nuclei without surrounding cytoplasm are abundant (fig. 2, 5, 6). The mitotic rate is reduced shortly after treatment, but later rises again. The increased occurrence of multinucleated giant cells in treated gliomas, showing a lower labelling index and multiplication capacity than spontaneously arising giant cells [17] is suggested to result from previous actions of radiation or drugs on cell kinetics [12, 21, 53]. On the other hand, the frequency and intensity of perivascular mononuclear infiltrates considered as an expression of cell-mediated

Table 4 Vaiation of histological findings in anaplastic gliomas in relation to therapy and survival time

Therapy Group	Operation + Conv. Care						Operation + Radiotherapy						Operation + CCNU						Operation + Radiother. + COMP					
Survival after first biopsy	< 6 mos			> 6 mos			< 6 mos			> 6 mos			< 6 mos			> 6 mos			< 6 mos			> 6 mos		
N. of cases	45			10			21			38			7			9			30			31		
Histology	↑	↓/=	0	↑	↓/=	0	↑	↓/=	0	↑	↓/=	0	↑	↓/=	0	↑	↓/=	0	↑	↓/=	0	↑	↓/=	0
Cellularity	9	36	–	4	6	–	4	17	–	14	24	–	–	7	–	4	5	–	–	30	–	9	–	21
Pleomorphism	9	36	–	4	6	–	2	19	–	10	18	–	1	6	–	3	6	–	5	25	–	8	–	23
Giant cells	11	23	11	3	7	–	*10**	7	3	13	17	8	*6**	–	1	*6**	3	–	*21**	3	6	15	8	8
Bizarre nuclei	7	35	3	3	7	–	8	11	2	12	24	2	*6**	–	1	*7**	2	–	*18**	8	4	11	11	2
Nucl. inclusion	–	4	31	2	2	6	2	1	18	1	6	31	3	–	4	5	1	3	10	5	15	8	8	18
Mitoses	12	33	–	6	4	–	2	19*	–	23	15	–	–	7*	–	2	7*	–	–	*30**	–	11	20	–
Mecroses	25	20	–	*8**	2	–	*18**	3	–	*37**	1	–	*6**	1	–	*8**	1	–	*29**	1	–	*27**	4	–
Vasc. prolif.	26	29	–	*8**	2	–	*18**	3	–	*38**	–	–	*5**	2	–	*8**	1	–	*30**	–	–	*28**	3	–
Lymphocyt. inf.	–	12	33	5	3	2	3	6	12	2	9	27	–	1	6	1	2	6	–	11	19	–	5	26
Mening. invas.	20	17	23	*10**	–	–	5	8	8	15	11	12	1	1	5	3	1	5	10	7	13	14	9	8
Calcification	–	1	44	–	–	10	3	–	18	–	–	38	1	–	6	–	–	9	2	–	28	–	–	31

* Difference $p < 0,01$

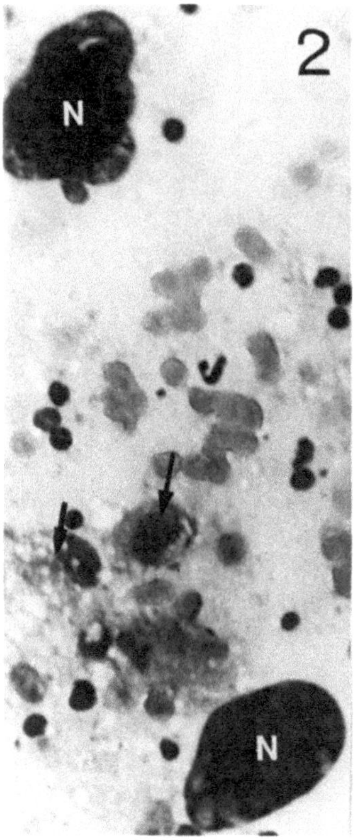

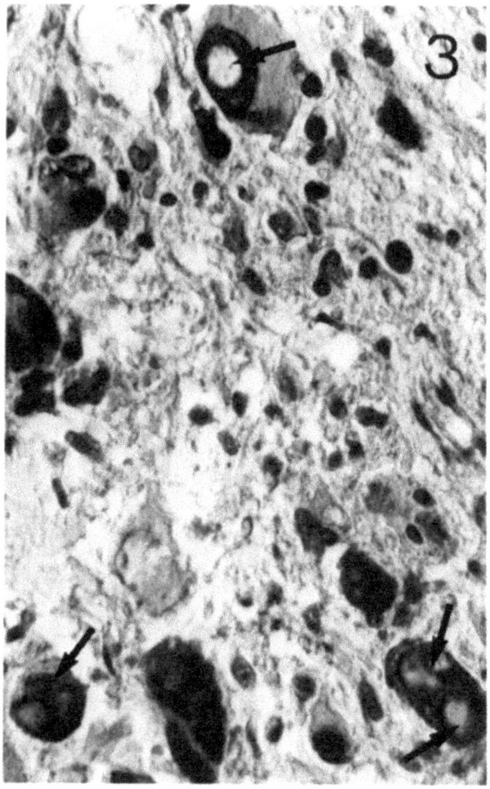

Fig. 2 Imprint cytology of glioblastoma after chemotherapy. Two hyperchromatic giant nuclei without cytoplasm (N) and large cells vith vacuolar degeneration of cytoplasm (arrows). M.G.G. × 300.

Fig. 3 Autopsy specimen of anaplastic astrocytoma after radiation and chemotherapy. Monstrous cells with intranuclear cytoplasmic inclusions (arrows). H. E. × 300.

immunity, often decreases in patients with long survival and their slight, but non-significant reduction after antitumour treatment may indicate some immunosuppressive effects of therapy [12, 21, 43].

The possible relations of some histological features of malignant gliomas with therapy and survival time are summarized in table 5. Wide necroses, cellular pleomorphism and vascular proliferation generally increase with total duration and after antitumour treatment. The increase in the number of giant cells and bizarre nuclei, and of small necroses is related to shorter survival, while the mitotic rate, after a transient post-treatment decrease, later increases again.

Recurrent gliomas show a tendency towards *dedifferentiation* characterized by an increase in cellularity, anaplasia, and other signs of malignancy. Primary anaplastic gliomas with short progression intervals show less spontaneous anaplastic changes than isomorphic gliomas with longer progression-free intervals. Comparison of con-

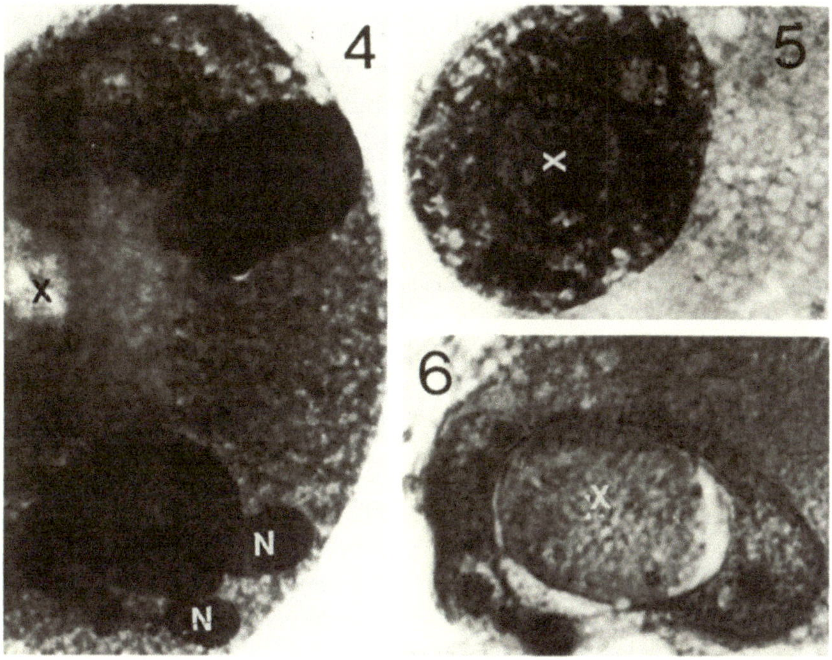

Fig. 4 Cytology of irradiated glioblastoma. Binuclear giant cell with nuclear protrusions (N) and reticular degeneration of cytoplasm (×). M.G.G. × 1000.

Fig. 5,6 Giant cells with nuclear cytoplasmic invagination (×) and degenerating cytoplasm. M.G.G. × 1200.

secutive biopsy and autopsy specimens show the same malignancy grade in 20–45% of recurrent isomorphic gliomas, 45–66% or anaplastic tumours and in 70% of grade III anaplastic gliomas [20]. Post mortem specimens of anaplastic gliomas compared with those of biopsies usually reveal enhanced anaplasia with increased cellularity and a preponderance of small-sized cells without appreciable changes in the general architecture of the tumour [7, 19, 39, 55].

There may be a small number of gliomas at risk of an adverse response to antitumour treatment with *rapid anaplasia* which, however, may also occur spontaneously in supratentorial gliomas of adolescents and young adults [39, 42]. Among 63 cases of anaplastic gliomas treated with adjuvant radio- and chemotherapy, Budka et al. [5] reported three young adults with increasing preponderance of small medulloblastoma-like cells. In our autopsy series of 100 aggressively treated anaplastic gliomas, we observed such a change of phenotype in three cases: one grade III astrocytoma showed overgrowth of a primitive, small-cell population 20 months after operation and 5 COMP cycles. Similar dedifferentiation was seen in biopsy specimens of the second and third operation in two other grade III astrocytomas 9 to 17 months after adjuvant radio-chemotherapy. The occasional anaplastic change of phenotype due

Table 5 Possible relationship between histological features of malignant gliomas and treatment (modified after Schiffer [43])

Histology Features	Increase related to	Decrase related to
Wide necroses	total duration any treatment	
Small necroses		total duration
Polymorphism	total duration distance from radiation	
Monstrous cells	dosage of/distance from radiation chemotherapy	distance from radio/chemotherapy
Mitoses	total duration distance from radiation	short distance from radio/chemotherapy
Vessel degeneration	short distance from radio-/chemotherapy	distance from radio- and/or chemotherapy
Vascular proliferation	total duration distance from radiation dosage of radiation	
Macrophage areas		distance from radio-/chemotherapy No of chemother. cycles total duration

to "focal progression" in tumour or selection of a primitive cell population with enhanced proliferation capacity is considered to result from changes of the genetic expressivity with "cloning" of anaplastic tumour cells which may occur both spontaneously or secondary to treatment [42].

Malignant gliomas have a tendency towards invasion of the meninges and ventricles, seen in 10–15% of the biopsy specimens and in more than onethird of the autopsies [19, 39]. Despite aggressive treatment, with increasing survival time, they may show diffuse invasive or multifocal growth and generalized spread via the CSF spaces. Burger et al. [7] reported ventricular dissemination in three of five glioblastomas treated with chemotherapy, and in two of 20 autopsies after radio-chemotherapy. In our autopsy series, CSF dissemination in malignant gliomas with 8 spontaneous course (17%) was less frequent than in all treatment groups (26–42%), but its incidence was not related to survival time or the type of treatment (tab. 2). On the other hand, the extremely low incidence of remote extracranial metastases of anaplastic gliomas may increase with prolonged survival. Among about 2000 gliomas, we observed 13 cases (0,65%) with metastases outside the neuraxis (lymph nodes, lungs, liver, bone), five of which were among the present series of 218 autopsies (2.3%). Only four patients had operation alone, all others had adjuvant radiation and/or chemotherapy; survival ranged from 7 to 31 months.

Zülch [55] suggested the danger of "malignization of gliomas by irradiation". However, in view of the well-established tendency of supratentorial gliomas towards progressive anaplasia and transliquoral spread, a therapeutic induction or enhancement of such changes may occur rarely, but cannot be substantiated in the majority of cases, while the danger of remote extraneural metastases may increase with therapy-induced prolongation of survival of the tumour host.

Changes in the tumour bed and adjacent brain

The marginal proliferation zone and the brain adjacent to the tumour (BAT) are important for both the tumour growth (regrowth after therapy) and the efficacy of chemotherapy from cell-kinetic and pharmacokinetic considerations. BAT is the major site of tumour growth and reproliferation, and contains the majority of the "silent" compartment B of tumour cells showing the potential for future growth [16]. On the other hand, due to a concentration gradient of drug delivery ("sink-effect") the tumour edge shows the highest level of systemically administered antitumour drugs [26]. After radiation and chemotherapy, a variety of morphological changes occur in the marginal zone of the tumour and the adjacent brain tissue that are related to the intensity of treatment and the time interval between therapy and histological examination (fig. 7):

a) Low radiation doses below 10 Gy hardly induce any changes either in the tumour or in the BAT that shows a highly cellular proliferation zone with nuclear pleomorphism, abundant mitoses, circumscribed necroses with pseudopalisading, and vascular proliferation with bands of glomeruli.

b) When death occurs during radiation (45 Gy), giant cells nuclear monstrosities and necroses are more frequent, while typical mitoses, circumscribed necroses and endothelial proliferation are almost absent. The BAT shows oedema, spongiosis, reactive astroglial proliferation with bizarre nuclei, and hypervascularity with fibrinoid or hyalin degeneration of small vessels.

c) At death within six months of irradiation (60 Gy), the large central necrosis, often including most of the tumour, is surrounded by a larger proliferation zone. Nuclear polymorphism, cell monstrosities and small necroses with pseudopalisading become more numerous, and typical mitoses reappear. There are abundant vessels with fibrinoid necrosis, endothelial proliferation and bizarre endothelial nuclei. The BAT shows oedema and an intense glial hyperplasia with giant cells, bizarre nuclei and mitoses, and an increase in small vessels with or without fibro-hyaline degeneration, and endothelial proliferation (figs. 8, 10).

d) After longer survival following irradiation, the less sharply deliminated central necrosis contains islands of proliferating tumour cells and is surrounded by a wide proliferation zone with high cellularity, pleomorphism, abundant circum-

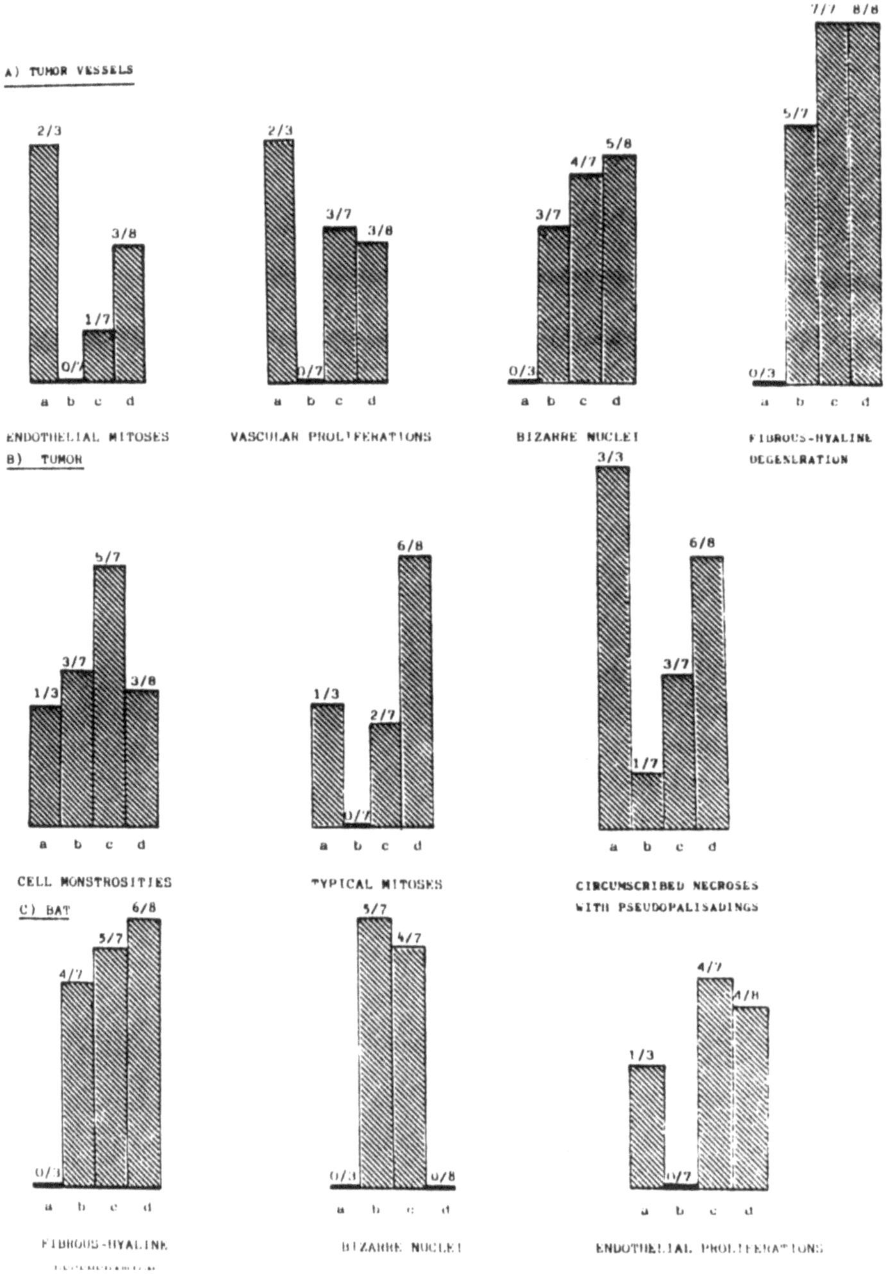

Fig. 7 Variations of histologic parameters in different treatment groups (from 45): a) Radiotherapy (10 Gy); b) Death during radiation (45 Gy); c) death less than 6 months after irradiation (60 Gy); d) death more than 6 months after radiation.

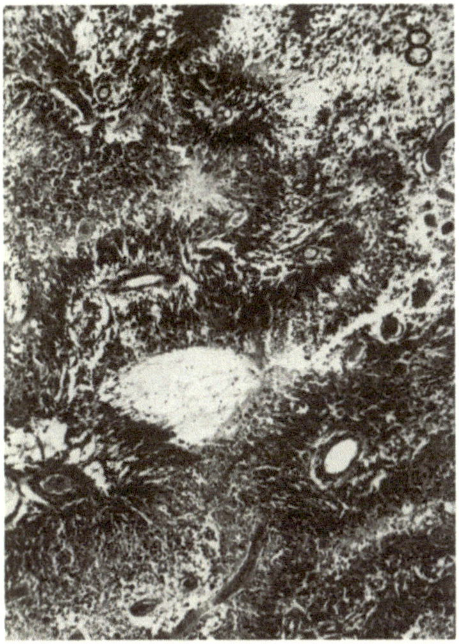

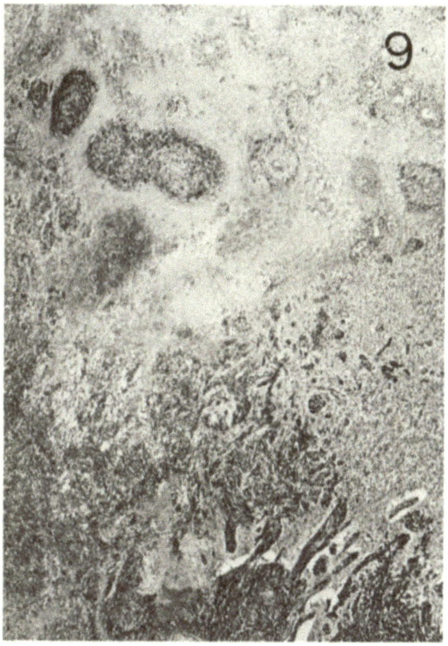

Fig. 8 Circumscribed necroses with pseudopalisading in irradiated glioblastoma. C.V. × 35.

Fig. 9 Transition between central necrosis (upper right) and proliferation zone in treated glioblastoma. H.E. × 200.

scribed necroses and mitoses, but reduced number of nuclear monstrosities. Vessels are abundant with endothelial proliferation and frequent glomeruli. The BAT ist often interrupted by tumour and radionecrotic areas, with high vascular density, and/or fibrohyaline degeneration (fig. 9). In the surrounding gliomatosis containing abundant mitoses, a distinction between reactive hyperplasia and blastomatous transformation is often impossible. Rapid increase in tumour cell density, and the occurrence of neoplastic cells and mitoses in the BAT indicate tumour progression and regrowth, although the BAT in treated cases has a variable morphology and can be masked by peritumoral reactive glial proliferation and radionecroses (fig. 9, 11).

e) After radiotherapy and chemotherapy, completed a short time before death, the tumour shows extensive dry coagulative necrosis, prominent vascular proliferation with fibrinoid necrosis and telangiectasias, and perivascular fibrosis with or without residual or recurrent tumour which is often less prominent than that following chemotherapy alone or longer survival. The peritumoral zone shows abundant proliferation of hyperplastic astroglia with bizarre giant cells and nuclear monstrosities. The BAT is characterized by diffuse oedema, sponginess, myelin pallor or demyelination with vesicular myelin disintegration and axonal

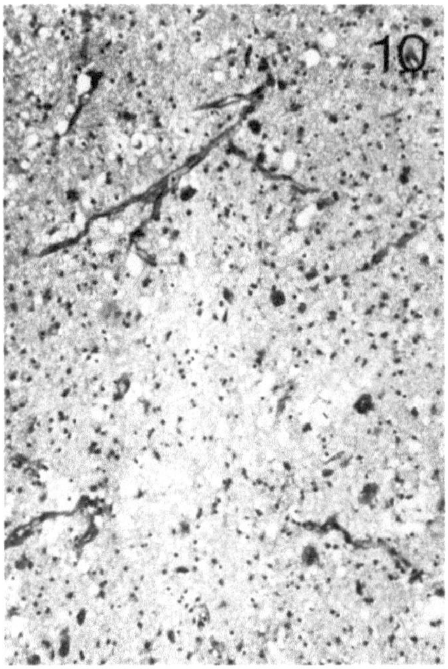

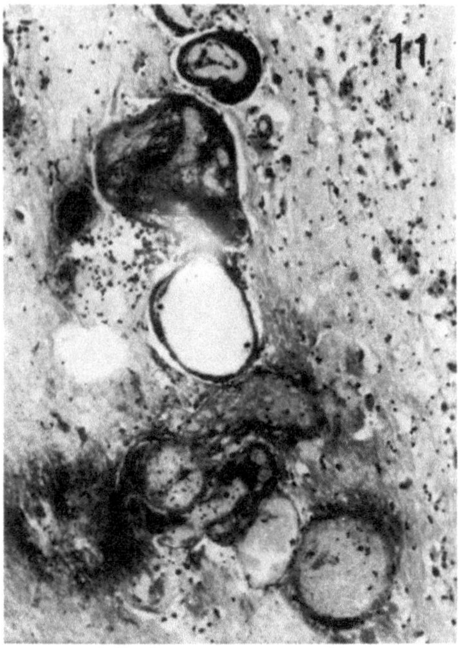

Fig. 10 Hyperplastic astrocytes in BAT of glioma. H.E. × 200.

Fig. 11 Delayed radionecrosis with telangiectasis, fibrinoid vascular necrosis, and plasma exudation. C.V. × 90.

damage, hyaline degeneration of vasculature, and marked astrogliosis with bizarre and multinucleated giant cells. The diffuse changes surrounding the BAT, corresponding to hypodense areas in the CT, may range from sponginess to focal demyelination, necrosis or cyst formation.

Large *space-occupying cerebral cysts* in malignant gliomas may occur spontaneously or after operation [19, 39], but are more frequent following irradiation and radiochemotherapy with an incidence of 12–16% [52]. In our series, their occurrence, after radiation or combination treatment was demonstrated by CT in 7 and 14%, respectively, and in 16 to 22% of all autopsies. Developing 4 to 12 months after treatment, clinically and at CT they may mimic tumour recurrence and other complications, such as brain abscess. Grossly, the fluidfilled cysts are limited by necrotic tissue, scars with or without residual tumour or superficially by the dura, or they communicate widely with the enlarged ventricles. Histology shows coagulative necrosis at or adjacent to the operation site; the walls are formed of glio-mesenchymal, hypervascularized tissue with or without fibrinoid vascular necrosis or recurrent tumour (figs. 12, 13). These cysts are considered to result from radiogenic and drug-induced necrosis of tumour and adjacent brain tissue with surrounding scar formation and increased influx of fluid from the highly vascularized wall containing vessels with increased permeability [7, 21, 52]. The tumour bed of irradiated gliomas

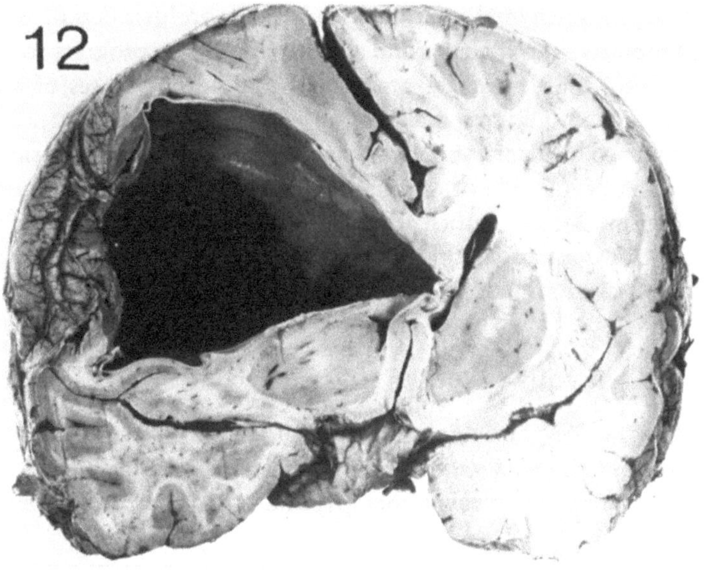

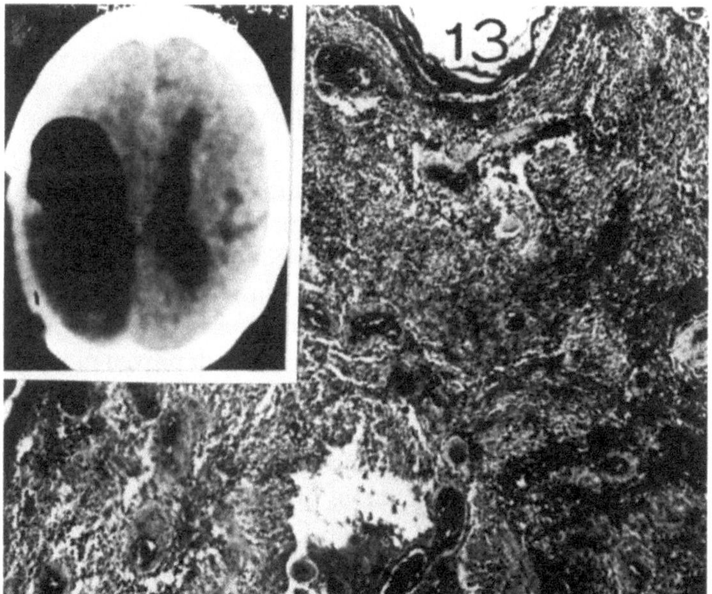

Fig. 12 Large fluid-filled cyst in left hemisphere without macroscopically detectable tumour; C.T. (inset); 30 months after multimodal treatment of grade III astrocytoma.

Fig. 13 Gliomesenchymal wall of tumour cyst with glioma tissue. H. E. × 35.

often shows strong mesenchymal reaction with fibrosis, proliferation of vessels and perivascular fibroblasts with high mitotic activity that rarely progress to sarcomatous transformation [7, 18]. In three among our 100 autopsy cases of malignant gliomas, development of "gliosarcoma" was observed 9–24 months after aggressive radio-chemotherapy, which corresponds to the spontaneous occurrence rate of gliosarcomas, accounting for 2–3% of malignant gliomas [19, 39]. Most patients with malignant gliomas do not live sufficiently long to implicate radiation as a cause of any sarcomatous transformation. On the other hand, meningeal and dural sarcomas are not uncommon after radiation for various neoplasms [7, 18, 39].

Changes in the Nervous tissue

The advance of aggressive brain tumour treatment has increased the risk of damage to the CNS and has created a variety of complications that include a) radiation damage, b) brain damage from chemotherapy, and c) sequelae of combined treatment.

Radionecrosis of the brain

The incidence of brain damage after radiotherapy for intracranial tumours ranges from 1.5 – 20%, and was 15 – 20% in recent autopsy series of malignant gliomas treated with megavoltage radiation [7, 29, 44, 49]. In our autopsy series of 100 aggressively treated glioms, the incidence of radionecrosis after irradiation and multimodality treatment was 13 and 6%, respectively; 6 of 8 cases who had received 66.5 Gy with misonidazole (tab. 2). The incidence of radionecrosis of the CNS depends on the total dose, fractionation pattern and the number of treatments, and is closely related to the tolerance level of the brain that is suggested to be 1600–1800 ret ED (equivalent dose), corresponding to conventional dose schemes of about 60 Gy given in 30 fractions over 6 weeks [28, 49]. However, radiation damage may occur at lower doses, particularly when addition of chemotherapy may increase brain sensitivity to irradiation. Analysis of 83 patients with proven radionecrosis of the brain showed that 54% had received total doses exceeding 70 Gy, and 22% those exceeded 50 Gy, while in 17% the daily fraction ranged from 2.5–3.5 Gy, and only in 9% from 1.8 to 2.25 Gy [49]. The incidence of radionecrosis is considered 4% after total dose of 50 Gy given in fractions of 180 cGy/day, and rises to 14.3% after doses of 60 Gy given in fractions of 200 cGy/day. Adverse CNS reactions to radiation can be divided into three groups according to the time of appearance, namely acute or early, subacute, and delayed reactions, the late damage showing early and delayed manifestation.

Acute reactions with total necrosis of the tumour and adjacent brain are occasionally seen after brachytherapy (implantation of radionuclides) and irradiation with heavy particle beams (proton beam and neutrons) [1, 8, 48]. Acute reaction, occuring during the course of conventional radiotherapy, is due to oedema caused by breakdown of the BBB, and amenable to corticosteroid therapy for symptomatic relief. Recovery is generally spontaneous.

Subacute postradiation leucoencephalopathy, with progressive clinical symptoms beginning weeks to 2–3 months after radio-chemotherapy of malignant gliomas [7], cranial irradiation and intrathecal or systemic chemotherapy of childhood leukemias [3], is characterized pathologically by multiple spongy focal lesions and coagulation necrosis in the brain and brain stem, and largely corresponds to the "disseminated necrotizing leukoencephalopathy".

Delayed reactions include rare instances of *"early" delayed* effects with disseminated patches of spongy demyelination occuring 2–3 months after radiation [18, 25], and *late delayed radionecrosis* constituting the major hazard of high-dose CNS irradiation. The latency interval ranges from six months to three years with an average of 15 months [49]. The earliest autopsy-proven radionecrosis occurred after 4–5 months [44].

Delayed radionecrosis, defined as a clinico-tomographic recurrence while the "major finding at operation or autopsy is necrosis with little or no persistent tumour" [32], appears as an intracranial mass lesion at the primary tumour site or in remote brain areas presenting as a ring structure with marginal enhancement in the CT scan. However, since radionecrosis may occur also in association with tumour recurrence, and since tumour regrowth often affects nervous tissue damaged by radiation, their clinico-radiological and even morphological separation may be difficult if not impossible. Distant radionecrosis occuring in the contralateral hemisphere of the irradiated tumour may mimic multicentric glioma. In our autopsy series, two patients with progressive clinical deterioration 6–11 months after operation on an anaplastic glioma with adjuvant 66.6 Gy radiatio with misonidazol, at autopsy revealed extensive radionecrosis without or with only small remnants of tumour. Another patient developing progressive dementia after postoperative irradiation of a right temporal glioma (60.7 Gy) and 3 COMP cycles, at death 33 months after operation, in addition to a small tumour recurrence showed left parietal radionecrosis and considerable internal hydrocephalus. The pathological features of delayed radiation damage are coagulation necrosis with collagen formation, astroglial proliferation and vascular changes ranging from acute fibrinoid necrosis with extravasation of plasma to fibrous thickening and formation of telangiectasias, associated with deposition of protein and amyloid-like substances with or without mineralization, and reactive, often tumour-like astrogliosis (fig. 11). Localized radionecrosis may terminate in cystic defects or fibro-collagenous scars with protein deposition and calcification, as was seen in both temporal lobes of a man who for suspected glioma had received repeated X-irridiation with estimated total dose of 133 Gy for 24 years [18]. Peritumoral necrosis, with sharply deliminated dry coagulation is often surrounded by macrophage-filled areas, spongy lesions and oedema with myelin damage, loss of oligodendroglia, peritumoral or distant reactive gliosis with bizarre giant cells and hyperchromatic nuclei, and disseminated foci of tissue necrosis. Most of the lesions, in particular radionecrosis, peritumoral necrosis, vascular pathology, perifocal oedema, myelin damage, and distant astroglial reaction, are positively related to total radiation dose and survival time [44]. The strong predilection of this tissue response for the white matter adjacent to the neoplasm suggests a local sensitivity which may have been enhanced by cerebral oedema, but changes of diffuse oedema are also noted in many of the radiated brains.

CNS damage as a result of chemotherapy

After intra-arterial (carotid) perfusion with bleomycin and BCNU sudden seizures and fatal coma were observed. There was oedematous necrosis with angionecrosis or necrotizing angiolitis and haemorrhages in the ipsilateral hemisphere [4, 36]. Systemic high-dose BCNU therapy without cranial radiation (1.4–3.5 g/sqm) may not result in any CNS lesions [15], or may induce acute progressive encephalomyelopathy, with multiple small focal necroses with swollen axons and myelin vacuolation, and larger symmetrical areas of oedema with white and grey matter necrosis, fibrinoid vascular necrosis and fibrin microthrombi, similar to "MTX encephalopathy" and delayed radionecrosis [6].

Misonidazole-encephalopathy, occasionally observed after cummulative doses of 18 g/5 weeks, is characterized by similar focal cortical necroses and demyelination with haemorrhages [24]; the reported CNS toxicity of misonidazole in the RTOG glioma study was 3% [34]. The cause of neurotoxicity of these drugs is unknown, but the common pathology of BCNU encephalopathy after intra-arterial and systemic administration with fibrinoid necrosis suggest a primary damage of the cerebrospinal vasculature, while misonidazole is considered to cause dehydration. *5-fluorouracil* and related drugs which cause encephalopathy in up to 40% of the patients, with lethargy, coma, parkinsonism, visual disorders and cerebellar dysfunctions [54], experimentally induce spongy CNS lesions with myelin vacuolation similar to that produced by triethyltin or hexachlorophene [35]. While high doses of MTX, BCNU and 5-FU cause damage of the BBB, most of these neurotoxic effects show a complete reversibility [21].

Encephalopathy associated with radiation and chemotherapy

After radio-chemotherapy, a variety of acute and progressive CNS lesions occur:

1. *Disseminated necrotizing leukoencephalopathy* (DNL) clinically featured by insidious or rapidly progressive neurological signs, intellectual impairment, dementia or fatal coma, with onset 3–15 months after cranial irradiation with intrathecal or various combinations of oral, IT and systemic chemotherapy for leukemia, lymphomas, other systemic neoplasia and brain tumours has an estimated inci-

dence of 2–45% [3, 21, 31, 40]. CT shows periventricular hypodensity. Morphological changes range from small disseminated spongy areas with demyelination and axonal swelling to multiple foci of coagulative necroses with mineralization and occasional fibrinoid vascular necrosis, with diffuse perifocal oedema and reactive gliosis. Similar disseminated lesions were seen in the brain stem after radio-chemotherapy of malignant gliomas [3, 7]. Since the spongy lesions of DNL, also referred to as "MTX-encephalopathy" closely resemble early delayed radionecrosis, a multifactorial pathogenetic mechanism is suggested, in that increased permeability of the BBB induced by cytostatic drugs may add to the manifestation of latent radiation damage.

2. *Diffuse brain damage:* Progressive cerebral atrophy and internal hydrocephalus are the most frequent, and most debatable late sequelae of long-term treatment of systemic malignancies [13, 21]. Of long-surviving patients with malignant gliomas, about two years after multimodal treatment, in the absence of tumour recurrence, 10–30% develop progressive neuro-psychiatric dysfunctions and dementia with cerebral atrophy, internal hydrocephalus or bilateral hypodense CT lesions, similar to those seen in one to two thirds of long-term survivors of aggressively treated leukemia in remission [13, 21]. Autopsy reveals diffuse spongy white matter degeneration with or without demyelination and diffuse astroglial hyperplasia and fibrillary gliosis in the affected or in both cerebral hemispheres [37, 44]. These and other diffuse cerebral lesions also observed in 10–65% of all autopsies of aggressively treated leukemias [10, 21] are interpreted as chronic sequelae of brain oedema (post-oedematous lesions) and are to be distinguished from DNL and postradiation damage (figs. 14, 15).

Many pathological changes within the white matter ipsilateral and contralateral to the tumour are more pronounced after multimodal treatment than after irradiation alone, suggesting synergistic or overlapping mechanisms of neural toxicity [3, 7, 21, 37, 44]. In spite of the well established beneficial effect of corticosteroids on perifocal oedema and BBB permeability [50], their protective efficacy against radionecrosis suggested from the autopsy studies by Burger et al. [7] is not supported by experimental data [30] and other human case series showing no relationship between the occurrence of iatrogenic CNS lesions and non-treatment with steroids, although peritumour necrosis after radio-chemotherapy more often occurs in patients without additional steroid treatment [45]. The possible protective effect of steroids against radionecrosis and other adverse effects of antitumour treatment on the CNS remains to be further elucidated.

Common complications of antitumour treatment

Rather rare CNS complications of antineoplastic treatment are haemorrhages into the tumour or brain, related to haemototoxic effects and CNS infections due to radiogenic and cytotoxic immunodepression. These complications are less frequent

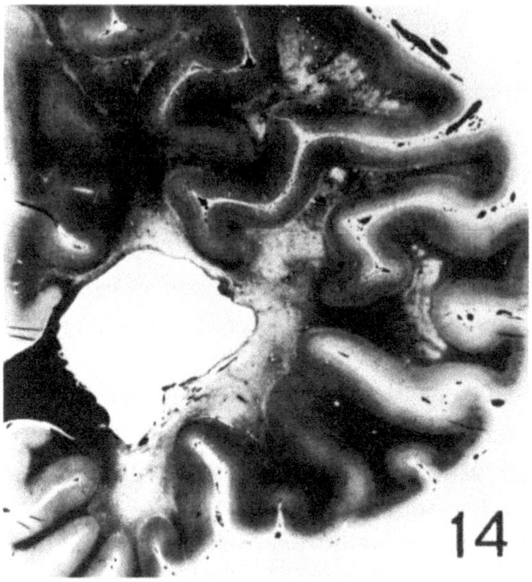

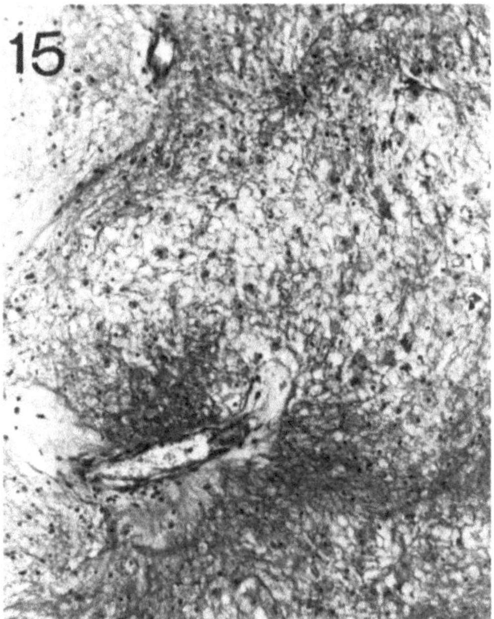

Fig. 14 Internal hydrocephalus and spongy demyelination in contralateral hemisphere of glioblastoma after multimodal treatment (survival 33 months with progressive dementia).

Fig. 15 Spongy changes of white matter with vascular fibrosis and astroglial hyperplasia. H. E. × 100.

in glioma patients than after chemotherapy of systemic neoplasms, leukemias and lymphomas [4, 14, 22], while in the latter group direct antitumour-related CNS lesions are less frequent than in glioma patients: in a large autopsy series of leukaemia-lymphoma cases we observed diffuse gliosis in 20% and other secondary CNS lesions (radionecrosis, DNL etc.) in only 7.5% [22].

Finally, the development of secondary malignancies observed with increasing frequency after radiation and chemotherapy of neoplasms has to be considered. While development of dural and meningeal sarcomas is not uncommon after radiation of various extra- and intra-cranial tumours [18, 19, 39], acute leukaemia complicating therapy of malignant glioma has been observed only in five documented cases [9, 11, 51] and therefore appears to be much less frequent than following aggressive chemotherapy of lymphomas and other neoplasms.

In conclusion, aggressive radiation and chemotherapy as they are presently employed cannot completely destroy or eradicate the majority of malignant gliomas, that often continue to grow until the patient's death, but they severely damage the tumour and even my stop tumour progression, and thus improve the prognosis and survival. On the other hand, radio- and chemotherapy with the dosages and techniques commonly employed for malignant gliomas carry a considerable risk of a variety of injuries to the surrounding cerebral tissues that may impair the quality and even the duration of survival. Some of these adverse reactions become increasingly apparent only as a result of therapy-induced prolongation of survival and may explain progressive nervous and mental dysfunctions occuring without tumour recurrence. In view of the poor prognosis of malignant gliomas, however, the incidence and severity of adverse effects of antitumour therapy are less severe than for other solid and systemic neoplasms, and their calculable risk may be further minimized by greater sophistication and optimization of multimodal treatment techniques.

Summary

The morphologic effects of antitumour treatment on human glioma tissue and its proliferative zone (tumour bed and adjacent brain), and on both the surrounding and intact brain are reviewed. General, but non-specific morphological sequelae of treatment are an increase within and around the tumour tissue of degenerative and regressive changes and a variety of cytologic and histologic alterations (increase of necrosis, vascular proliferation, giant cells, nuclear monstrosities etc.) indicating increased cell kill and transient slowing of tumour growth. Most of these changes are time-related, and may also occur spontaneously in the natural course of tumours. In the tumour bed, there is increased glial proliferation and progressive tumour regrowth. Both total destruction of malignant gliomas with currently used dosages and forms of treatment and therapy-induced enhancement of anaplasia are extremely rare, but there is an increased risk of adverse reaction in the CNS (local and diffuse), the separation of which from tumour progression and regrowth may be difficult. Radiogenic and drug-related lesions affecting both the tissue surrounding the tumour, remote or diffuse brain areas, range from spongy white matter damage with gliosis to focal demyelination, coagulation necrosis or cyst formation. Radionecrosis (early and delayed) seen in about 15% of the treated glioma-brains, and large fluid-filled cysts resulting from necrosis of tumour and adjacent brain (occurring in 12–20%) may mimic tumour recurrence. Multifocal lesions, similar to disseminated necrotizing leucoencephalopathy, and diffuse brain damage (atrophy, internal hydrocephalus, diffuse sponginess and gliosis of white matter) resulting from chronic oedema are similar to those seen after aggressive treatment of systemic neoplasm. Most local and diffuse CNS changes are more pronounced after multimodal treatment than after irradiation alone, suggesting synergistic and overlapping mechanisms. Adverse CNS reactions become increasingly apparent with therapy-induced prolongation of survival and may cause progressive cerebral dysfunction and impairment of quality of survival even without tumour recurrence. In view of the poor prognosis of malignant gliomas the risk of iatrogenic CNS damage has to be considered by designing more effective and less harmful therapeutic strategies.

References

[1] Ashbury, A. K., R. G. Ojemann, S. L. Nielsen, et al.: Neuropathology of 14 cases of malignant gliomas treated by boron-10 slow neutron capture radiation. J. Neuropath. exp Neurol. **31** (1972) 278–302.

[2] Bleyer, W. A.: Neurologic sequelae of methotrexate and ionizing radiation: A new classification. Cancer Treat. Rep. **65**, Suppl. 1 (1981) 89–98.

[3] Breuer, A. C., N. K. Blank, W. C. Schoene: Multifocal pontine lesions in cancer patients treated with chemotherapy and CNS radiotherapy. Cancer **4** (1978) 2112–2120.

[4] Budka, H.: Pathology of encephalopathies induced by treatment or prophylaxis of neoplastic lesions of the nervous system. In: Treatment of Neoplastic Lesions of the Nervous System (J. Hildebrand, D. Gangji, eds.), pp. 45–50. Pergamon Press, Oxford–New York 1982.

[5] Budka, H., I. Podreka, F. Zaunbauer: Overgrowth of a primitive cell population in operated recurrent gliomas: the possible role of chemo- and radiotherapy. In: Multidisciplinary Aspects of Brain Tumor Therapy (P. Paoletti, M. D. Walker, et al., eds.), pp. 357–362. Elsevier-North Holland, Amsterdam–New York 1979.

[6] Burger, P. C., E. Kamenar, C. Schold, et al.: Encephalomyelopathy following high-dose BCNU therapy. Cancer **48** (1981) 1318–1327.

[7] Burger, P. C., M. S. Mahaley, L. Dudka, et al.: The morphologic effects of radiation administered therapeutically for intracranial gliomas. Cancer **44** (1978) 1256–1272.

[8] Catterall, M., H. J. G. Bloom, D. V. Ash, et al.: Fast neutrons compared with megavoltage X-rays in the treatment of patients with supratentorial glioblastoma. Int. J. Rad. Oncol. Biol. Phys. **6** (1980) 261–266.

[9] Cohen, R. J., P. H. Wiernik, M. D. Walker: Acute non-lymphocytic leukemia associated with nitrosurea chemotherapy. Report of two cases. Cancer Treat. Rep. **60** (1976) 157–261.

[10] Crosley, C. J., L. B. Rorke, A. Evans, et al.: Central nervous system lesions in childhood leukemia. Neurology (NY) **28** (1978) 678–685.

[11] Genot, J.-Y., M. Krulik, M. Poisson, et al.: Two cases of acute leukemia following treatment of malignant glioma. Cancer **52** (1983) 222–226.

[12] Gerstner, L., K. Jellinger, W.-D. Heiss, et al.: Morphological changes in anaplastic gliomas treated with radiation and chemotherapy. Acta neurochir. (Wien) **36** (1977) 117–138.

[13] Habermalz, E., H. J. Habermalz, U. Stephani, et al.: Cranial computed tomography: 64 children in continuous complete remission of leukemia. Neuropaed. **3** (1983) 144–148.

[14] Henson, R., H. Ulrich: Cancer and the nervous System. Blackwell, London–Edinburgh–New York 1982.

[15] Hochberg, F. H., L. M. Parker, T. Tokvorian, et al.: High-dose BCNU with autologous bone marrow rescue for recurrent glioblastoma multiforme. J. Neurosurg. **54** (1981) 455–460.

[16] Hoshino, T., H. Townsend, I. Muroako, et al.: An autoradiographic study of human gliomas: Growth kinetics of anaplastic astrocytoma and glioblastoma multiforme. Brain 103 (1980) 967–984.

[17] Hoshino, T., C. B. Wilson, W. G. Ellis: Gemistocytic astrocytes in gliomas. An autoradiographic study. J. Neuropath. exp. Neurol. **34** (1975) 263–281.

[18] Jellinger, K.: Human central nervous system lesions following radiation therapy. Zbl. Neurochir. **38** (1977) 199–220.

[19] Jellinger, K.: Glioblastoma multiforme: morphology and biology. Acta neurochir. (Wien) **42** (1978) 5–32.

[20] Jellinger, K.: Histologische Klassifikation und therapiebedingte Veränderungen. In: Therapie maligner Neoplasien des Gehirns (P. Krauseneck, H. G. Mertens, eds.), pp. 13–25. Perimed, Erlangen 1983.

[21] Jellinger, K.: Pathologic effects of chemotherapy. In: Oncology of the Nervous System (M. D. Walker, ed.), pp. 285–340. M. Nijhoff, Boston–Hague–Dordrecht–Lancaster 1983.

[22] Jellinger, K.: Primäre und sekundäre Lymphome des ZNS. In: Verh. Dtsch. Ges. Neurol. (D. Seitz, P. Vogel, eds.), pp. 14–48. Springer, Berlin–Heidelberg–New York 1983.

[23] Kretzschmar, K., K. H. Schicketanz: Measurement of the volume and density of intracranial tumors by CT following therapy. Neuroradiol. **23** (1982) 175–184.

[24] Kun, L. E., K.-C. Ho, J. E. Moulder: Fatal misonidazole-induced encephalopathy An RTOG case report. Cancer **49** (1982) 423–426.

[25] Lampert, P. W., R. L. Davis: Delayed effects of radiation on the human nervous system. Neurology (Minn.) **14** (1964) 912–917.

[26] Levin, V. A., M. S. Edwards: Chemotherapy of malignant gliomas: In: Brain Tumours (D. G. T. Thomas, C. I. C. Graham, eds.), pp. 344–358. Butterworth, London–Boston 1980.

[27] Lieberman, A. N., S. H. Foo, J. Ransohoff, et al.: Long term survival among patients with malignant brain tumors. Neurosurg. **10** (1982) 450–453.

[28] Marks, J. E., R. J. H. Baglan, S. C. Prassad, et al.: Cerebral radionecrosis: Incidence and risk in relation to dose, time, fractionation and volume. Int. J. Rad. Oncol. Biol. Phys. **7** (1981) 243–252.

[29] Marsa, G. W., D. R. Goffinet, L. J. Rubinstein, et al.: Megavoltage irradiation in the treatment of gliomas of the brain and spinal cord. Cancer **36** (1975) 1681–1689.

[30] Martins, A. N., R. E. Severance, J. M. Henry, et al.: Experimental delayed radiation necrosis of the brain. I. Effects of early dexamethasone treatment. J. Neurosurg. **51** (1979) 587–596.

[31] Mena, H., J. H. Garcia, F. Velandia: Central and peripheral myelinopathy associated with systemic neoplasia and chemotherapy. Cancer **48**, 1724–1737.

[32] Mikhael, M. A.: Dosimetric consideration in the diagnosis of radiation necrosis of the brain. In: Radiation damage to the nervous system (H. A. Gilbert, A. R. Kagan, eds.), pp. 59–92. Raven, New York 1980.

[33] Nakamura, N., H. Ogawa, T. Kumanishi: Pathological investigation of radiation necrosis. Complete necrosis of brain tumors observed in autopsy cases. Neurol. Surg. **2** (1974) 213–220.

[34] Nelson, D. F., D. Schoenfeld, A. S. Weinstein, et al.: A randomized comparison of misonidazole sensitized radiotherapy plus BCNU and radiotherapy plus BCNU for treatment of malignant glioma after surgery. Preliminary results of an RTOG study. Int. J. Rad. Oncol. Biol. Phys. **9** (1983) 1143–1151.

[35] Okeda, R., T. Karakama, S. Kimura, et al.: Neuropathologic study on chronic neurotoxicity of 5-fluorouracil and its masked compounds in dogs. Acta neuropath (1983) in press.

[36] Omojola, M. F., A. J. Fox, R. N. Auer, et al.: Haemorrhages encephalitis produced by selective non-occlusive intracarotid BCNU injection in dogs. J. Neurosurg. 57 (1982) 791–796.
[37] Poisson, M., J.-J. Hauw, R. Mashaly, et al.: Status spongiosus in the course of treatment of malignant gliomas. J. Neuro-Oncol. 1 (1983) 29–37.
[38] Rosenblum, M. L., K. D. Knebel, U. W. Kaquez, et al.: Brain tumor therapy: Quantitative analysis using a model system. J. Neurosurg. **46** (1977) 145–157.
[39] Rubinstein, L. J.: Pathology of the tumors of the central nervous system. Atlas of Tumor Pathology, FAsc. 2nd ed. Armed Forces Inst. Pathology, Washington 1972.
[40] Rubinstein, L. J., M. M. Herman, T. F. Long, et al.: Disseminated necrotizing leukoencephalopathy. A complication of treated CNS leukemias and lymphomas. Cancer 35 (1975) 291–305.
[41] Salazar, O. M., P. Rubin, J. V. McDonald, et al.: High dose radiation therapy in the treatment of glioblastoma multiforme. Int. J. Rad. Oncol. Biol. Phys. 1 (1976) 717–727.
[42] Schmitt, H. P.: Rapid anaplastic transformation of gliomas in childhood. Neuropaed. 3 (1983) 137–143.
[43] Schiffer, D., M. T. Gioradana, P. Paoletti, et al.: Pathology of human malignant gliomas after radiation and chemotherapy. Acta neurochir. (Wien) 53 (1980) 205–216.
[44] Schiffer, D., M. T. Giordana, R. Soffietti, et al.: Radio- and chemotherapy of malignant gliomas. Pathological changes in the normal nervous tissue. Acta neurochir. (Wien) 58 (1981) 37–58.
[45] Schiffer, D., M. T. Giordana, R. Soffietti, et al.: Histological observations on the regrowth of malignant gliomas after radiotherapy and chemotherapy. Acta neuropath. (Berl.) 58 (1982) 291–299.
[46] Schold, S. C., D. B. Biogner: A review of animal brain tumor models that have been used for therapeutic studies. In: Oncology of the Nervous System (M. D. Walker, ed.), pp. 31–64. M. Nijhoff, Boston–Hague–Dordrecht–Lancaster 1983.
[47] Seiler, W.: Die undifferenzierten Astrozytome des Großhirns. Springer, Berlin–Heidelberg–New York 1982.
[48] Shaw, C.-M., S. M. Sumi, E. C. Alvord, et al.: Fast-neutron irradiation of glioblastoma multiforme. Neuropathological analysis. J. Neuropath. exp. Neurol. 49 (1978) 1–12.
[49] Sheline, G. E.: Radiotherapy of adult primary cerebral neoplasms. In: Oncology of the Nervous System (M. D. Walker, ed.), pp. 223–245. M. Nijhoff, Boston–Hague–Dordrecht–Lancaster 1983.
[50] Selker, R. G.: Corticosteroids: their effect on primary and metastatic brain tumors. In: Oncology of the Nervous System (M. D. Walker, ed.), pp. 167–191. M. Nijhoff, Boston–Hague–Dordrecht–Lancaster 1983.
[51] Vogl, S. E.: Acute leukemic complicating treatment of glioblastoma multiforme. Cancer **41** (1978) 333–336.
[52] Volc, D., K. Jellinger, H. Flament, et al.: Cerebral space occupying cysts following radiation and chemotherapy of malignant gliomas. Acta neurochir. (Wien) 57 (1981) 177–193.
[53] Willson, N., P. E. Dauffy: Morphologic changes associated with combined BCNU and radiation therapy in glioblastoma multiforme. Neurology **24** (1974) 65–471.
[54] Young, D. F.: Neurological complications of chemotherapy. In: Neurological Complications of Therapy (A. Silverstein, ed.), pp. 57–113. Futura Publ. Comp., Mount Kisco 1982.
[55] Zülch, K. J.: Biology and morphology of glioblastoma multiforme. Acta radiol. Ther. **8** (1969) 65–77.

Microsurgical management of gliomas

W. Haßler, A. Harders, W. Seeger

Introduction

Since the first operative treatment of a glioma [2] was performed in 1884, the prognosis of "brain tumours" has not changed. Although the surgical mortality has decreased considerably, there is still no cure for malignant gliomas, in spite of radical macrosurgical or microsurgical techniques, in spite of cytostatics and irradiation [3, 12, 13, 16, 19]. These procedures have had only a slight effect on the survival time. Glioma patients therefore have to be operated upon as radically and as carefully as possible so that they are able to live out the rest of their lives in a good clinical condition [1, 14].

We have performed microsurgery on gliomas for the last eight years. The method allows gliomas – even those located in the depths of the brain, in the dominant hemisphere, and in highly vascularized areas – to be removed without the risk of severe neurological deficits [14]. We do not support the practice of tumour resection by lobectomy [9, 10, 11, 15].

Surgical indication

We remove all gliomas that are located close to the brain's surface and that are clearly delineated from the surrounding brain (tab. 1), provided only one hemisphere is affected. If pre-existing neurological and psycho-organic disorders tend to diminish under treatment with dexamethasone, we also operate on gliomas in the speech centre, the central region, the Sylvian fissure, the corpus callosum, and the thalamic region.

Table 1 Indication and contraindication for microsurgery of gliomas

Indication	Contraindication
– relationship to surface	– deep seated in basal ganglia
– circumscribed	– not circumscribed
– location in one hemisphere	– location in both hemispheres
– good effect of dexamethason	– no effect of dexamethason

Surgical principles and strategy of approach

The exact location, the extent of the tumour, and thus the topography in relation to the surrounding brain structures are shown in the CT scan. Deep-seated tumours must be projected onto the brain surface in such a way that the shortest approach is possible and that the white matter connections are carefully protected [6, 17, 18]. This is of particular importance in the parietal region. A rostral or occipital approach is used, following the white matter fibres of the pyramidal tract (fig. 1).

If the tumour does not reach the surface of the brain (tab. 2), an approach via a sulcus is used in which the arachnoid layers are spread. Utilizing the various axis settings of the microscope, one provides a good view so that even larger tumours can be removed piecemeal through tiny, 2 cm cortical incisions. When the cerebral cortex is thin and tumours are located in or near a ventricle, they must be operated on by the transcortical approach. An interhemispheric transcallosal approach is only used für intraventricular location (tab. 3). With tumours which reach the surface, the affected gyrus is removed and dissected from the healthy brain under magnification. Tumours which are delineated by sulci can often be fairly well dissected by a subpial exposure. Veins in the area of approach are spared. If multiple gyri are infiltrated with tumour, the affected gyri are resected while sparing arteries and veins in the sulci (fig. 2). After the tumour is projected onto the surface of the skull and skin, exact measurements are taken to provide individually tailored incisions and craniotomy [6].

Operative technique

For the microsurgical glioma operation, the surgeon must have a clear view of the anatomical structures and therefore an operative technique, which keeps bleeding at a minimum is mandatory. As in all microsurgical operations, the assistant is only necessary for irrigating. Self-retaining retractors and a set of simple instruments (aspirator, forceps, dissector) are sufficient. In most cases we prefer the "aspirate-dissect-cut technique" for intratumoral mass reduction [17]. Tough tumours of the

Table 2 Principle of microsurgery of gliomas

– exact topographical localization in the brain and projection on the skull and skin	
– appropriate approach	through gyrus
	through sulcus
	through interhemispheric fissure or sylvian fissure
	sparing white matter connections
– small incision – sparing uneffected brain	
– sparing arteries and veins in approach area	

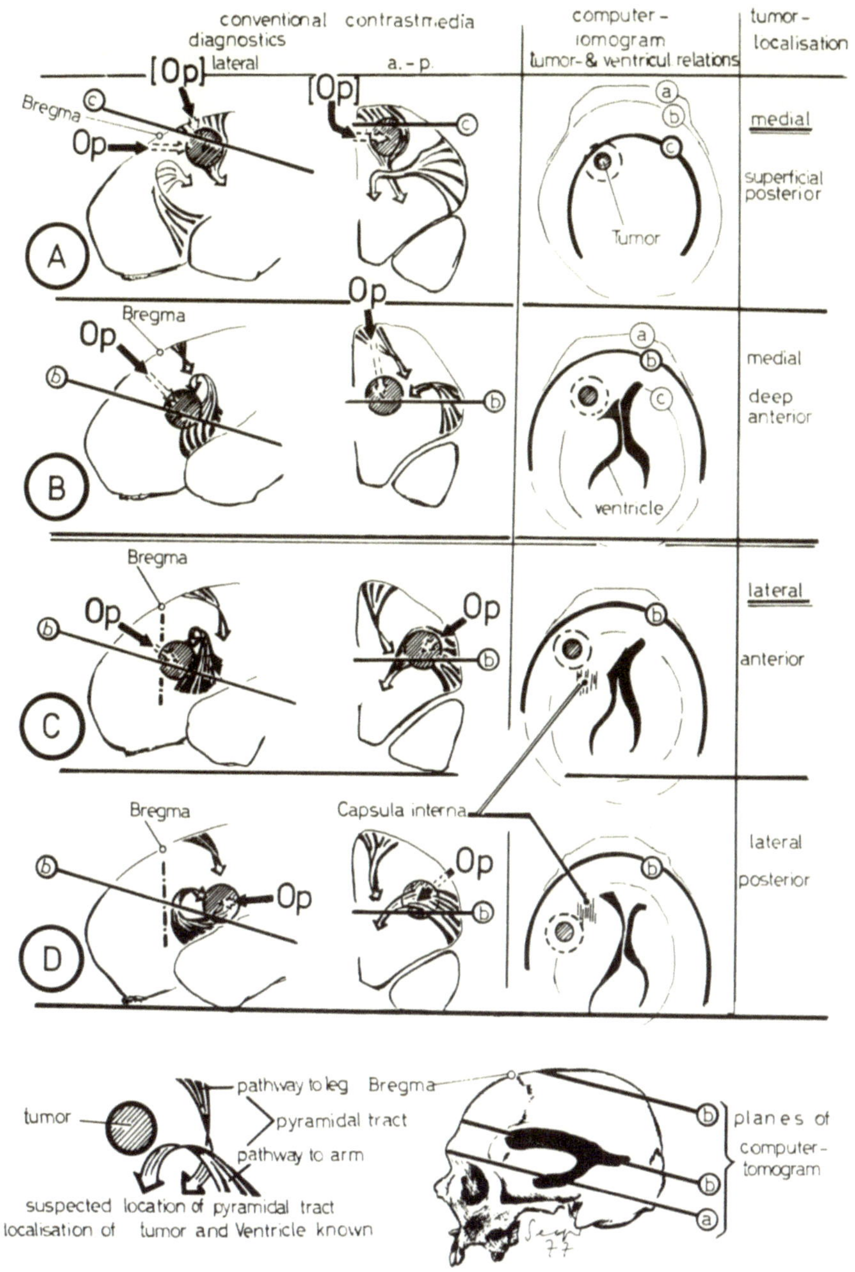

Fig. 1 Approaches to deep seated gliomas in frontal or parietal region. The fibres of the pyramidal tract are dislocated in different ways and must be spared.

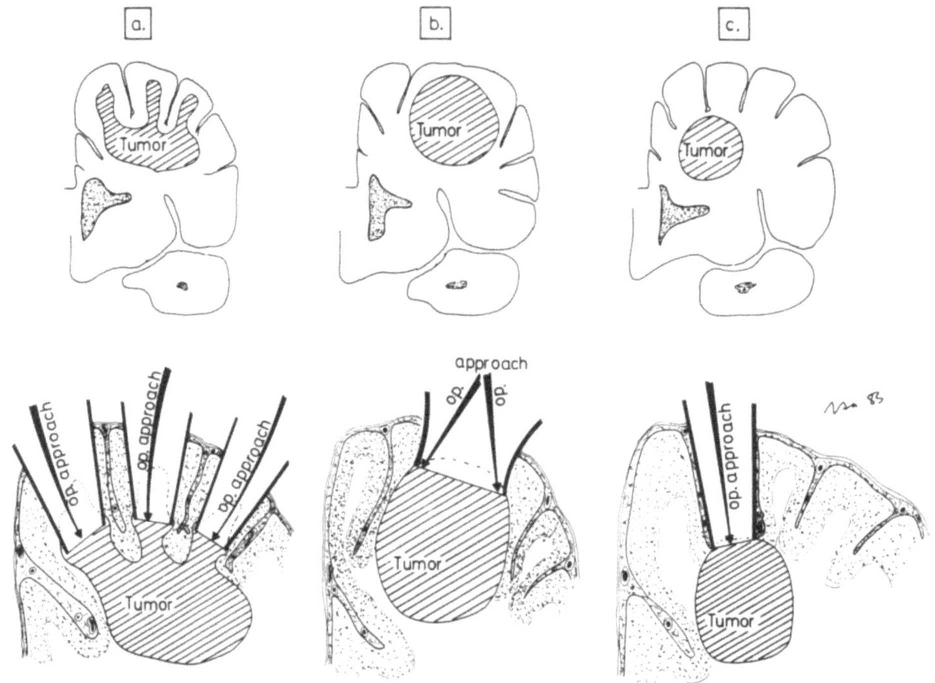

Fig. 2 Transgyral and trans-sulcal approach to gliomas:
a) infiltration of several gyri: approach via several gyri. Surface vein drainage not affected;
b) tumour situated in enlarged gyrus: resection of gyrus;
c) trans-sulcal approach to deep-seated gliomas protecting the brain cortex and vessels.

white matter such as astrocytomas and oligodendrogliomas can be reduced to small pieces with a dissector or with sharp forceps and removed through narrow approaches.

The surgeon must have exact knowledge of the topographic anatomy using major landmarks and borderlines for orientation in order to proceed safely in the white matter. This is a pre-requisite for the careful treatment of vital brain structures. The following examples illustrate our concepts and procedures.

Table 3 Approach to gliomas of and near by ventricle

interhemispheric-transcallosal	→ rostral corpus callosum		→ anterior part of third ventricle
	→ occipital corpus callosum		→ lateral ventricle and trigone
transcortical (thin cortex)	→ transgyral	parietal	→ lateral ventricle and trigone
	→ transsulcal	temporal	→ temporal horn

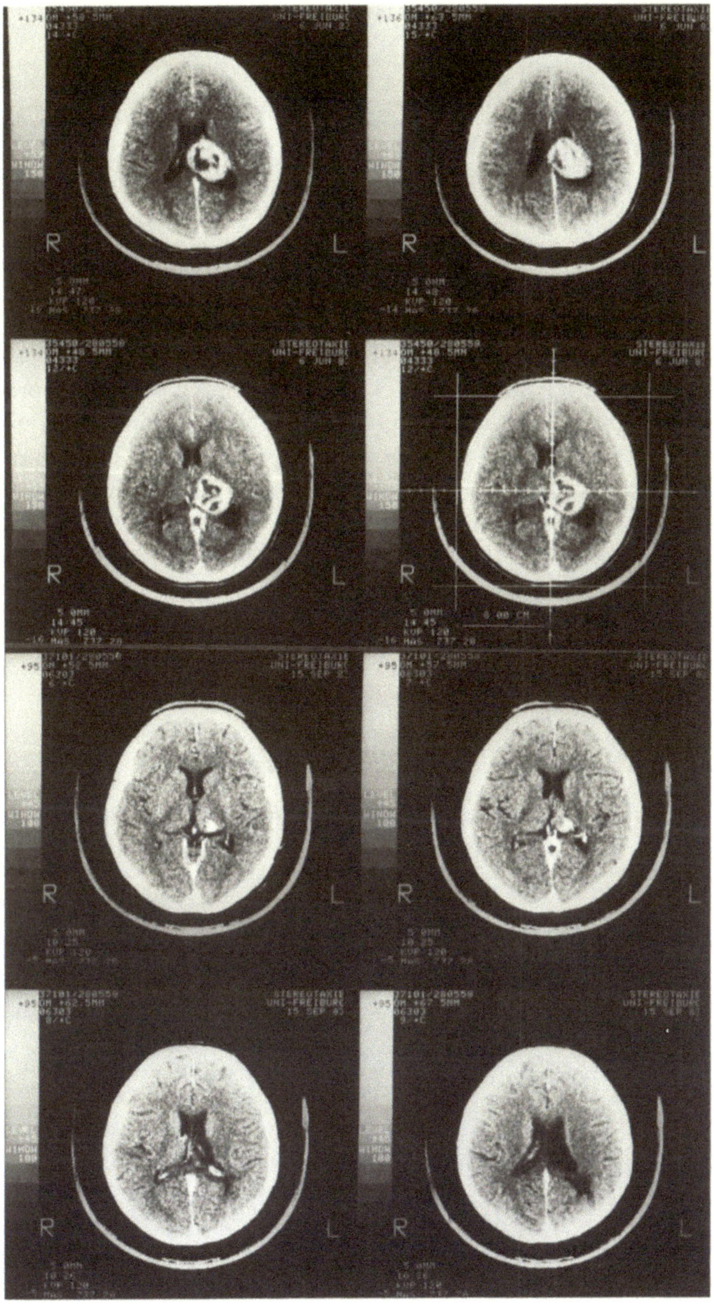

Fig. 3 a) Glioblastoma of left thalamus;
b) three months after transcortical trans-sulcal resection of tumour: excellent condition of patient with only incomplete hemianopia.

Gliomas in and closely related to ventricle

Depending on the location and nature of a tumour, we select an interhemispheric transcallosal approach through the rostral or posterior corpus callosum or a transcortical approach via a gyrus or sulcus [5].

a) We use a transcortical approach via a sulcus for a glioma of the thalamus (fig. 3). In the area of the trigone, the tumour is approached between the stria terminalis and the insertion of the plexus. The tumour mass is reduced subependymally and the perforating arteries from the transverse fissure are protected.

b) For plexus papillomas we always use an interhemispheric approach [5, 12]. Before he begins the operation, the surgeon has to know exactly where the cerebral veins lead into the sagittal sinus in order to determine the possible approaches (fig. 4). For this purpose, tilted angiographies are performed, which determine the terminal course of the cerebral veins [16, 17]. Depending on the distribution of the cerebral veins the surgeon can decide whether the interhemispheric approach and the callosal dissection should be wide or narrow. When detaching the tumour from the plexus, one has to distinguish between the tumour arteries and the perforating arteries to the thalamus. That is the major difficulty with this operation, however, it can usually be overcome when the tumour mass is sufficiently excavated and the attachment of the papilloma is resected at the end of the operation.

Gliomas in the central region and the dominant hemisphere

For these tumours we use an approach through a gyrus and remove the affected gyrus if the tumour reaches the surface of the brain. If the tumour is deeper, an

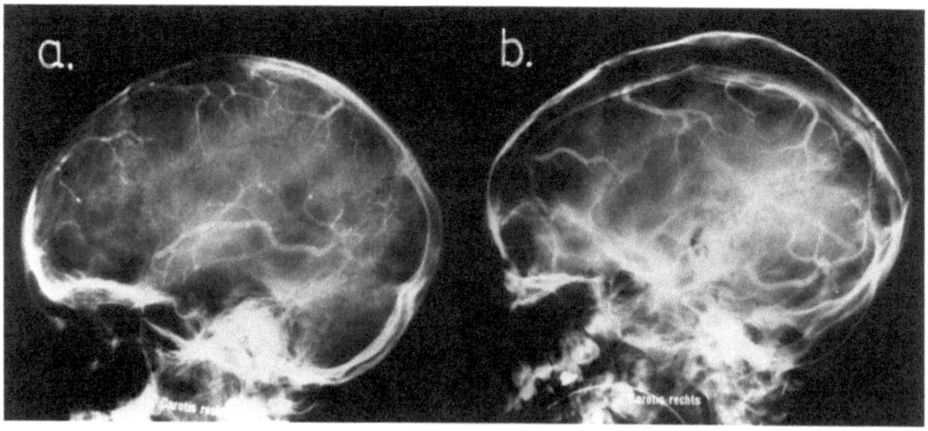

Fig. 4 a) Normal lateral projection of veins in angiogramms;
b) tilted lateral projection of venous angiography: exact location of where the veins lead into the sagittal sinus: interhemispheric approach can be planned.

approach is used through a sulcus or through the interhemispheric fissure or Sylvian fissure (tab. 4).

a) For deep-seated parietal tumours in the central region the approach has to be adapted to the white matter fibres of the pyramidal tract. These lesions have to be approached either fronto-dorsally at the level of the bregma or parieto-occipitally with a starting point at the junction of the lambda and sagittal sutures (fig. 1).
b) Lesions within the pars orbitalis of the frontal lobe can be removed without the risk of additional neurological deficits, provided that vessels, particularly the opercular arteries, remain intact and the insular structures are not damaged. This can be achieved by subpial evacuation of the tumour up to the surface of the insula while protecting the arachnoidea layers of the insular surface and of the temporal lobe.
c) Tumours in the depths of the angular region (fig. 5) should be approached via a parieto-occipital route in order to prevent damage to the corona radiata and the basal ganglia. Such damage can occur if erroneously the approach is chosen too far rostral. A good orientation will be achieved if the ventricle is reached in the region of the trigonum.

Temporal gliomas

Problematic temporal gliomas are those which are located in the medial posterior temporal lobe, i.e., in the area of the uncus and the hypocampus. Since the uncus (fig. 6) is surrounded by a number of important vessels (rostral from the carotid artery and the middle cerebral artery, occipital from the basilar artery cerebral artery, and the posterior cerebral artery, medial from the posterior communicating artery and the anterior choroidal artery with perforating arteries), a lack of caution could cause severe neurological deficits. The uncus which is enlarged by the infiltration of the tumour often extends so far over the tentorium edge towards the midline that its medial surface is in direct contact with the oculomotor nerve, the infundibulum, and the midbrain.

We prefer the trans-sylvian approach to these tumours because it provides a clear field of vision and we can aspirate the tumour subpially while keeping the medial arachnoid intact. In contrast to the subtemporal approach, the temporal veins remain intact. The limits of the tumour resection should not exceed anteriorly the level

Table 4 Operative approach to gliomas of central region

extending to the surface	→ direct approach with resection of the gyrus
not related to cortical surface	→ intersulcal approach → interhemispheric approach (trans-sylvian approach) → approach taking note of white matter connections

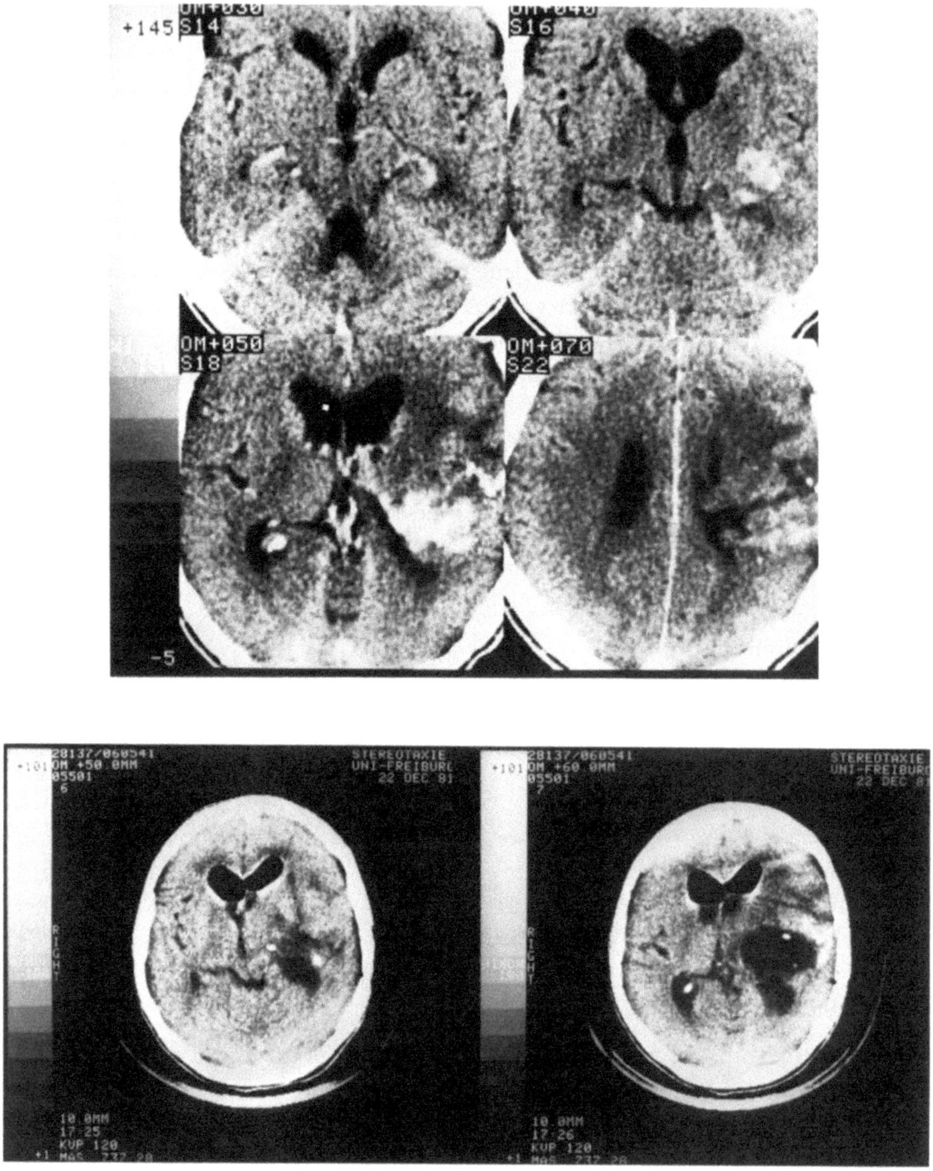

Fig. 5 a) Oligodendroglioma of the left angular region;
b) CT immediately after resection: air in tumour bed, no neurological deficit.

of the insula and posteriorly the ventricle roof of the temporal horn. Damage to the roof of the temporal horn means damage to the putamen and optic fibres, which results in hemiparesis and hemianopsia. Medially, if the arachnoid is preserved it acts as a protective shield for the optic tract.

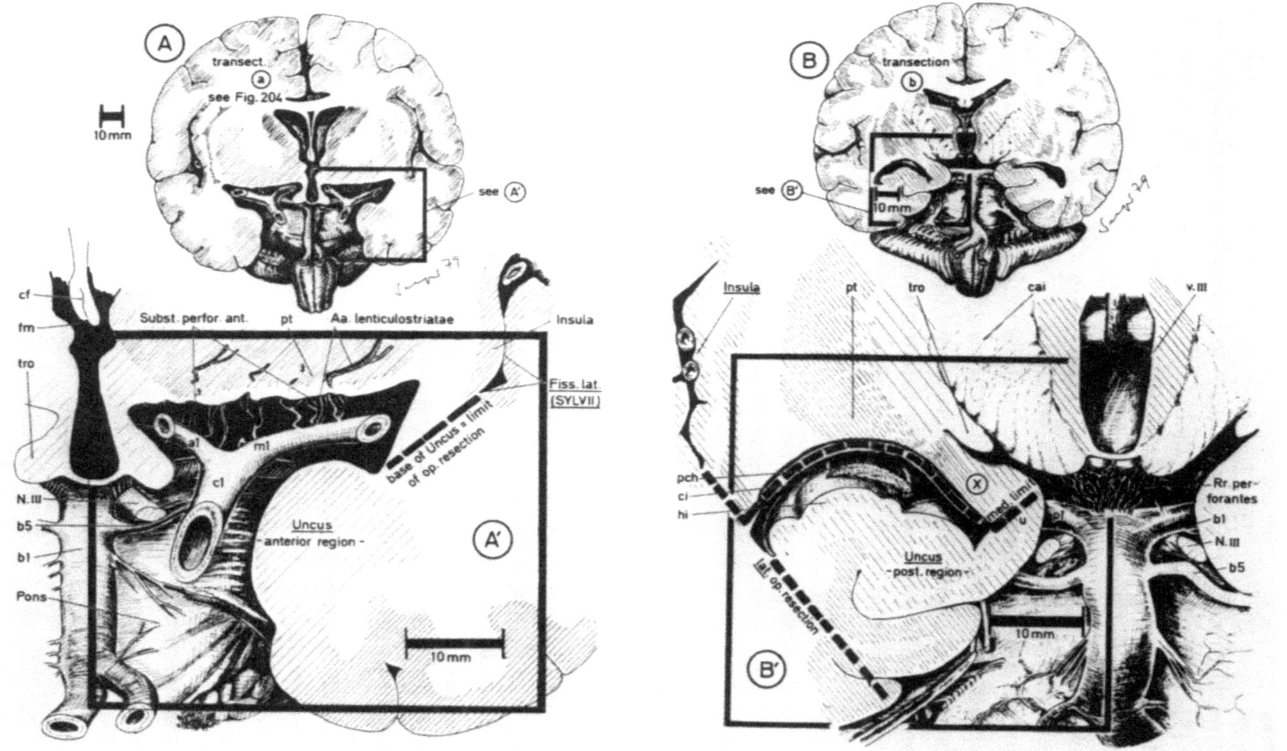

Fig. 6 Borderlines of resection of tumours in the medial temporal lobes. A: anterior region of uncus B: posterior region of uncus

Frontal gliomas

In removing frontal gliomas, it is essential that the critical limits of the resection must be respected [8]. Fronto-basal and medial gliomas can also then be removed. The limits should be the anterior insular region, the corpus callosum and the bifurcation of the carotid artery. In tumours located frontolaterally, notice should be taken that the pre-central region begins approximately 3 cm behind the bregma. Frontolaterally the precentral gyrus extends within the coronal suture. The fibres of the cortico-spinal tract for the arms and hands curve frontally in the depths of the white matter and are thus particularly endangered. These fibres can be protected by exposing the anterior surface of the insula. In these white matter tumours the border lines of the resection should therefore run between the anterior horn of the lateral ventricle and the anterior part of insula.

Discussion

The most cautious operative technique should not only be employed for benign tumours but also and to the same degree for malignant tumours [8, 17]. For this purpose an exact surgical plan has to be worked out before the operation. This is possible by means of the precise information given by CT. The radical lobectomy [11] should be abandoned, because the rate of recurrence associated with this method is not lower when compared with that of tumour extirpation alone. The early postoperative course as well as the mortality are also worse [4]. The microsurgical operation makes it possible to retain more functionally important brain tissue at the boundary surfaces of the tumour.

The approach to the tumour should be made via an anatomically pre-existing route such as the interhemispheric fissure, the Sylvian fissure and the sulcus. These natural fissures have to be opened wide to prevent neighboring structures from damage caused by continous strong spatula retraction.

To maintain the function of the brain in the approach area, the arteris and the veins must be protected. Large cerebral veins are isolated from the tumour and retained. The microscope provides an optimum view, even in narrow deep fissures, which allows the approach to be kept small. If the surgeon uses the microscope regularly, the operation will not take any longer than a macro-surgical operation. The survival time is the same, but the operative mortality is considerably lower [4], the immediate postoperative clinical course is better, and the hospital stay shorter. A further factor in the microsurgical technique of glioma operations which must not be underestimated is the training of the surgeon, who can apply his acquired technique on difficult benign tumours.

Summary

The principle of microsurgical glioma operation is based on the exact topical localization in the brain and the projection of the tumour of the skull surface and the skin. Individually worked out approaches (via sulcus, gyrus, sylvian fissure or interhemispheric fissure) are used while the white matter fibres are protected. Tiny approaches prevent damage to neighbouring brain structures as well as to arteries and veins in the approach area and at the boundary. Our surgical experience with more than 600 gliomas encourages us to continue using this method.

References

[1] Bartal, A. D., et al.: Extensive resection of primary malignant tumors of the left cerebral hemisphere. Surg. Neurol. **1** (1973) 337–342.

[2] Bennett, A. H., R. J. Godlee: Case of cerebral tumor. Proc. Roy. Med. and Chir. Soc. London, ns. **1**, 438, 1885; and Lancet 1884 II, 1090, (cited after G. Jefferson).

[3] Bucy, P. C.: Treatment of supratentorial gliomas. In: Gliomas – Current concepts in Histology, Diagnosis and Therapie (J. Hekmartpands, ed.). Springer, Berlin 1975.

[4] Eggert, H. R., J. Gilsbach, M. Sprich, et al.: Quality of Life following microsurgical removal of glioblastomas. In: The chemotherapy of gliomas (D. Voth, P. Krauseneck, eds.). Walter de Gruyter, Berlin – New York 1984.

[5] Geffen, G., et al.: Comparision of the effects of transcortical and transcallosal removal of intraventricular tumors. Brain **103** (1980) 773–788.

[6] Hassler, W., J. Gilsbach, W. Birg, et al.: Computertomographic findings of brain tumors projected on x-rays and scalp. Advances in Neurosurgery **10** (1982) 11–15.

[7] Hassler. W., J. Gilsbach, W. Seeger: Surgical treatment of supratentorial ventricle tumors in children. 8. Kongress Europeen society for Paediatric Neurosurgery 28. 6.–2. 7., Rennes, France, 1982.

[8] Hassler, W., W. Seeger: Microsurgery of tumors of the frontal white matter. Acta Neurochir. **44** (1978) 11–47.

[9] Jelsma, R., P. C. Bucy: The treatment of glioblastoma multiforme of the brain. J. Neurosurg. **27** (1967) 388–400.

[10] MacCarthy, C. S.: Surgical treatment of gliomas of the brain. J. Internat. Coll. Surg. **23** (1955) 290–297.

[11] Olivecrona, H. A.: Die Gliome der Großhirnhemisphären. Dtsch. Z. f. Nervenheilkunde (1932) 128.

[12] Raimondi, A. J., F. A. Gutierrez: Diagnosis and surgical treatment of choroid plexus papillomas. Childs Brain **1** (1975) 81–115.

[13] Ramsey, R. G., W. N. Brand: Radiotherapy of glioblastoma multiforme. J. Neurosurg. **39** (1973) 197–202.

[14] Ransohoff, J., A. Liebermann: Surgical therapy of primary malignant brain tumors. Clin. Neurosurg. **25** (1978) 403–411.

[15] Ray, B. S.: Surgery of recurrent intracranial tumors. Clin. Neurosurg. **10** (1964) 1–30.

[16] Rubinstein, L. J.: Tumors of the Central Nerves System. The Armed Forces Inst. of Pathology, Bethesda, Maryland 1972.

[17] Seeger, W.: Microsurgery of the Brain. Vol. I. Springer, Wien 1980.

[18] Seeger, W.: Atlas of topographical anatomy of the brain and surrounding structures. Springer, Wien 1978.

[19] Young, B., et al.: Reoperation for glioblastoma. J. Neurosurg. **55** (1981) 917–921.

Management of malignant gliomas. A ten year survey at the Neurosurgical Department of Rennes

J. Pecker, M. Chatel, J. M. Scarabin, F. Darcel, M. Ben Hassel

Introduction

This paper deals only with clearly malignant supratentorial gliomas (anaplastic astrocytomas and glioblastomas).

The pessimism concerning these types of brain tumour has been stressed by two famous neurosurgeons:

"about the group of gliomas, it is difficult to say anything intelligent concerning them" (Percival Bailey 1926) and later
"a cure of gliomas is still not possible today, even while using the most modern surgical techniques, radiotherapy and chemotherapy" (Paul Bucy 1978), as if nothing had happened during more than fifty years.

Nevertheless, in spite of a striking improvement in the accuracy of diagnosis, the final outcome of treatment is still disappointing.

All the cases included in our review were submitted to one or more pathological examinations [16] conducted either on surgical specimens or on biopsy samples. The few cases treated without histological control, because of the potential risk of biopsy in an angioblastic tumour, especially in elderly patients, are not included in this study.

In the field of malignant gliomas, the main concern is oncological. So we will not take into consideration any functional problems such as the treatment of epilepsy which is prominent in the case of low grade tumours.

We will successively consider, the place of stereotaxy in confirming diagnosis [30, 33], improvements in the understanding of the tumour biology [35] and our treatment strategy.

The stereotactic approach to diagnosis

Since 1973 we have developed a special stereotactic room prompted by the method used for many years by Talairach and the Ste Anne school [34]. The stereotactic frame is the most important element. It provides the plane of reference and allows a precise threedimensional approach. Stereotactic radiology is based upon the use of a focus film distance of 5 metres. The axis of the X-rays is perpendicular to the plane of the film and passes through the median plane of the contention system. Among the improvements carried out we shall mention the use of an isocentric chair equipped with a wheel which enables the chair to move in a complete circle: by means of a remote control system it can be set in motion according to various angular and linear movements (fig. 1). It can also be used in a horizontal position to allow retrograde catheterization of the femoral artery (fig. 2). Whatever the movements are, the centre of the contention system is always maintained in the same place. This technique allows us to obtain in the same session a collection of unmagnified and undistorted vascular, ventricular, and cisternal data, all super-imposable and reproducible from one session to another [23]. This "radiological morphogram" can be compared with others, for the purpose of statistical studies, by means of an electronic system which normalizes the radiological data by anamorphosis [28, 31, 37, 38].

Another technique which allows a true threedimensional reconstruction of the normal and pathological structures of the brain is stereo-angiography which enables us to see the relief. With photogrammetry the threedimensional coordinates of a point are automatically provided by the electronic system [11] (fig. 3).

Since the CT scan is available, we have developed a common referential procedure to transfer CT data onto stereo-angiographic films (fig. 4). Using information from the "radiological morphogram", a whole series of investigations can be safely and precisely carried out: stereo-electroencephalographic recording; impedance measurements. Above all, staggered biopsies can be performed securely and reliably by inserting a cannula through the double grid of the frame (fig. 5).

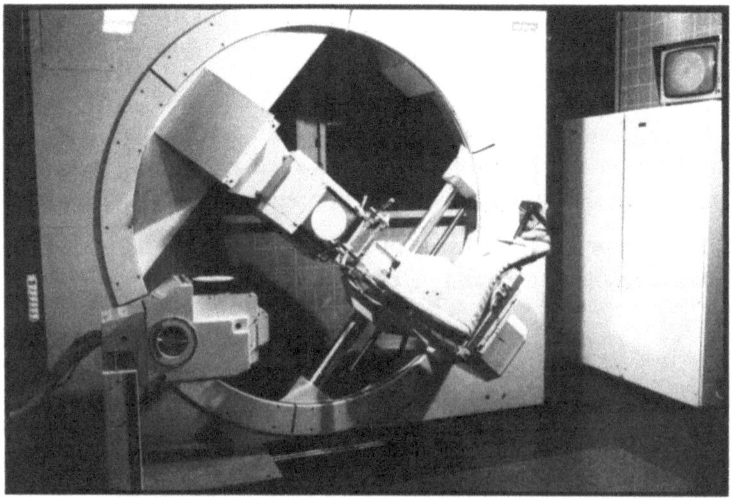

Fig. 1 *Stereotactic room:* the isocentric chair with its wheel.

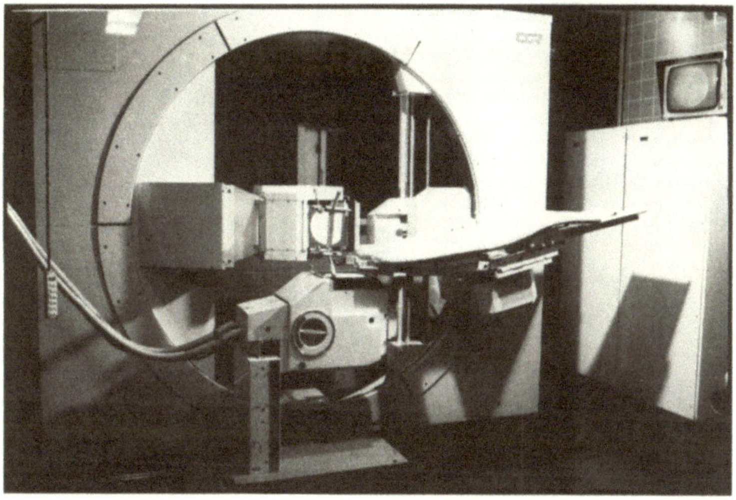

Fig. 2 Chair in the horizontal position (for femoral catheterization).

We call "individual morphogram" the sum of anatomical, physiological and histological data collected in a given patient. It is a true identity document, highly useful for treatment planning (radiotherapy) (fig. 6).

The advent of the CT scan did not fundamentally alter this procedure, especially as far as biopsy is concerned. In the first place we do not trust CT criteria in assessing the nature and particularly the grading of a tumour. Secondly, we prefer to obtain

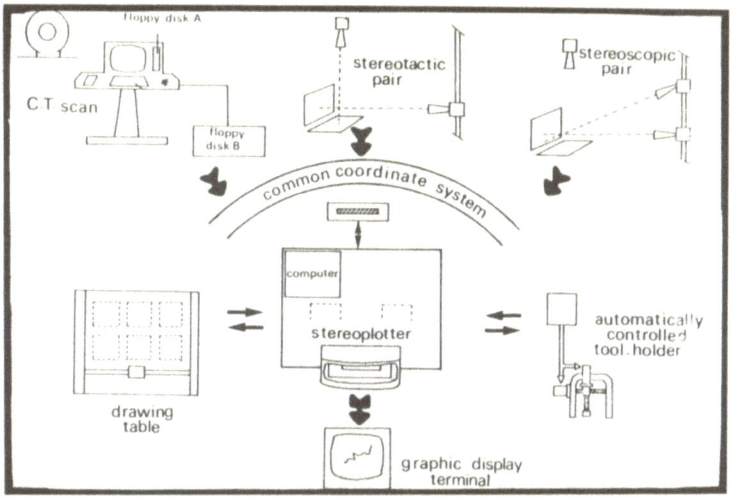

Fig. 3 *Photogrammetry:* the common coordinate system integrating the data from CT scan and stereotactic neuroradiology. The computer of the stereoplotter controls the drawing-table and a tool-holder.

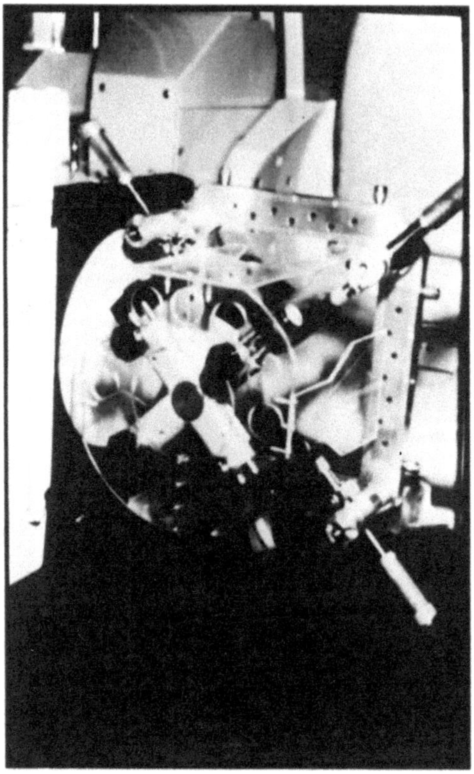

Fig. 4 *The common referential helmet* adapted to the stereotactic frame.

exact knowledge of the trajectory of the vessels even if some authors advocate only a CT-guided biopsy [6, 19, 26].

However, the transfer of CT data onto the stereoscopic morphogram is, of course, essential for biopsy [9, 11].

Like many others, we use smear biopsies during the approach to the tumour: these smears studied extemporaneously confirm the accuracy of the tumour site. They give a good idea of the cytology and indicate whether the tumour is anaplastic or not. The biopsy sample is embedded in paraffin and the pathological report is then completed. In spite of the moderate size of the biopsy samples, we rarely observe significant differences between the histological results after biopsy and tumour removal.

To improve the harmlessness of the procedure, the number of specimens taken is always limited to an average of three per patient. We know that we sometimes deprive ourselves of the possibility of spatially delimiting gliomas, which is advocated as useful by others [10]. We do not think that this lack of information alters the prognosis and treatment of malignant gliomas.

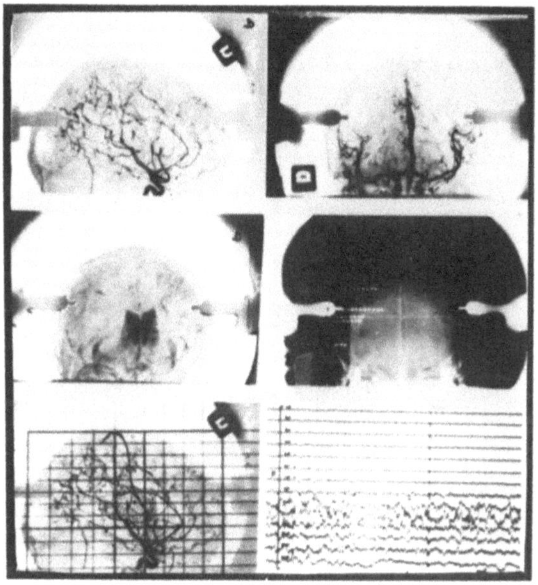

Fig. 5 *Morphogram of a rolandic* tumour with stereo-electro-encephalographic recording.

Understanding tumour biology: our present trends

Currently, our therapeutic decisions are based on the morphological diagnosis alone. We believe that if progress is to be made in understanding the causes and evolution of gliomas, more is to be expected of a biological than a pathological approach. In this line of thought we are looking for new criteria to define prognosis factors better and for more appropriate therapeutic measures.

NMR studies

Unfortunately, we still do not have NMR imaging facilities. But for the last few years, we have been studying *in vitro* NMR data obtained from brain tumours [3]. Our prospective goal is to establish correlations between T1, T2 relaxation times, accurate preoperative histological diagnosis, and topographical extension of the lesion based on NMR images when available. Up to now we have studied 137 specimens (36 meningiomas, 45 gliomas – 11 grade II – 23 grade III – 15 glioblastomas, 5 medulloblastomas, 12 metastases) from 98 patients. The samples are measured soon after tumour removal, then fixed and embedded. The spectrometer is a Bruker P 20 and the physical parameters: 20 M.H.Z., 22 °C Meiboum – Gill – Carr – Purcell sequence for T1, and 180 90 pulse sequence for T2.

Our results may be summarized as follow:

1. Every intracranial tumour whatever its histology and grading may be, has proton

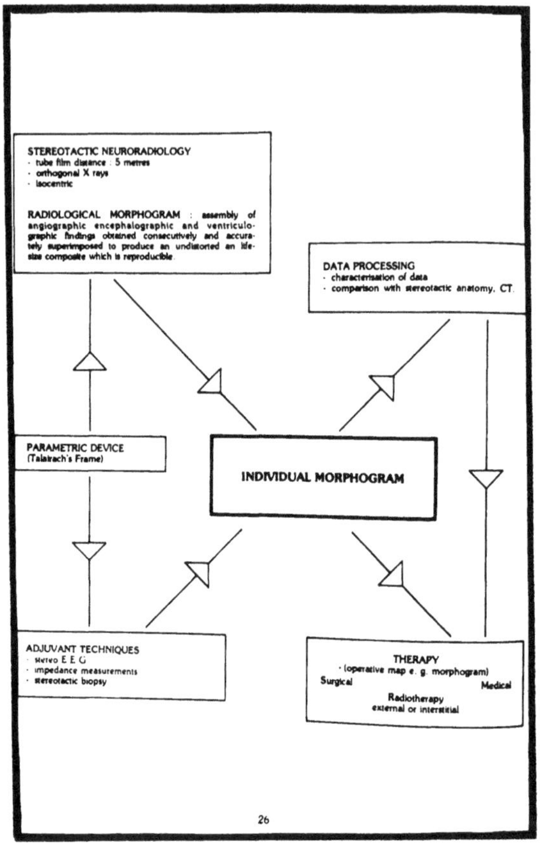

Fig. 6 *The individual morphogram*, sum of radiological data, physiological recordings and pathological examination.

relaxation times greater than those of normal brain tissue. This coincides with the good quality imaging obtained by proton NMR tomography.

2. Highly cellular tumour tissues tend to have lower relaxation time values: meningiomas, metastases, medulloblastomas (cluster below 800 milliseconds).
3. As for neuro – epithelial tumours, the range of glioma values is wide: grade II and grade IV gliomas may have a high T1 and T2. Such a dispersion may be related to the variability of both the water content and the molecular environment (oedema, microcystic formation, necrosis . . .). This applies even if the tumours belong to the same histological group and whatever their grade.
4. It should be noticed that T1 and T2 do not express the degree of malignancy when a metastasis is suspected. They share the same range of T1 and T2 values as benign highly cellular meningiomas.
5. A differential diagnosis between benign and malignant intracranial tumours based upon proton relaxation times does not seem relevant.

These results are partially in agreement with others [17] and our project is to extend these studies to other paramagnetic nuclei. In a more basic orientation, we are simultaneously running experimental protocols with established human glial cell lines *in vitro* observing NMR data variations according to cell cycle phases.

Polyamines metabolism

Polyamines are present in any normal or neoplastic tissue. Their existence has been known for several centuries (1678) but they were disdained as secondary bacterial putrefaction products and it is only during the last two decades that searchers have pointed to their major biological roles in cell proliferation and differentiation. Among the polyamines, three are relevant to human tumour proliferation:

- putrescine, whose level increases with cell multiplication;
- spermidine, which is related to cell hypertrophy and metabolism;
- spermine, which reflects cell differentiation.

In brain tumours Marton et al. [18] has shown that polyamine levels in cerebrospinal fluid could be used as criteria of evolution for monitoring therapeutic strategies. More recently Scalabrino et al. [27] showed a close correlation between Ornithine Decarboxylase levels and the degree of glioma malignancy (O.D.C. is the enzyme needed for polyamine synthesis from ornithine).

Our own studies attempted to establish a relation between tumoural free polyamines and histology, and to look for a correlation between tumour, cerebrospinal fluid, and red blood cell polyamine levels. We may summarize our results in a few words:

1. Cerebrospinal fluid putrescine levels are higher in all patients suffering from brain tumours than in those of controls.
2. Polyamine levels are higher in medulloblastomas than in any other type of tumour.
3. Red blood cell spermidine levels are higher in glioblastoma patients.
4. The ratio between tumour/cerebrospinal fluid/red blood cells is statistically significant in glioblastomas and medulloblastomas.
   - In medulloblastomas: putrescine and spermidine levels are linked in tumour and cerebrospinal fluid.
   - In glioblastomas: the sum of putrescine, spermidine, spermine tumoral levels is linked to that of cerebrospinal fluid, and there is a highly significant correlation between spermidine/spermine ratio in tumour and red blood cells.

These findings need to be expanded. In our opinion, this break-through in understanding the role played by polyamine metabolism in brain tumour pathology has improved its biological approach. It has opened the way to the use of a new generation of drugs, the anti-polyamines which act as inhibitors on the synthetic polyamines pathway.

Positron emission tomography

Positron emission tomography (PET) seems to be the most promising method apart from NMR, imaging, which is not available in Rennes. We have had a short but interesting experience with PET jointly undertaken with the Neurosurgery Department of the University of Caen and the Department of Nuclear Medicine of the Orsay Hospital. The studies carried out by others with PET concern cerebral oxygen and glucose metabolism showing a reduction of oxygen extraction in tumours although the glucose extraction rate is close to normal. This suggests an anaerobic metabolism inside the gliomas [36]. We have just begun a study with 11 C labelled Methionine. It already appears that malignant gliomas show an increase of protein synthesis whereas low grade gliomas show hypometabolism (figs. 7 and 8) [39].

Therapeutic management

Surgery

For superficial tumours which do not involve highly functional areas of the hemispheres, we advocate a direct surgical approach with the most complete removal possible. In these cases a previous stereotaxic morphogram is not necessary. The extemporaneous histological diagnosis is performed on a biopsy sample at the start of the operation.

For tumours which involve eloquent areas of the cortex (e.g. the motor area), we think that surgical removal can be performed without permanent major neurological

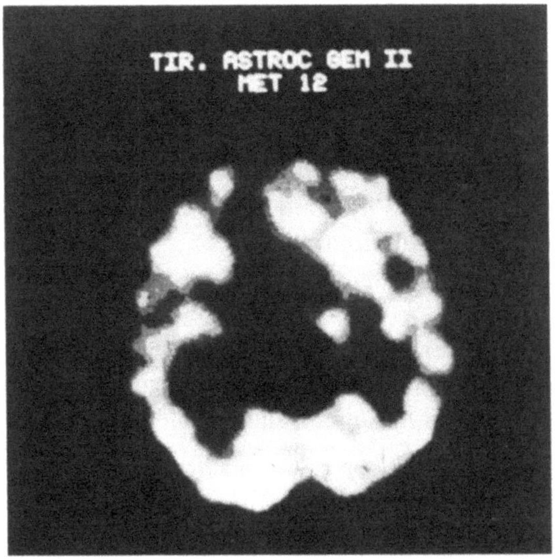

Fig. 7 *PET* with 11 C labelled methionine in a case of malignant astrocytoma: area of hypermetabolism in right frontal lobe.

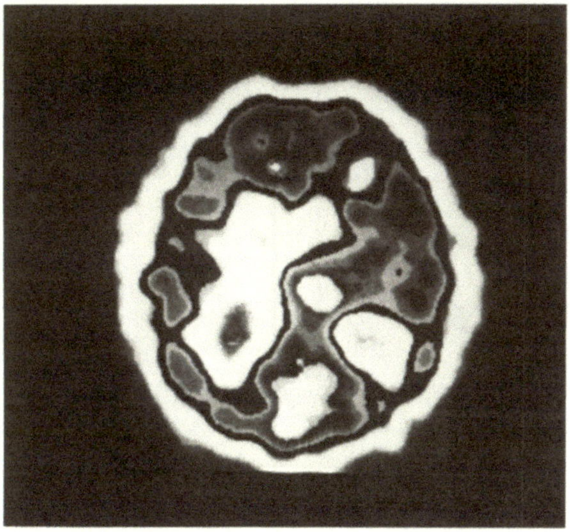

Fig. 8 *PET* with 11 C labelled Methionine in a low grade astrocytoma: long lasting hypometabolism (46‘) in left rolandic zone.

deficit provided that the feeding vessels are untouched. A complete radiological tridimensional morphogram is the best way to plot the structural landmarks, i.e., the vessels whose trajectory is often deviated [25, 32] (fig. 9).

Radiotherapy

Of course we cannot believe in a surgical cure for gliomas. What we do know, however, is that the biology of these tumours indicates that the use of nonsurgical methods, especially radiotherapy, has a more decisive effect on the length and quality of patient survival [24].

Interstitial curie therapy

Deep seated tumours are often not unsuitable for removal. Between 1973 and 1979 we used interstitial curie-therapy according to protocols established by other centres [21, 22]. Our results were published as a contribution to a cooperative study on this technique [28]. This interstitial radiation therapy associates a sharply circumscribed high dose volume and the potential biological advantages of low dose rates (fig. 10).

Since 1979, we have restricted 192 Iridium wire brachytherapy [29] to strictly selected cases (tumour volume less than 3 cm in diameter). A comparison with external radiotherapy was tried. The results did not favour Iridium implant techniques.

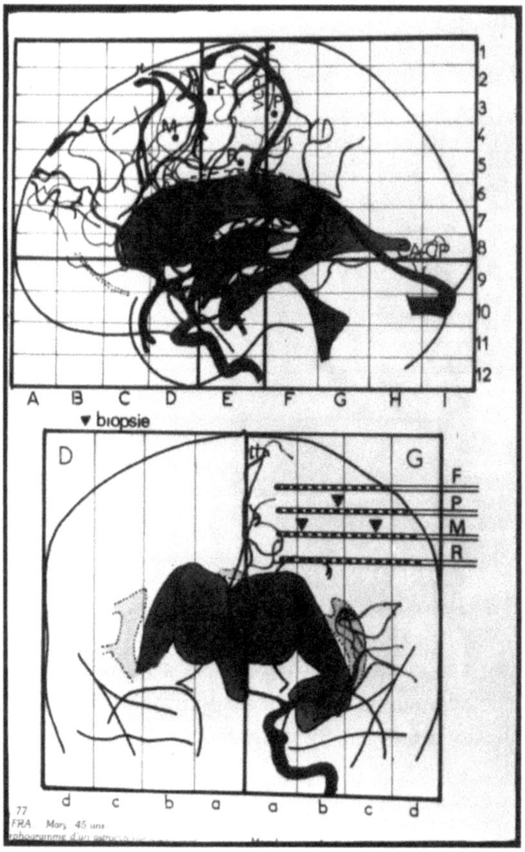

Fig. 9 *Operative map* in case of rolandic glioma.

External radiotherapy

External radiotherapy has improved mean survival time [5]. Progress in radiation therapy equipement (linear accelerators, radiologic threedimensional morphograms, CT scan and computerized treatment planning systems, simulators) has rendered the delivery of an optimum dose to a definite volume, efficient.

These technological advances with megavoltage equipment generating high dose rate beams but with low Linear Energy Transfer have made no further progress while using a conventional fractionation.

We tried, in a cooperative study [2], a combination of shorter overall treatment time, a split course of treatment, and hyper-fractionation. For the whole patient population (73 patients with and without tumour removal) the median survival time was 34 weeks. Fifteen percent of the patients survived 77 weeks. Given the poor mean survival times this altered fractionation schedule was chosen to shorten treatment

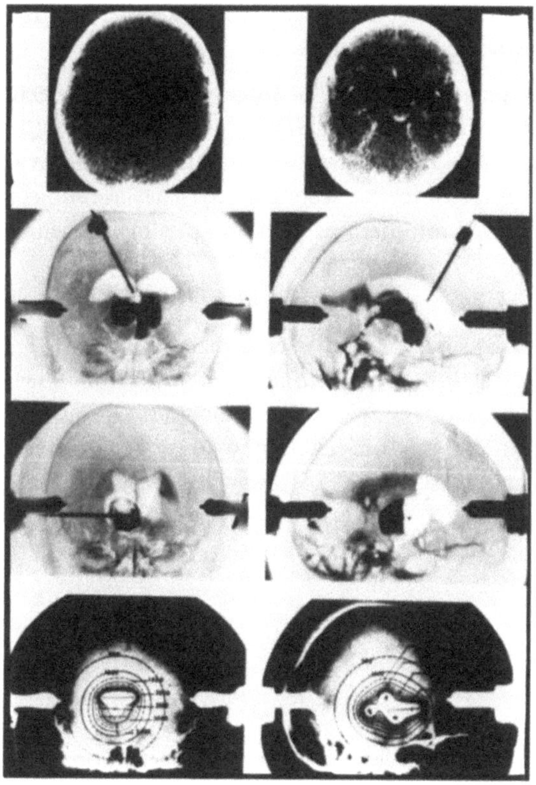

Fig. 10 *Interstitial irradiation* with 192 Iridium for a deep malignant cystic astrocytoma.

time and thus to preserve the survival quality of our patients. Awareness of the increasing incidence of brain radiation damage verified by 7 post mortem studies led us to reconsider conventional fractionation as safe while waiting for end results of EORTC trials. Our participation in a trial using misonidazole as a hypoxic cell radiosensitizer was short and rather disappointing (EORTC 26 781).

Despite a lack of new and striking improvements in our results linked to a different modality of radiotherapy, postoperative irradiation remains however the only means prolonging survival and of producing a significant difference in the outcome of malignant gliomas without altering the quality of life.

Chemotherapy

A French Cooperative study (Caen-Paris-Rennes-Tours) was started in 1975 to assess the value of immediate post-operative chemotherapy and delayed radiotherapy versus immediate post-operative radiotherapy followed by chemotherapy. Preliminary results clearly favoured immediate post-operative chemotherapy [8]. They were good enough to prompt a randomized protocol within the EORTC Brain Tumour

Group (EORTC 26 812 Trial). Final results are not yet available, but the trend observed so far does not confirm the initial study.

Independently, we are running phase II trials; 1° – In cases of tumour recurrence, High Dose Costicosteroid Therapy (HDC) versus HDC + Antipolyamines (difluoromethylornithine) is being tested. 2° – Patients whose tumour is not removable but who have undergone biopsy are selected for the second study. They are subjected to a combined use of Cisplatinum and Radiotherapy. Follow up is insufficient for any results to be given.

To sum up we think that the drugs currently available give rise to numerous side effects that impair the quality of the survival. However as these protocols [13, 14, 20, 40] demand an improved medical follow up, we are convinced that they are of benefit to both patients and their relatives. We expect much more of new drugs or carriers such as monoclonal antibodies. Completely new approaches, for example combined laser beam surgery and porphyrines [15], may also provide greater relief for patients.

Results

Operative mortality

Cases previous to 1973 were not retained for the present study. Postoperative mortality in the first month was then slightly above 20%, in agreement with most author's series [24]. Over the last ten years, postoperative mortality has decreased to below 5%. We do not know whether this drop is due to a better selection of patients suitable for operation, to advances in radiological techniques, or to improvements in operation and/or anaesthesia.

Latest results

Of 448 treated between 1973 and 1980, 87 have been lost to follow-up for various reasons. The mean survival time for the remaining 361 patients after operation and radiotherapy is 9,2 months. The best results were obtained when macroscopic tumour removal was total. Like other authors, we had some striking cases where survival lasted several years. The pathological diagnosis was carefully checked out in all longterm survivors. In our series, the mean survival rate after treatment is 71% after 6 months, falling to 35% after one year.

Conclusion

We do not believe that the alternative methods [7, 13] currently at our disposal with a combination of operation, postoperative low LET ionizing radiation therapy with conventional time-dose factors and/or cytotoxic chemotherapy with the drugs available today – can improve on these poor results [1, 4]. Our research aims at improving treatment and prognosis by:

- extensive screening of new drugs or therapeutic techniques on glial cells *in vitro* and on human glial cells grafted into immune-deficient mice;
- basic analysis of polyamine metabolism in brain tumour patients to obtain biological criteria for evolution and guidelines to efficient chemotherapy;
- NMR and PET studies to acquire highly detailed information on tumour metabolism and pharmacokinetic data;
- developing a broad range of monoclonal anti brain tumour antibodies.

Summary

The present study is based on 628 cases of malignant glioma treated in our Department during the past ten years. We emphasize the value of a stereotactic approach to diagnosis leading to a more precise radiological work-up, the radiological morphogram. Several new devices have been developed: an isocentric chair, a referential tool for the transfer of CT data onto the stereo-angiographic films and a photogrammetric device allowing a three dimensional reconstruction of the normal and pathologic structures of the brain. The pathological diagnosis is ensured by a stereotactic biopsy.

We hope the diagnosis may be improved by a better understanding of the tumour biology. Our present trends include NMR studies, research on metabolism of polyamines and positron emission tomography with 11 C labelled methionine. For therapeutic management we advocate operation whenever it seems feasible but even if its hazards are reduced, its limitations are well known and we cannot dream of a surgically cured glioma. The indications for interstitial irradiation are restricted to selected cases. External radiotherapy still plays a pre-eminent part with low LET ionizing radiations and conventional or altered fractionation schedules. Promising high LET beams, are under study. Many rather disappointing trials have been carried out with combinations of ionizing radiation and drugs.

Future prospects are new drugs (anti-polyamines, combination of cis platinum and radiotherapy) and new carriers (monoclonal antibodies).

The latest results are given for 361 patients with a adequate follow-up. The mean survival rate after six months is 71% and falls to 35% after one year.

References

[1] Baurand, Ch., G. Lena: Quel traitement pour quel malade? Organisation d'une stratégie. Neurochirurgie 27 (1981) 325–329.

[2] Ben Hassel, M., et al.: High grade astrocytomas: radiotherapy with a three fraction per day regimen in a split course of irradiation. (Presented as a free communication: 3rd annual meeting British Glioma Group – Bristol 8 April 1983).

[3] Benoist, L., M. Chatel, F. Menault, et al.: Variations des temps de relaxation du Proton dans les tumeurs humaines intracraniennes – Premiers résultats. J. de Biophysique et Médicine Nucléaire 6 (1981) 143–145.

[4] Bloom, H. J. G.: Combined modality therapy for intracranial tumours. Cancer 35 (1975) 111–120.

[5] Bloom, H. J. G.: Intracranial tumours: response and resistance to therapeutic endeavors, 1970–1980. Original contribution: 4th del Regato lecture, New Orleans, USA, May 1980.

[6] Boethius, J., M. Bergstrom, T. Greitz: Stereotaxic computerized tomography with a G.E. 8800 scanner. J. Neurosurg. 52 (1980) 794–800.

[7] Chatel, M., F. Menault: Bases biologiques des stratégies thérapeutiques des gliomes malins. Données oncologiques générales, place des moyens actuels et résultats, perspectives. Neurochirurgie 27 (1981) 299–303.

[8] Chatel, M., D. Dresse, P. Huguenin, et al.: Gliomes malins hémisphériques de l'adulte. Intérêt de la radiothérapie "seconde" dans les protocoles combinés: chimiothérapie (VM 26-CCNU) – radiothérapie. Etude coopérative sur 137 cas. Sem. Hôp. Prais 57, n° 5–6 (1981) 225–228.

[9] Cohadon, F., A. Rougier, D. Da Silva Nunes, et al.: La tomodensitométrie en conditions stéréotaxiques. Neurochirurgie 23, 6 (1977) 433–452.

[10] Daumas-Duport, C., G. Szikla: Délimitation et configuration spatiale des gliomes cérébraux. Données histologiques, incidences thérapeutiques. Neurochirurgie 27 (1981) 273–284.

[11] Gibaud, B., J. M. Scarabin, B. Lorig, et al.: Accurate use of CT scanner, stereotaxis and photogrammetry for diagnosis and treatment of cerebral lesions (tumours). Internat. Arch. of Photogrammetry (London) 24, 5 (1982) 225–234.

[12] Gullotta, F., W. Bettag: Long survival in glioblastoma. Acta Neurochir. (Wien) 16 (1967) 122–128.

[13] Hatlevoll, R., et al.: Combined modality treatment of operated astrocytomas grade 3 and 4 7th European congress of neurosurg. Abstract, p. 195 (Brihaye, ed.) 1983.

[14] Hildebrand, J.: The results of the EORTC brain tumour group in Multidisciplinary aspects of brain tumours therapy. (Paoletti, ed.), pp. 235–245. Elsevier North Holland Publ. 1979.

[15] Hryntiw, J., T. Origitano, S. Stokowski, et al.: Total gioma kill by hematoporphyrin and laser. Reprinted from American College of Surgeons 1982. Surgical Forum volume XXXIII, p. 514–516.

[16] Jacque, C. M., C. Vinner, M. Kujas, et al.: Determination of glial fibrillary acidic protein (GFAP) in human brain tumours. J. Neurol. Sci. 35 (1978) 145–155.

[17] Jezernik, M., M. Sentjure, M. Schara, et al.: Proton magnetic resonance characterization of brain tumours. 7th European congress of neurosurg. Abstract, p. 60 (Brihaye, ed.) 1983.

[18] Marton, L. J., M. S. Edwards, V. A. Levin, et al.: CSF polyamines: A new and important means of monitoring patients with medulloblastomas. Cancer 47 (1981) 757–760.

[19] Mennel, H. D., C. Ostertag: Stereotactic intraoperative cytological diagnosis of brain tumours. Inserm Symposium n° 12 (Szikla, ed.), pp. 43–49. Elsevier North Holland Publ. 1979.

[20] Müller, H., M. Brock: Long term survival and recurrence free interval in combined surgical, radio and chemotherapy (CCNU) of malignant brain gliomas. 7th European congress of neurosurg. Abstract, p. 193 (Brihaye, ed.) 1983.

[21] Mundinger, F.: Brain tumour therapy by interstitial application of radioactive isotopes. In: Radionucleide applications in neurosurgery and neurology. C. C. Thomas, Springfield 1970.

[22] Mundinger, F.: Rationale and methods of interstitial iridium 192 brachytherapy and Iridium 192 or Iodine 125 protracted long term irradiation Inserm Symposium n° 12 (Szikla, ed.), pp. 101–115. Elsevier North Holland Publ. 1979.

[23] Pecker, J., J. M. Scarabin, J. M. Brucher, et al.: Stereotactic approach to diagnosis and treatment of cerebral tumours. Edit. Medic. P. Fabre, Paris 1979.
[24] Pecker, J., J. M. Scarabin, M. Dekkiche, et al.: Place de la chirurgie dans le traitement des gliomes malins supratentoriels. Neurochirurgie 27 (1981) 287–293.
[25] Raybaud, Ch., P. Michotey, W. Bank, et al.: Angiographic – anatomic study of the vascular territories of the cerebral convolutions. In: Advances in Cerebral Angiography (Salomon, ed.). pp. 2–9. Springer, Berlin–Heidelberg–New York 1975.
[26] Russel, A., Brown: A computerized tomography computer graphics approach to stereotaxic localization. J. Neurosurg. 50 (1979) 715–720.
[27] Scalabrino, G., D. Modena, M. E. Ferioli, et al.: Degrees of malignancy in human primary central nervous system tumours: ornithine decarboxylase levels as better indicators than adenosyl-methionine decarboxylase levels. JNCI, vol. 68, n° 5, May 1982, p. 751–754.
[28] Scarabin, J. M., J. Pecker, J. Simon, et al.: Stereotaxic angiography in cerebral tumours. In: Advances in Cerebral Angiography (Salamon, ed.), pp. 251–261. Springer, Berlin–Heidelberg–New York 1975.
[29] Schlienger, M., H. Bouhnik, O. Missir, et al.: Association of temporary interstitial 192 Ir implantation and external radiotherapy in the management of supratentorial tumours. Technique and dosimetry. Inserm Symposium n° 12 (Szikla, ed.), pp. 117–121 Elsevier North Holland Publ. 1979.
[30] Sedan, R., J. C. Peragut, Ph. Farnarier, et al.: Place de la biopsie en condition stéréotaxique dans la tactique thérapeutique des gliomes malins. Neurochirurgie 27 (1981) 285–295.
[31] Suetens, P., J. Gybels, A. Haegemans, et al.: A global 3 D image of the cerebral blood vessels, tumour and simulated probe. 7th European congress of neurosurg. Abstract, p. 177 (Brihaye, ed.) 1983.
[32] Szikla, G., T. Hori, G. Bouvier: The third dimension in cerebral angiography: a stereotactic study on cortical localization and hemispheric asymmetry in living man. In: Advances in Cerebral Angiography (Salamon, ed.), pp. 236–250. Springer, Berlin–Heidelberg–New York 1975.
[33] Szikla, G., O. Betti, L. Szenthe, L'experience actuelle des irradiations stéréotaxiques dans le traitement des gliomes hémisphériques.Neurochirurgie 27 (1981) 295–298.
[34] Talairach, J., J. C. Peragut, Ph. Farnarier, et al.: The role of stereotaxic radiographic exploration in the neurosurgical intervention. In: Advances in Cerebral Angiography (Salamon, ed.), pp. 215–261. Springer, Berlin–Heidelberg–New York 1975.
[35] Thomas, D. G. T., D. I. Graham: Brain tumours – Scientific basis, clinical investigation and current therapy. Butterworths Ltd., London 1980.
[36] Thomas, D. G. T., R. J. S. Wise, R. Beaney, et al.: PET scan in patients with cerebral glioma: mismatching between cerebral oxygen and glucose metabolism. 7th European congress of neurosurg. – Abstract, p. 59 (Brihaye, ed.) 1983.
[37] Vignaud, J., P. Rabischong, J. P. Yver, et al.: Multidirectional reconstruction of angiogram by stereogrammetry and computer. Neuroradiology **18** (1979) 1–7.
[38] Vigneron, C.: Traster 77: Matra analytical stereoplotter. Photogrammetric engineering and remote sensing. **43**, 11 (1977) 1391–1397.
[39] Volkow, N., S. Goldman, E. S. Flamm, et al.: Labelled putrescine as a probe in brain tumours. Science **221** (1983) 673–675.
[40] Walker, M. D., E. Alexander, W. E. Hunt: Evaluation of BCNU and/or radiotherapy in the treatment of anaplastic gliomas: a cooperative clinical trial. J. Neurosurg. **49** (1978) 333–343.

Re-operating on malignant gliomas: Indications, problems and results

R. Brenner, G. Wöber

Introduction

Numerous questions are raised when one has to undertake a further operation on a malignant glioma and it is perhaps fitting to reflect on the general and the particular considerations raised by the surgical treatment of malignant tumours. One thing is certain, namely that no neurosurgeon is very enthusiastic about performing such an operation. We are permanently overworked in our Dept. of Neurosurgery and have to show reservations as regards the indications in a great number of neurosurgical diseases, especially in the case of gliomas which have recurred. We hope to justify our decision to operate on glioma recurrences, and will refer to a group of cases dealt with in our department in the last five years or so.

Material

Our study is based on 225 histologically verified malignant gliomas (grades worse than II), mainly astrocytomas, some glioblastomas and a few ependymomas. All these patients were operated on in the years 1977–1982. The primary mortality (within the first 4–7 weeks postoperatively) was 10.6% (24 patients out of 225), including all internal complications. Of the 201 patients discharged, 101– exactly a half – were operated on a second time. The increase in mortality to 12% within the first seven weeks was only insignificantly higher. We had to operate on 33 patients a third time, with a mortality of 25% and five patients were operated on a fourth time, of whom one died within the period mentioned above. Altogether 364 tumour resections were performed in 225 patients with a total postoperative mortality of 12.3%.

Results

From these figures it appears that the mortality is no significantly higher for the first operation for recurrence than for the primary operation. Why are the postoperative chances of those patients operated on three or more times, and how long are they likely to survive. We know that 147 patients had died in the meantime and an analysis of these patients yielded the following information:

The Median Survival Time (MST) of discharged patients was

with patients operated on once	7.1 months (max. 33 months)
with patients operated on twice	13.0 months (max. 60 months)
with patients operated on three times	20.7 months (max. 68 months)
with patients operated on four times	16.0 months (max. 25 months)

We will not discuss the statistical failures which result from the fact that we have only listed those persons whose death has been recorded. Definite information could only have been obtained if a continual follow-up examination of all the discharged patients had been possible, so as to record their most recent condition.

It seems to us of greater significance that a further operation was only indicated when it was considered that there was a chance of preserving or restoring the patient to a good neurological and psycho-organic condition. A malignant glioma with extensive recurrences has never been submitted to a further operation when the neurological findings definitely showed a hopeless anatomical situation. In other words we tried to avoid surgically prolonged invalidism.

When we compare the Median Survival Time (MST) of operations performed one to four times, with the other relevant supporting and therapeutic measures, we found some interesting results (tab. 1).

It was apparent that:

1. A considerable number of patients (23%) were operated on only once and these had the shortest MST (5.5 months). Obviously those with the most severe neurological picture deteriorated without any chance of recovery.
2. Combined supportive treatment (irradiation and chemotherapy) were used in most of the cases.
3. In this combined group most of the repeat operations were performed (56%) and the best MST was reached, with 17.7 months. Among this group there are also those who died after the longest period of survival (60 and 68 months).

Finally, the question may be raised as to whether there is a higher rate of postoperative complications in the reoperated cases. In this respect we considered damage to the tissue around the tumour, and to the skin- and bone-flap, as well as haematological and immunological complications. The review showed that in all the operations (364) for malignant gliomas there was postoperative haemorrhage in 13

Table 1 Middle Survival Time (MST) in the various patients groups

	without supportive care	irridiation	chemotherapy	irridiation and chemotherapy
operated once	n = 27 MST: 5.5 month (max. 12 month)	n = 1 15 month	n = 5 MST: 6 month (max. 9 month)	n = 11 MST: 11 month (max. 33 month)
operated twice	n = 13 MST: 8.2 month (max. 19 month)	n = 3 MST: 6.6 month	n = 1 11 month	n = 26 MST: 16.1 month (max. 60 month)
operated three times	n = 4 MST: 18.5 month (max. 24 month)	n = 5 MST: 14.8 month (max. 30 month)	n = 3 MST: 10.3 month	n = 13 MST: 26 month (max. 68 month)
operated four times	n = 2 11.5 month			n = 1 25 month

(3.5%), and infection of the operation area in only four cases (1.1%). These figures were too small to be regarded as significant.

Treating a malignant glioma – one of the commonest problems in our special field – needs a wide and comprehensive concept of therapy. A part of this therapy must be a carefully indicated operation and further operation if indicated. The indications and timing depend on the clinical findings and on the reaction of the patient and his relatives. It depends on the site, extent, malignancy and vascularity of the tumour. It is also necessary to consider the problem of toxic brain oedema, the rate or tumour growth and finally the sensitivity of the tumour to the supplementary treatment.

Summary

A study of 225 patients with histologically verified gliomas (worse than grade II) during the years 1977–1982 compares the results of repeated operations, with and without supplementary treatment, and supportive care.

The Ommaya reservoir and its significance for intrathecal cytostatic treatment. Surgical aspects and complications

G. Keßel, M. Schwarz, D. Voth

Introduction

In 1963 Ommaya first reported on the system named after him, with which access is rapidly available to the CSF spaces, at any time [4]. By this means new possibilities were opened up for the intrathecal administration of cytostatics, as for example was undertaken in the treatment of leukaemic meningiosis and neoplastic diseases of the central nervous system [5, 7]. In addition there was the possibility of intermittent drainage of intracranial cysts, as for example when dealing with a primary inoperable malignant tumour with a cystic component [3]. We also mentioned the possibility of intrathecal administration of antibiotics, as was described for the treatment of fungal meningitis [2].

Method

The technique of implanting an Ommaya reservoir is simple and standardised. If access to the ventricular system is required, the right frontal, parasagittal and precoronal position is usually preferred. Should it follow the extirpation of a tumour, in view of the imminent radiotherapy the subgaleal layer is chosen as far as possible from the site of the craniotomy. A selection of models of the Ommaya reservoir is available according to the requirements of any particular case (fig. 1).

In the literature [1, 6] a whole range of complications is mentioned, in connexion with the insertion and use of the Ommaya-system. Apart from skin ulceration and infection, fluid fistulas and displacement of the catheter are described. In individual cases cerebral convulsions and intracerebral haemorrhages have actually occurred, after the insertion of the system. Finally one should also mention methotrexate leuco-encephalopathy.

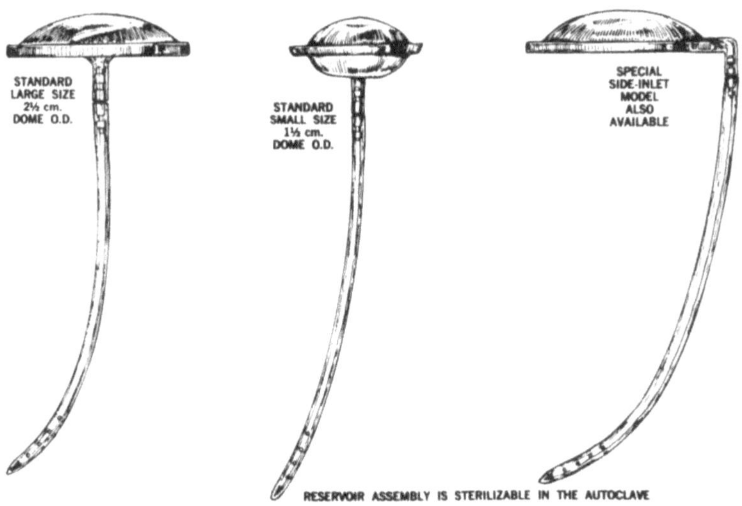

Fig. 1 Schematic diagram of various models of the Ommaya system.

In our patients we check the position and function of the Ommaya system by scintigraphy after the injection of 300–500 micro Curies of Indium 111 DTPA into the reservoir. Measurement of activity then follow, one, 24 and 48 hours after the injection (fig. 2).

Results

We report here on 22 patients in whom an Ommaya-reservoir was inserted. These are not all the patients operated on by us, as some remain for example, in the further care of the haematologists. The majority were glioblastomas, followed by three astrocytomas of grade II–III, as well as two ependymomas grade III. Besides these there was one each arachnoid sarcoma, astroblastoma, a metastasis from an adenocarcinoma as well as a cystic malignant tumour. In the latter case after puncturing the cyst no utilisable could be recovered for histological examination (tab. 1). The implantation usually took place at the time of the first operation but in two of the

Table 1 Twenty-two patients with the Ommaya reservoir – Summary of the diagnoses

Diagnosis	Numbers
Glioblastoma multiforme	13
Astrocytoma II–III	3
Ependymoma III	2
Astroblastoma III	1
Arachnoidal sarcoma	1
Malignant cystic tumour	1
Metastasis from an adenocarcinoma	1

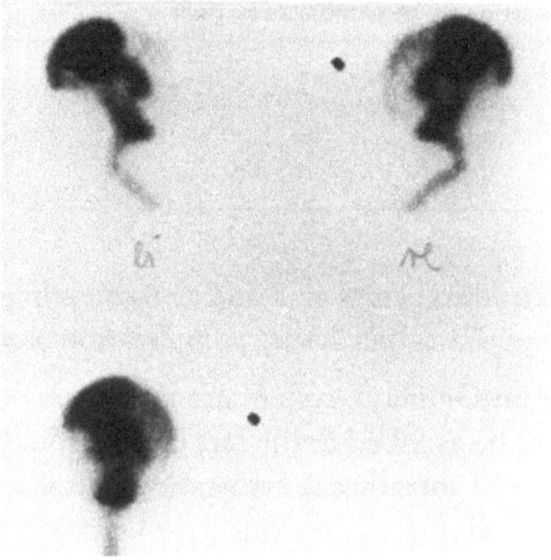

Fig. 2 Testing of the position and function of the Ommaya-system by scintigraphy with Indium 111.

patients during operation on a recurrence. With one exception postoperative radiation was given to all the patients. Oral and intravenous chemotherapy was administered to all the patients.

Each patient received 60–80 mg methotrexate intrathecally, divided into weekly doses of 10 mg. In one patient the treatment had to be stopped after the second puncture on account of intolerance.

Not all of the complications mentioned at the beginning have been observed in our patients. Thus, we saw no convulsions or intracerebral haematoma. Also, we saw fluid fistulas as infrequently as methotrexate leuco-encephalopathy.

As a late complication, one patient developed three years after the implantation a tension over the Ommaya reservoir with phlegmonous infiltration of the skin flap, followed by five cutaneous perforations with escape of purulent secretion. A straight X-ray and CT examination showed osteomyelitis of the bone flap with an extradural empyema. When the empyema was drained and the bone flap removed, the Ommaya system was also removed.

In a second patient only one week after putting in the device a reddening and subsequent formation of purulent fistulae developed over the reservoir. Here also, when the system was removed involvement of the bone flap and epidural space was found. In both cases Staphylococcus epidermidis was identified as the cause.

Summary

We can summarise our observations in 22 patients with an Ommaya reservoir as follows (tab. 2): Of the previously mentioned complications we saw infection in only two patients, which corresponds to an incidence of 9%. Nevertheless in both cases it

Table 2 Summary of the complications after insertion of an Ommaya reservoir

Frequency: Two out of 22 patients = 9%
Infection + perforation over the reservoir
Osteomyelitis of the bone flap
Epidural empyema

followed a very severe course with an extradural empyema and also osteomyelitis of the bone flap. The method therefore shows a rather lower complication rate.

The indications for the implantation of an Ommaya-system are becoming progressively fewer at present. This is not least to be ascribed to the fact that various groups of workers are doubtful about the value of intrathecal cytostatic treatment, especially as regards malignant gliomas. However, just as previously the Ommaya system is being used during the treatment of meningeal manifestations of malignant diseases of the haematopoietic system, and also occasionally for particular tumours of a high grade of malignancy e.g. glioblastomas, astrocytomas and ependymomas. Finally one should not overlook the indication when there is a primary inoperable cystic malignant tumour, less commonly also with cystic craniopharyngiomas and spongioblastomas, where very easily repeatable punctures can be carried out with intermittent drainage for the relief of increased intracranial pressure.

References

[1] Bleyer, W. A., Ph. A. Pizzo, A. M. Spence, et al.: Ommaya-Reservoir. Newly recognized complications and recommendations for insertion and use. Cancer **41** (1978) 2431–2437.
[2] Diamond, R. D., J. E. Bennett: A subcutaneous reservoir for intrathecal therapy of fungal meningitis. New Engl. J. Med. **288** (1973) 186–188.
[3] Fox, J. L.: Intermittent drainage of intracranial cyst via the subcutaneous Ommaya reservoir. J. Neurosurg. **27** (1967) 272–273.
[4] Ommaya, A. K.: Subcutaneous reservoir and pump for sterile access to ventricular cerebrospinal fluid. Lancet **2** (1963) 983–984.
[5] Ommaya, A. K., R. C. Rubin, E. S. Henderson, et al.: A new approach to the treatment of inoperable brain tumours. Medical Annals of the District of Columbia **34/10** (1965) 455–458.
[6] Roosen, K., W. Hawers, J. Schaaf: Indications and experiences with the Ommaya-Reservoir for treatment of CNS neoplasms in childhood. In: Tumours of the Central Nervous System in Infancy and Childhood (D. Voth, P. Gutjahr, C. Langmaid, eds.). Springer-Verlag, Berlin–Heidelberg–New York 1982.
[7] Spiers, A. S. D., B. L. Firth: Treating the nervous system in acute leukaemia. Lancet **1** (1972) 433.

The significance of age as a factor in the prognosis of surgically treated cerebral gliomas
(Brief communication)

M. Brandt, Th. Herter

Between the years 1977–1981 200 patients were operated on for cerebral glioma, 19% of these patients were over 60 years old.

Of those patients over 60, 34% had an extensive resection of the tumour, 58% a partial resection, and in 8% emptying of a cyst and the taking of a biopsy specimen.

The operational lethality rate (patients dying within 30 days p.o.) was for all glioma patients under 60 years 10%, for patients over 60 years 23%. A further analysis of the mortality rate related to the histopathology is in progress.

It is evident, that increased age is detrimental for survival (fig. 1). This negative influence is more marked in cases of astrocytoma and oligodendroglioma (fig. 2) than in cases of glioblastoma. A further analysis of the mean survival time in relation

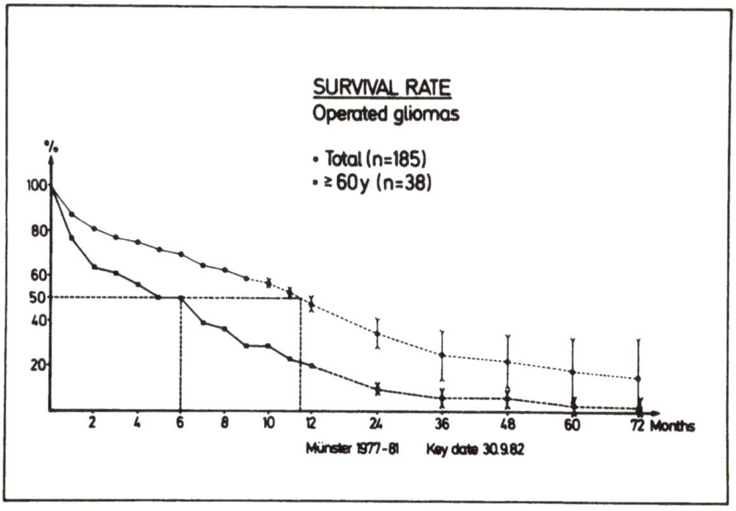

Fig. 1 Survival rate of all surgically treated cerebral gliomas (above) and of those over sixty (below).

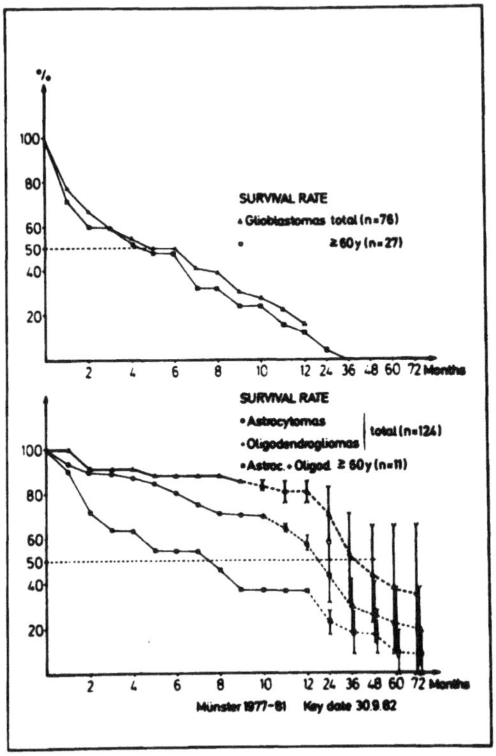

Fig. 2 Survival rate of all surgically treated cerebral gliomas and of those over sixty according to the histological diagnosis (glioblastoma above, astrocytoma and oligodendroglioma below).

to the extent of resection of tumour tissue and additional radiotherapy is in progress. Obviously this is a retrospective and not a randomised study and has certain limitations. One point, however, has already emerged, namely that the pre-operative level of consciousness influences the average survival time considerably.

Quality of life following microsurgical removal of glioblastomas
(Brief communication)

H. R. Eggert, J. Gilsbach, M. Sprich, C. Schandelmaier

Despite numerous advances in the fields of diagnosis and perioperative management in neurosurgery, the surgical treatment of glioblastomas is still unsatisfactory. Since microsurgical methods have been used in intracranial and spinal lesions, the mortality and morbidity of these lesions have been significantly reduced. Microsurgical methods used in intrinsic brain tumours have been recently described but there are no reports dealing with results of microsurgical treatment of glioblastomas. The present study reports on the results of microsurgical treatment in 77 patients with glioblastomas operated on between 1976 and 1980.

Patients and methods

The series consisted of 77 patients suffering from histologically confirmed glioblastomas, on whom adequate data on the postoperative course could be collected. The patients had been operated on between 1976 and 1980. The information about the postoperative course had been accumulated up to November 1, 1982. The series included 39 women and 38 men. The age at operation ranged from 22 to 75 years (average 53.7). Most of the tumours were located in the frontal and temporal lobes (tab. 1). Patients with severe psychopathological and neurological deficits which were estimated to be irreversible were not operated on. Tumours primarily located in the brain stem, basal ganglia and limbic system were also excluded as well as glioblastomas spreading through both cerebral hemispheres. All other glioblastomas, even though they were located in areas of high functional significance, were operated on using microsurgical techniques. These techniques included surgical approaches adapted to the individual location of each tumour, removal of all tumour tissue, as far as the tumour location allows up to the visible borderline of normal brain tissue, and sparing all vessels not feeding or draining the tumour. Normal brain tissue not affected by the tumour was not removed.

Results

Mortality and survival time

Operative mortality was 6.5% (n – 5) including all patients who died within one month of the operation. At the end of the follow-up period no patient was alive. Mean survival time was 6.7 months in female and 8.0 months in male patients (mean 7.5 months). In patients younger than 14 years of age (n = 6) a mean survival time of 12.2 months was found, whereas on an average the older patients (n = 71) survived for 6.9 months. The survival time seemed to be significantly increased by postoperative radiation therapy. On an average, radiated patients survived 10.5 months, whereas in patients not radiated a mean survival time of 3.7 months was noted. However, it has to be considered that radiation therapy was not recommended in patients who were in poor condition for several weeks after the operation. The mean survival time also depended on the location of the tumours. Patients suffering from temporal glioblastomas showed the worst prognosis (mean survival time 5.7 months), whereas patients with tumours of the occipital lobe survived for more than ten months (tab. 1).

Summary

From 1976 to 1980 77 patients suffering from histologically confirmed glioblastomas of the cerebral hemispheres were operated on. No restrictions according to the location in areas of high functional significance were made. Information on survival time and postoperative quality of life was collected and compared with data obtained from the literature. Our results do not differ from other studies in terms of

Table 1 Location and mean survival time in 77 microsurgical treated glioblastomas

location	patients n (%)	mean survival time (months)
occipital	9 (11.7)	10.3
fronto-parietal	2 (2.6)	9.0
parieto-occipital	8 (10.4)	7.6
temporo-parieto- occipital	6 (7.8)	7.6
parietal	11 (14.3)	7.2
frontal	24 (31.2)	6.9
temporal	17 (22.1)	5.7

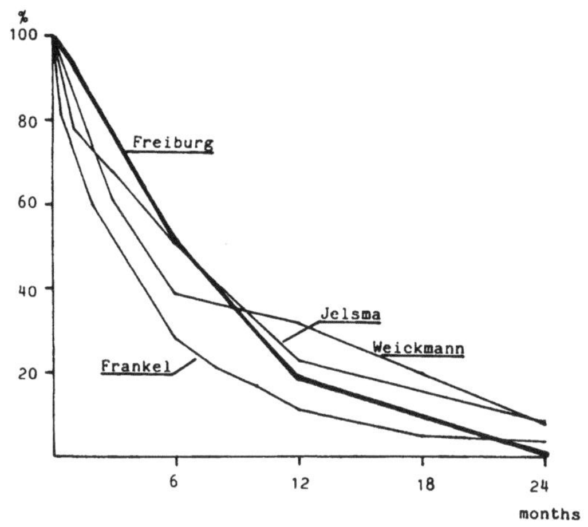

Fig. 1 Survival time of surgically treated glioblastomas reported by different authors.

survival times (fig. 1) and quality of life attributable only to the microsurgical technique. This may be due to the rather rough criteria used to estimate the quality of life in every study as well as to the differently selected groups of patients.

Neuropsychological studies under the therapy of malignant gliomas

H. Wilhelm

Introduction

If the effectiveness of treatment for malignant tumours of the brain is to be properly assessed it must not only report on the duration of survival, but also on its quality. This latter can be objectively determined by psychometric methods in the same way that the other factors are demonstrated by the neurological and neuropsychiatric assessments. Our concern was to find out how the necessary treatments of tumours of the brain do affect the patient's subjective condition and his intellectual efficiency. Within the scope of a prospective study, we carried out psychometric examinations in temporal dependence on operation, radiation and chemotherapy.

Material and methods

The random sample:

The random sample comprises 40 patients. The ratio between male and female is 28:12. The youngest patient was 14 at the time of diagnosis, the oldest was 64 years old. The mean age is 45.6; the standard deviation is 12.5. Astrocytomas comprised 60%, gliomastomas 25% and oligodendroglias 7.5% of the total and another 7.5% could not be definitely classified.

Methods of examination

The patients had a clinical-neurological, a neurophysiological as well as a neuropsychological examination. This was done either before of the neurosurgical intervention or before the radiation, according to the course of the treatment. Further examinations followed between the operation and the begin of the radiation, between radiation and CCNU-dose, before every further chemotherapeutical phase of treatment and also every six months after the end of chemotherapy.

Findings before of the operation

Only two patients reached in all tested intellectual functions the expected results in the psychometric tests used according to age and education [2, 3, 5]. Of the patients 95% showed organic-brain disorders which can be subdivided like this: 19 patients (47.5%) were aphasic at the time of the first psychometric inquiries. Because of serious organic-brain impairment five patients (12.5%) were unable to carry out the instructions, which were given to test their mental efficiency; this also includes the patients with serious speech disturbances. The memory disturbances of the remaining 33 patients were proved by the Benton-test [1]. These disturbances could be graduated by calculating the difference between the formerly expected results and the patient's actual achieved performance. A slight disturbance (difference of 2 or 3 points) was seen in 12 patients, 8 patients had 4–6 points of difference (medium disturbance) and 13 patients had more than 6 points of difference (tab. 1).

The patients' subjective condition before the operation

The single characteristics of condition are marked in their quantitative measurement on a bipolar scale. The 24 determined profiles all carried high charges on the dimensions "sensitivity" and "excitement". According to Janke [3] this is a hint as regards emotional lability and irritation. In their quantitative measurement the scales "anxiety" and "depression", which express on the one hand actually witnessed fear and on the other hand a general listlessness, are the next to follow. Finally, there predominates a physically perceived reduction of activity, which is accompanied by a general passivity and which is reflected on the scale "tiredness".

Table 1 Organic brain impairment before the operation and the radiation

Kind of impairment	no disturbance	slight disturbance	medium disturbance	serious disturbance	not to be examined
Aphasia (Token-test)	21 (52.5%)	8 (20.0%)	7 (17.5%)	4 (10.0%)	0
Disturbances of memory (Benton-test)	2 (5.0%)	12 (30.0%)	8 (20.0%)	13 (32.5%)	5 (12.5%)
	PR 25	PR 10–24	PR 10		
Disturbances of concentration (d2-test)	7 (17.5%)	16 (40.0%)	4 (10.0%)		13 (32.5%)

Findings after the operation

One third of all the patients who were examined after their operation showed an increase of organic brain disturbances. In three cases, patients with a tumour in the left hemisphere showed an increase of disturbances concerning memory and concentration. Aphasic disturbances of medium seriousness also occurred so that in these cases a qualitative change of the organic brain disturbances found out ahead of the operation exists. In another three cases, patients with a tumour in the left hemisphere showed after their operation a quantitative change of their speech disorders as well as of their disturbances of memory and concentration. Concerning the group of patients with a tumour in the right hemisphere the disturbances of memory increased in one case.

The patients' subjective condition after the operation

Beside a distinct relief of the factor "anger", which is composed of the dimensions "anxiety", "depression" and "dreaminess", there were subjectively perceived changes concerning the patient's inactivity to be found. This was especially to be noticed in the dimensions "numbness" and "tiredness" as well as in the dimensions "excitement" and "anger" with regard to the emotional irritation. As could be concluded from the patients' statements, simply the idea that the tumour was removed, led to a distinctly perceived ease and relief. The psychological profiles of ten patients contain no data which differ essentially from those of the first examination.

Findings after the radiation

The entire random sample of the remaining patients showed no qualitative changes of the organic brain disturbances compared to the preceding examinations. Functional disturbances, which had not existed before the operation, did not supervene. On the other hand, disturbances, which had existed before of the operation, also continued after that. Quantitative shiftings of the disturbances were to be found in 44% of the cases, 16% showed an improvement and 28% a deterioration of the previously discovered symptoms. The average range of variability amounted to 3–7 points of difference in the Benton-test.

The subjective condition after the radiation

More than one third of the patients showed a striking behaviour. When answering questions on psychopathologic phenomena, they appeared to be in a shallow euphoric mood with a diminished seriousness. The self-assessment of these patients by means of the list of adjectives [3] leads to a profile which shows the shallow euphoric mood, moreover the dimension "sensibility" shows in each case a deviation towards high sensibility. Three patients explained that their stay exclusively among patients suffering from cancer and the situation of radiation had been a mental strain. The other patients stated an unchanged condition compared to the first examination.

Findings after the chemotherapy

Systematic, organic-brain conditioned effects of the chemotherapy [4] on the intellectual efficiency could not be proved with the applied psychometric proceedings. An increase of organic brain disturbances appeared in the progress together with relapses. Regarding all psychometric factors of performance in the sequel, greater fluctuations of performance after having finished the radiation are striking, although there is no change of the patients' efficiency. Only one patient, a girl who was 14 at the time of operation, showed in the tested intellectual functions a measurable improvement of performance, which persisted for a longer period in its positive trend.

The subjective condition after the chemotherapy

The fluctuation of the patients' condition in the sequel up to a relapse can be attributed in the main to psychosocial problems, which affect the patients especially after their discharge from the clinic. In this connection keywords like problems in relations, financial problems as a pensioner, being a pensioner after the discharge from work should be mentioned.

Discussion

In order to estimate which positive chances of living patients with malignant gliomae have got, you should not renounce the use of factors, which make it possible to judge the patient's subjective condition and his organic brain disturbances regarding their quality and quantity in the progress. The findings presented here confirm this assumption. According to them, 46.4% of the patients had already noticed changes of their behaviour and/or of their perception before the diagnosis was made, 47.5% had shown central disturbances in speech and in 95% of the cases intellectual disturbances could be proved. Furthermore, the findings demonstrate that qualitative and/or quantitative changes of the organic brain disturbances, which existed at the time of diagnosis, are only to be expected in the progress of the treatment undertaken, if an operation has taken place. One third of the operated patients of our random sample showed an increase of symptoms. The shiftings of performance observed in the sequel after the radiation impress by a labilisation of the availability of intellectual functions: The capacities which existed before the radiation are still entirely present, but they get more easily exhausted. The patient's subjective condition and his intellectual efficiency prove to be two independantly varying factors. In this connection the relief after the operation, which affects the state of health, has to be mentioned. However, it becomes obvious that the patients' expectations concerning an operation are often too high. Psychosocial and economic changes, which are consequence of the patient's affection, often involve a lot of problems after his discharge from the protecting milieu of the clinic. In consideration of the patient's psychopathology [6] an early participation in the further care of persons who have been referred as far as a sound relation does exist, proves to be efficient.

Summary

In the scope of a multidimensional study we examined patients with malignant gliomas neuropsychologically in a temporal relationship to their operation, radiation and chemotherapy.

With the help of psychometric procedures disturbances of intellectual functions could already be shown in 95% of the cases at the time of diagnosis. One third of the patients who were examined after the operation showed an increase of mental disturbances. At the same time the operation caused a distinct relief of the patient's subjective condition in 52.4% of the cases. A reduction in the dimensions "anxiety", "depression" and "dreaminess" was especially to be found. While after the radiation fluctuations of the mental efficiency, which impressed with an increased disturbance of mental functions, were to be noticed, organic brain effects from the chemotherapy could not be elicited.

It appeared that intellectual efficiency and subjective condition are two independantly varying factors which are to be regarded as valid indicators of the estimation of the remaining quality of living in case of malignant tumours of the brain.

References

[1] Benton, A. L.: Der Benton-Test, Handbuch. Huber, Stuttgart 1972.

[2] Haas, G., G. Vogt, M. Schiemann, et al.: Aphasia and Non-Verbal-Intelliquence in Brain Tumor Patients. J. Neurol. 227 (1982) 209–218.

[3] Janke, W., G. Debus: Die Eigenschaftswörterliste EWL, Handanweisung. Hogrefe, Göttingen 1978.

[4] Jellinger, K., et al.: Ergebnisse der Kombinationsbehandlung maligner Gliome. Nervenarzt 52 (1981) 41–50.

[5] Orgass, B.: Eine Revision des Token Test II. Validitätsnachweis, Normierung und Standardisierung. Diagnostica 12 (4) (1976) 141–156.

[6] Paal, G.: Zur Psychopathologie des Hirntumorkranken. Fortschr. Neurol. Psychiat. 49 (1981) 265–274.

Quality of life in patients with malignant brain tumours

E. Keiper, P. Krauseneck

Introduction

As aggressive therapy usually prolongs the survival time of patients with malignant brain tumours only for some months the quality of life has to be considered thoroughly and critically.

The following aspects of quality of life (QL) can be differentiated in up-to-date trials measuring QL by standardized interviews:
- lack of physical complaints;
- lack of psychic complaints;
- ability to work and care for oneself;
- ability for social relations;
- subjective well-being

The EORTC study-group on QL [1] has developed a questionnaire containing 27 items referring to ability to work and care for oneself, ability to relate social, physical and psychic complaints and to general assessments of the last few weeks. As this questionnaire includes all these particular aspects we decided to translate it.

As experiential and emotional capability are essential factors besides these physical aspects [2, 3, 4] we also asked questions on these themes.

Methods

To supplement the EORTC questionnaire we developed a list of twenty questions on the subject of experiencing and emotions. Following a preliminary study using 23 members of the medical staff of the Neurological Department of the Würzburg University Clinic ten questions were chosen on the base of discrimination analysis and content.

These general questions were, for example:
- Have you been able to be very pleased about something in recent weeks?

- Has anything happened in recent weeks that has emotionally moved you greatly?
- Have you had the feeling of being needed?

These questions could be answered by "yes" (2 points), "somewhat" (1 point), or "no" (no points), so that a maximum of 20 points could be reached for this section. As a complete measure of subjective well-being we used a rating scale developed by the EORTC study group on quality of life [1], which ranges from +5 as the best time of life down to −5 as the worst time of life. In the evaluation no points were given for −5 and ten points for +5.

At the time of questioning the Karnofsky index was estimated in order to obtain, apart from the subjective answers of the patients, an objective measure for the study of QL.

Thus, the following procedures for the study of QL were used in the tumour ward of the Neurological Department of the Würzburg University Clinic on a total of four groups of patients (patients with malignant brain tumours, patients with MS, patients with other neurological complaints, and members of the medical staff):
subjective tests

1. a German translation of the questionnaire developed by the EORTC study group,
2. as complement, the above-mentioned ten questions on the aspect of experiential and emotional capability,
3. an full assessment of the well-being in comparison with a subjective scale of optimal well-being,

Objective evaluation

4. estimation using the Karnofsky index.

The results of our research refer to 26 patients of the Neurological Department of the Würzburg University Clinic; namely, ten patients with brain tumours (where not only primary brain tumours but also metastatic ones were included), eight patients with MS and eight patients with other neurological complaints. The answers from nurses, attendants and physicians were used as controls.

During the course of the research it was found that patients often had difficulty remembering in detail the time before the onset of their illness, if even remembering at all, so we did not use the questionnaire referring to this period. A general estimate of their well-being was, however, possible for all patients.

Results

A significant difference in average ($p<.01$) between the rating of QL at the time before the onset of the illness ($\bar{X} = 8{,}2 \pm 2{,}32$) and of the two weeks prior to questioning ($\bar{X} = 4{,}6 \pm 3{,}01$) was noticeable in the general estimate of well-being for the group of patients as a whole. This means that the time before onset of the present illness was rated at almost the best time of life, the past two weeks at almost the centre of the scale.

On the same scale of rating the comparison of average for the period of the last two weeks resulted in a significant difference ($p<.01$) between the group of staff members ($\bar{X} = 6,9 \pm 1,79$) and the group of patients as a whole ($\bar{X} = 4,9 \pm 2,80$).

In addition, the questions on experiencing and emotional capability for the period of the last two weeks were significantly ($p<.01$) less rarely answered by "yes" by the group of patients as a whole ($\bar{X} = 12,2 \pm 3,68$) than by the group of staff members ($\bar{X} = 16,0 \pm 2,46$).

Table 1 shows the average of the general feeling of well-being for the period of the last two weeks for the various groups of patients and the members of the medical staff.

Here only the largest difference in average between the staff members and the patients with other neurological complaints at the 5% level is significant.

To establish the existing tendency differences between the three procedures of self-estimate used here and the Karnofsky Index assessed by the researcher, the intercorrelation was calculated (fig. 1), in spite of statistic doubts, because of the small number of patients (N = 16).

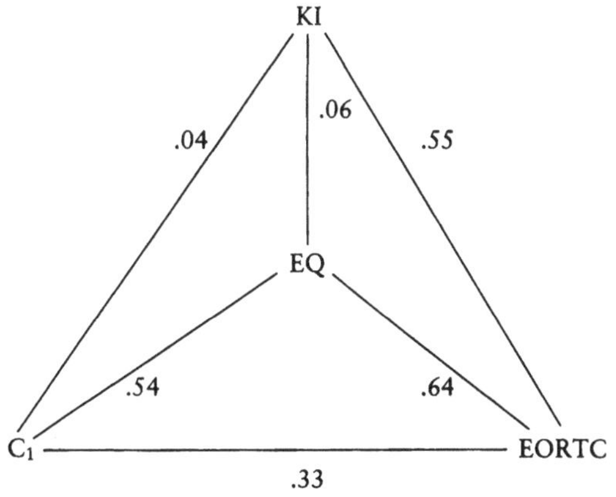

Fig. 1 Intercorrelation between instruments of measuring quality of life (n = 16).

C_1:	General rating-scale of well-being
EORTC:	Quality of Life questionnaire from EORTC
EQ:	Questions on experiential and emotional capability of quality of life
KI:	Karnofsky index

Product-moment-correlation coefficients statistically significant at the 5% level have been marked with an arterisk.

Discussion and conclusions

Because of the relatively small number of patients and the short period of time of our research results of changes in course cannot be given here.

Results given here, even if of statistical significance, are only to be interpreted as tendencies towards a specific direction. The relatively high estimates of the MS patients (tab. 1) may be explained by the circumstance that, at the time of the assessment they came as outpatients for follow-up examinations while the other group of patients were in hospital. Apart from the already described tendencies of patients with malignancies to ignore their illness [2], the lower assessment of our other NL-patients could also be attributed to the fact that a large number of these patients had psychological problems and were undergoing therapy.

Table 1 Mean values of C_1 (general rating of well-being)

	MS-pat (N = 8)	tumour-pat (N = 8)	other NL-pat (N = 8)	m. of med. staff (N = 33)
$\bar{X}$	5,9	4,6	3,3	6,9
S	± 2,0	± 2,9	± 2,7	± 1,8

A rating of 0 means the worst time in life, a rating of 10 means the best time in life.

In considering the correlation coefficients (fig. 1) one notices that the three procedures for subjective self-assessment not only do indeed interrelate (correlation of medium range), but also seem to include different aspects of QL. Regarding the extraneous estimate using the Karnofsky Index (KI), for the EORTC questionnaire alone a medium connection results ($r_{xy} = .55$; $p<.05$), which can probably be explained by the conformity of content of seven questions on ability to work and take care of oneself.

Thus far we can, however, say that the resulting differences between the procedures used here for studying the QL, seem to indicate different aspects of the QL.

References

[1] EORTC (European Organization for Research on Treatment of Cancer): "Quality of Life" Methods of Measurement and Related Areas. Proceedings of the Second EORTC Quality of Life Workshop held in Copenhagen, 1981. Published as an internal report of the Study Group on Quality of Life.

[2] Meerwein, F. (ed.): Einführung in die Psycho-Onkologie. Huber-Verlag, Bern–Stuttgart–Wien 1981.

[3] Simonton, O. C.: Wieder gesund werden. Rowohlt-Verlag, Reinbek 1982.

[4] Tausch, A. M.: Gespräche gegen die Angst. Rowohlt-Verlag, Reinbek 1981.

Postoperative rapid course irradiation of the glioblastoma

W. Hinkelbein, M. Wannenmacher, J. Gilsbach, G. Bruggmoser

Introduction

The glioblastoma (anaplastic astrocytoma and other dedifferentiated gliomas, grade IV according to WHO, 103) is the most frequent brain tumour of the adult. With its unfavourable prognosis – most patients die within the first year after diagnosis – this tumour has become a big challenge for oncology. There are great differences within the published results. Furthermore, many reports – especially from English speaking areas – do not make any distinction between grade III and grade IV tumours. This difference, however, is of considerable prognostic value [41, 50, 63, 76].

Compared to operation alone [8], postoperative radiotherapy leads to a significant prolongation (doubling) of the average survival time and an improvement in the quality of life [36] for the patients. There was a remarkable increase in the one-year and two-year survival rates [9, 88]. Radiotherapy alone seems relevant today only with puncture cytology and its efficiency is comparable to that of operation alone. Therefore, standard treatment today should comprise both, operation and radiotherapy [86]. Despite numerous efforts, additional measures have not brought any further improvement in the results of treatment.

Tests were made with chemotherapy in addition to operation and irradiation, e.g. with nitrosourea derivates such as BCNU that easily cross into the CSF [4, 26, 48, 53, 80, 94, 96], CCNU [2, 4, 12, 23, 32, 52, 56, 62, 96, 97], MeCCNU [91, 92, 96] and ACNU [51, 54, 67]. High doses of BCNU and CCNU were given followed by bone marrow replantation [14, 30, 33]. Furthermore, a number of cytostatic drugs were tested that do not penetrate the CSF, e.g. actinomycin D [2], methotrexate [85], vincristine [2, 45], bleomycine [3, 42, 43, 70, 82], DBD [2], DAG [2, 20], hydroxyurea [46], streptozotozine [57], DTIC [87], mithramycine [38, 93], procarbacine [99], VM 26 [78], and 5 FU [21]. Neither did this adjuvant polychemotherapy lead to any significant improvement of the therapeutic results [24, 35, 40, 47, 61, 70, 72, 74, 87, 91, 100].

Even the increase of the irradiation dose up to 80 Gy [65] or the introduction of high LET radiation were unsatisfactory measures. The use of high energetic neutrons [16,

25, 27, 44, 58] as well as mixed-beam-therapy [25, 44] were no great success. Up to now, there have not been many tests with 930 MeV-helium-ions [15]. Equally unsatisfactory were tests of pre-operative [39, 55, 71] and intraoperative [1] irradiation. No breakthrough was reached with a change of the fractions, neither with high individual fractions [49, 84] nor with superfractioning [34, 59, 60, 77]. Since therapy-resistence of the glioblastoma among others is the consequence of a tumour hypoxia, the introduction of radiosensitizing measures was the big hope. But irradiation under hyperbaric oxygen [17] or combined with the electron affinic sensitizers metronidazole [18, 19, 89] and misonidazole [6, 13, 18, 28, 34, 64, 83, 90, 95] led to disappointment, as well as radiosensitizing with bromodeoxyuridine [51, 68] and tri-iodothyronine [102]. Irradiation under hyperthermic [5, 29, 66, 73] or hypothermic [7] conditions showed no convincing results. All eforsts to improve the results with an adjuvant immunotherapy [98] were inefficient. These included the replantation of irradiated tumour cells [10] or the local infusion of autologious lymphocytes in combination with the non-specific immunopotentiator OK-432 [69] as well as the use of the immunopotentiators levamisole [11] and BCG [81].

It has to be pointed out that above measures – although they might bring a little prolongation of the survival time – can involve a deterioration in the quality of life.

With postoperative radiotherapy – that requires high doses of 50–60 Gy at a conventional fractioning of 5 × 2 Gy/week – the prolongation of survival time is to a large extent compensated by the therapy itself (it normally involves staying in hospital). Therefore, we tested the efficiency of rapid course irradiation with high fractions to reduce the treatment period and at the same time prolong the therapy-free survival time for the patient. Such a rapid course irradiation with high fractions was well known from the treatment of brain metastases, with individual fractions exceeding 5 Gy [31, 75, 101]. With glioblastoma patients, as well, a reduction of the treatment period [49] and the use of high individual fractions of 5 Gy [84] has been described, which did not involve any striking side effects.

Patients

From January 1980 until June 1983 70 patients with grade IV gliomas were treated with daily fractions of 3.5 Gy. The proportion of male to female was 1:1.4. The average age was 55.3 years, the youngest patient was 15 the oldest 78 years old (fig. 1). In all cases the diagnosis was confirmed histologically by operation or stereotactic puncture.

The histological examination in 11 patients revealed apart from the grade IV tissue (glioblastoma multiforme) portions with grade-III-gliomas, six patients had astrocy-

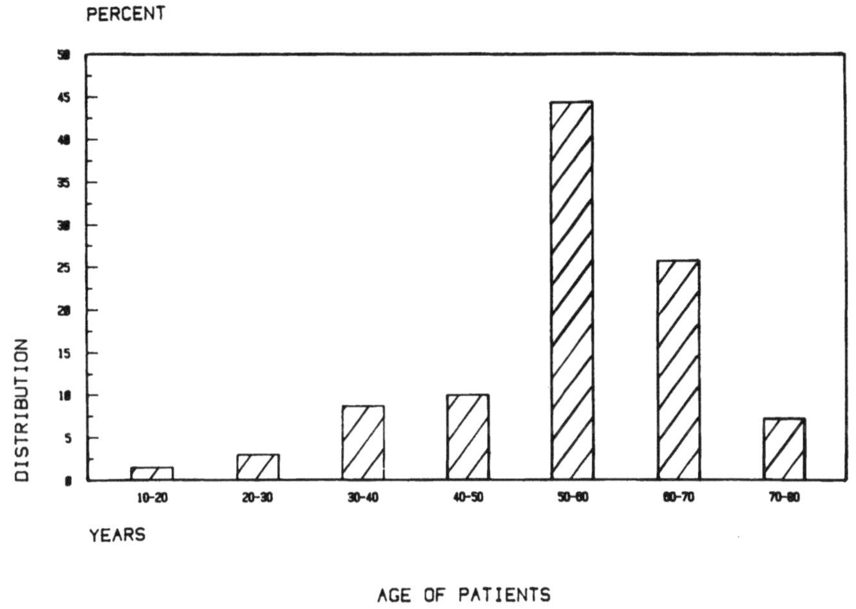

Fig. 1 A distribution of 70 patients with glioblastomas, treated with rapid course irradiation.

tomas, two had oligodendrogliomas and three were mixed-type gliomas. In 63 cases operation preceded radiotherapy, six patients had only a stereotactic biopsy and the latter was combined with a 125 iodine implantation in two cases. In 31 cases tumour was in the right hemisphere, in 33 cases in the left hemisphere, while in six patients the midline and brain stem were involved.

Methods

The whole brain was irradiated with lateral opposing fields, with 4 or 8 MeV photones from a linear accelerator. The daily fraction was 3.5 Gy based on the middle of the skull, 1.75 Gy from each side. The number of fractions was 4–6 per week. Initially the patients were treated with a total dose of 31.5 Gy.

Since the dose was well tolerated the total dose was increased to 35 Gy ending up with 38.5 Gy. On the average there was an interval of 14 days between the operation and radiotherapy, the range was between 7 and 15 days. The shortest interval was three, the longest 46 days. All patients were given dexamethasone at rapidly decreasing doses, starting with 8–16 mg/day during radiotherapy. As permanent medication they had diphenylhydantoin to prevent seizures. The calculation of the average survival times and rates were based on the Kaplan-Meier-method [37].

Results

All patients had an average survival time of 33.5 weeks. The six month survival rate was 62%, the one year survival rate was 16% and the two year survival rate was 11.5%. On the average, females had a significantly lower one and two year survival rate compared to the male group (tab. 1). The age was also of importance; the group aged 10–30 years had the highest average survival rate. The group aged 50–70 years had the lowest one year survival rate with 15% (tab. 1). The site of the tumour had no effect on the result of the treatment. Even the six patients with brain stem and midline tumours did not come up with significantly worse results. In this group was a 15-year-old boy who was excluded after 116 weeks. Without this patient the group had a remarkably lower survival rate (tab. 1).

The total dose was converted – according to the Ellis-formula [22] – into isoeffect doses of a conventional fractioning of 5 × 2 Gy/week. Three equal groups were formed with isoeffect doses of 30–46 Gy, 47–51 Gy and 52–60 Gy. Surprisingly the patients with the maximum exposure and the best six month survival rate of 68,4% died after that time very quickly. Figure 2 shows the survival rates of the three groups. We analysed all dead patients in two groups: 30–51 Gy and 52–60 Gy

Table 1 Results of treatment in 70 patients treated with rapid course irridiation at high fractions, correlated with the different marks of the collective

Group	Number	Average Survival (%)	Survival six months (%)	Survival 1 Year (%)	Survival 2 Years (%)
Total	70	33.5	62.0	16.0	11.5
Male	40	35.4	63.0	23.5	19.6
Female	30	31.0	60.7	11.4	3.8
10–30 Years	3	54.8	33.0	33.0	–
31–50 Years	13	31.0	63.6	36.4	–
51–70 Years	49	35.2	66.5	15.0	–
Location:					
right Hemisph.	31	33.2	62.7	23.4	–
left Hemisph.	33	33.8	65.0	11.1	–
Midline and Brain stem	6/5*	33.6/17.1	40.0/25.0	20.0/0	–
Total Dose:					
30–46 Gy**	20	26.7	56.1	5.6	–
47–51 Gy**	30	36.7	61.4	30.9	17.7
52–60 Gy**	20	35.6	68.4	10.5	10.5
Grade IV Tumours with Gr. III Parts					

* Explanation see text
** Isoeffect Dose for conventional fractioning according to Ellis Formula

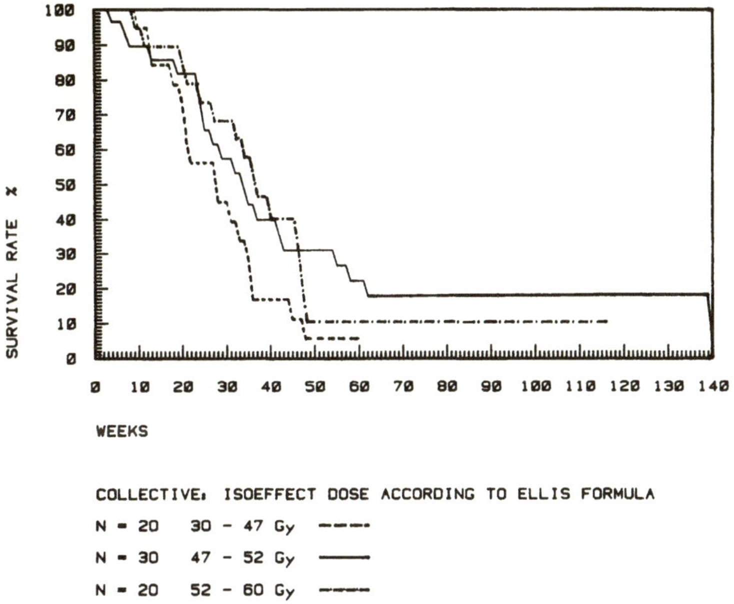

Fig. 2 Survival curves after rapid course irradiation. Isoeffect doses related to conventional fractioning of 5 × 2 Gy/week.

(fig. 3). Within the latter group most patients died between week 25–35. All other patients had a normal distribution concerning their survival time. This fact could possibly be a result of the therapy. Patients with parts of more differentiated glioma had an even more favourable prognosis than the group as a whole.

At the key-date on July 1, 1983, 13 patients were still alive: Within the group irradiated with 40–46 Gy one patient (14 weeks from end of treatment), within the group treated with 47–51 Gy seven patients (45.1 weeks average survival time) and within the group with the highest exposure five patients (56 weeks average survival time).

Five patients were "long-term-survivors" (more than 65 weeks): One patient was the above-mentioned 15-year-old boy with a grade III and IV tumour of the quadrigeminal region, who was still alive after 116 weeks. A 63-year-old patient (male, 50 Gy) was still alive after 72.5 weeks. The other three patients received intensive treatment of recurrences: the first patient was given irradiation with 20 Gy (5 × 2 Gy per week) and died after 140 weeks, the second patient had another operation and was still alive after 135 weeks. The third patient – chemotherapy (HeCNU) – was still alive after 66 weeks.

The quality of life – compared to patients with standard therapy – was better. Especially remarkable is the recovery after treatment with rapid disappearance of neurological signs and more often a change to a better performance state.

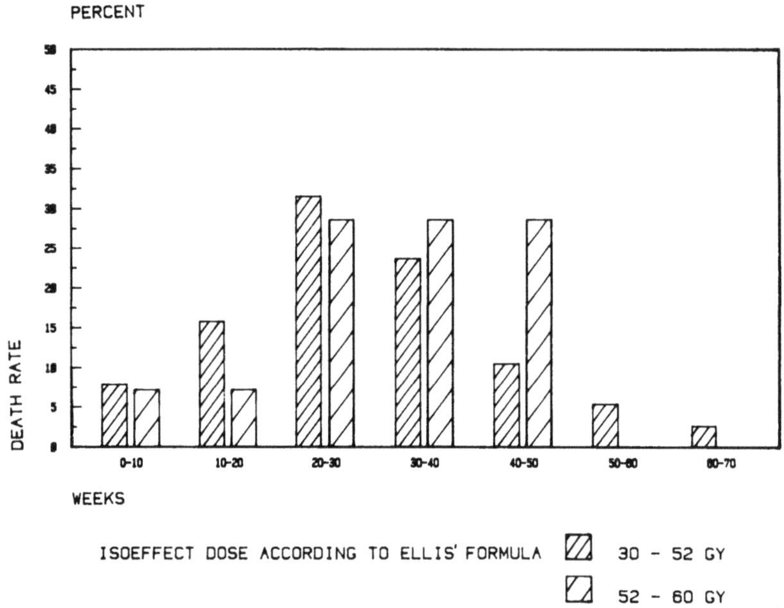

Fig. 3 Bar charts of patients who died after rapid course irradiation. Isoeffect doses related to conventional fractioning of 5 × 2 Gy/week.

Discussion

As expected, rapid course irradiation of glioblastoma (grade IV glioma) did not produce significantly better results than the standard postoperative radiotherapy. Compared to the published reports, however, this measure was satisfactory: An average survival rate of 33.5 weeks, a six month survival rate of 62%, and a one year survival rate of 16%. Thus it seems possible to achieve the most important aim, i.e. to prolong the therapy-free survival time for patients with glioblastomas. This is especially true for a total dose of 35 Gy. Since therapy with 38.5 Gy seems to involve a limitation of the survival time we will no longer use it. Our present treatment of glioblastoma (grade IV glioma) consists of postoperative radiotherapy with rapid course irradiation (6 × 3.5 Gy/week, total dose 35 Gy) versus superfractioning (3 × 1.5 Gy/day, 5 ×/week, total dose 40.5 Gy) in order to find out if compatibility can be improved still more with the latter. Our principle aim is the reduction of the treatment period and thus to prolong the therapy-free survival time.

Conclusion

The quality of life for glioblastoma patients treated with rapid course irradiation is similar to that with conventional fractioning, or even better. Postoperative rapid course irradiation with high fractions and a limited total dose (35 Gy) presently is – apart from the accelerated superfractioning – a successful measure for prolonging the therapy-free survival time for patients with grade IV gliomas.

References

[1] Abe, M., M. Takahashi: Intraoperative radiotherapy: The Japanese Experience. Int. J. Radiat. Oncol. Biol. Phys. 7 (1981) 863–868.

[2] Afra, D., E. Pasztor: Cytostatic drugs in the postoperative treatment of glioblastoma. Excerpta Medica Int. Congress Series **433** (1978) 420–422.

[3] Andersen, A. P., Scandinavian Blioblastoma Study Group: Combined modality therapy of operated astrocytomas grade III and IV. Confirmation of the value of postoperative irradiation and lack of potention of bleomycin on survival time. Cancer **47** (1981) 649–652.

[4] Band, P. R., B. K. Weir, R. C. Urtasun, et al.: Radiotherapy and CCNU in grade III and IV astrocytoma. Proc. Am. Assoc. Cancer Res. **15** (1974) 161.

[5] Bicher, H. J., T. S. Sandhu, D. W. Hetzel: Hyperthermia and radiation in combination: a clinical fractionation regime. Int. J. Radiat. Oncol. Biol. Phys. **6** (1980) 861–866.

[6] Bleehan, N. M., C. R. Wiltshire, P. N. Plowman, et al.: A randomized study of misonidazole and radiotherapy for grade III and IV cerebral astrocytoma. Br. J. Cancer **43** (1981) 436–442.

[7] Bloch, M., H. J. G. Bloom, J. Penman, et al.: Observations on patients with cerebral astrocytomas (Glioblastoma multiforme) treated by irradiation under whole-body hypothermia. Br. J. Cancer 20 (1966) 722–728.

[8] Bloom, H. J. G.: Combined modality therapy for intracranial tumors. Cancer 35 (1975) 110–120.

[9] Bloom, H. J. G.: Intercranial tumors: Response and resistance to therapeutic endeavours 1970–1980. Int. J. Rad. oncol. Bid. Phys. **8** (1982) 1083–111.

[10] Bloom, H. J. G., M. J. Peckham, A. E. Richardson, et al.: Glioblastoma multiforme: A controlled trial to assess the value of specific active immunotherapy in patients treated by radical surgery and radiotherapy. Brit. J. Cancer 27 (1973) 253–267.

[11] Caciagli, P., G. Acerbi, R. Ciccarelli, et al.: Surveys on the immune system in patients with glioblastoma. In: Multidisciplinary Aspects of Brain Tumor Therapy (P. Paoletti, M. D. Walker, G. Butti, R. Knerich, eds.). Elsevier/North-Holland Biomedical Press, Amsterdam 1979.

[12] Calliauw, L.: EORTC Brain Tumor Group Studies. In: Therapie maligner Neoplasien des Gehirns (P. Krauseneck, H. G. Martens, eds.), pp. 50–54. Perimed Verlag, Erlangen 1983.

[13] Carabell, S. C., L. A. Bruno, A. S. Weinstein, et al.: Misonidazole and radiotherapy to treat malignant glioma: A phase II trial of the RTOG. Int. J. Radiat. Oncol. Biol. Phys. 7 (1981) 71–77.

[14] Carekia, A. M., D. Giordano, G. Santini, et al.: High-dose BCNU with autologous bone marrow rescue for glioblastoma multiforme. 12th ICC, Florence 1981.

[15] Castro, J. R., J. M. Quivey: Clinical experience and expectations with Helium and heavy ion irradiation. Int. J. Radiat. Oncol. Biol. Phys. **3** (1977) 247–253.

[16] Catterall, M., H. J. G. Bloom, L. Walsh, et al.: Fast neutrons compared with negavoltage x-rays in the treatment of patients with supratentorial glioblastoma: A controlled pilot study. Int. J. Radiat. Oncol. Biol. Phys. **6** (1980) 261–266.

[17] Chang, C. H.: Hyperbaric oxygen and radiation therapy in the management of glioblastoma. Modern Concepts in Brain Tumor Therapy. Laboratory and Clinical Investigations NCI Monograph No **46** (1977) 163–169.

[18] Dische, S.: Hypoxic cell sensitizers in radiotherapy. Int. J. Radiat. Oncol. Biol. Phys. **4** (1978) 157–160.

[19] Dische, S.: Hyberbaric oxygen and hypoxic cell sensitizers in clinical radiotherapy: present state and prospects. In: High-LET Radiations in Clinical Radiotherapy (Proceedings of the 3rd meeting on fundamental and practical aspects of the application of fast neutrons and other High-LET particles in clinical radiotherapy, held at The Hague, Netherlands, 13–15 Sept. 1978, TNO Rijswijk. G. W. Barendsen, J. J. Broerse, K. Breur, eds.). Pergamon Press, Oxford 1979.

[20] Eagan, R. T., D. S. Childs, D. D. Layton, et al.: Dianhydrogalactitol and radiation therapy. J. Am. Med. Assoc. **241** (1979) 2046–2050.

[21] Edland, R. W., M. Javid, F. J. Ansfiels: Glioblastoma multiforme. An analysis of the results of postoperative radiotherapy alone versus radiotherapy and concomitant 5-FU. AJR **111** (1971) 337–341.

[22] Ellis, F.: Dose, time and fractionation: a clinical hypothesis. Clin. Radiol. **20** (1969) 1–7.

[23] EORTC, BTG: Effect of CCNU on survival rate of objective remission and duration of free interval in patients with malignant brain glioma. Eur. J. Cancer **14** (1978) 851–856.

[24] EORTC, BTG: Evaluation of CCNU, VM 26 and procarbazine in supratentorial brain gliomas. Final evaluation of a randomized study. J. Neurosurg. **55** (1981) 27–31.

[25] Geraci, J. P.: Efficacy of neutrons in radiotherapy. Health. Phys. **40** (1981) 41–53.

[26] Giunta, F., G. Gatta, B. Tanghetti, et al.: Surgery, radiotherapy and BCNU in supratentorial malignant glioma. Int. Symp. On Multidisciplinary Aspects of Brain Tumor Therapy, Brescia 1979.

[27] Griffin, R., J. Blasko, G. Laramore: Results of fast neutron beam radiotherapy pilot studies at the University of Washington. In: High-LET Radiations in Clinical Radiotherapy (Proceedings of the 3rd meeting on fundamental and practical aspects of the application of fast neutrons and other High-LET particles in clinical radiotherapy, held at The Hague, Netherlands, 13–15 Sept. 1978, TNO Rijswijk, G. W. Barendsen, J. J. Broerse, K. Breur, eds.). Pergamon Press, Oxford 1979.

[28] Gutin, P. H., W. M. Wara, T. L. Phillips, et al.: Hypoxic cell radiosensitizers in the treatment of malignant brain tumors. Neurosurgery **6** (1980) 567–576.

[29] Herbst, M., R. Sauer: Hyperthermie als strahlensensibilisierendes und cytotoxisches Adjuvans zur Strahlentherapie – Klinische Erfahrungen. Verh. Dtsch. Krebs-Ges. **4** (1983) 79–88.

[30] Hildebrand, J., R. Badjou, E. Collard-Ronge, et al.: Treatment of brain gliomas with high dose CCNU and autologous bone-marrow transplantation. Biomedicine **32** (1983) 71–73.

[31] Hindo, W. A., et al.: Large dose increment irradiation in treatment of cerebral metastases. Cancer **26** (1970) 138–141.

[32] Hochberg, F. H., R. Linggood, Wolfson, et al.: Quality and duration of survival in glioblastoma multiforme. J. Am. Med. Assoc. **241** (1979) 1016–1018.

[33] Hochberg, F. H., L. M. Parker, T. Takvorian, et al.: High-dose BCNU with autologous bone-marrow rescue for recurrent glioblastoma multiforme. J. Neurosurg. **54** (1981) 455–460.

[34] Horiot, J. C., W. Bogaert, K. K. van den Ang, et al.: EORTC Experience with misonidazole combined with a multiple daily fractionated (MDF) radiotherapy. Inaugural meeting of the Europ. Soc. for Therap. Rad. and Oncol., London (meeting abstract) 1982.

[35] Jellinger, R., P. Kothbauer, D. Volc, et al.: Combination Chemotherapy (COMP Protocol) and radiotherapy of anaplastic supratentorial gliomas. Acta Neurochir. (Wien) **51** (1979) 1–13.

[36] Jelsma, R., P. C. Bucy: The treatment of glioblastoma multiforme of the brain. J. Neurosurg. **27** (1967) 388–400.

[37] Kaplan, E. L., P. Meier: Non-parametric estimation from incomplete observation. J. Amer. Statist. Assoc. **53** (1958) 457–481.

[38] Kennedy, B. J., J. H. Brown, J. W. Yarbro: Mithramycin therapy for primary glioblastomas. Cancer Chemother. Rep. **48** (1965) 59–62.

[39] Kondo, T., M. Yoshioka, I. Muraoka, et al.: Preoperative radiotherapy and radical removal of malignant brain tumors. The U.S.-Japanese Conf. On Brain Tumor Therapy, Nikko, Japan 1981.

[40] Kono, T., N. Shitara, K. Takakura, et al.: Synchronized chemo-radiotherapy with vincristine and ACNU for malignant brain tumors. Int. Symposium on multidisciplinary aspects of brain tumor therapy, Brescia 1979.

[41] Kramer, S.: Radiation therapy in the management of malignant gliomas. 7th National Cancer Conf. Proc., pp. 823–826. Lipincott Co., Philadelphia 1973.

[42] Kristiansen, K., S. Hagen, T. Kollevold, et al.: Preliminary report on a scandinavian multicenter investigation on the effect of combined radio- and chemotherapy in patients operated for glioblastoma multiforme. Excerpta Med. Int. Congr. Ser. **433** (1978) 65–69.
[43] Kristiansen, K., S. Hagen, T. Kollevold, et al.: Combined madality therapy of operated astrocytomas grade III and IV. Confirmation of the value of postoperative irradiation and lack of potention of Bleomycin on survival time: A prospective multicenter trial of the scandinavian glioblastoma study group. Cancer **47** (1981) 649–652.
[44] Laramore, G. E., T. W. Griffin, A. J. Gerdes, et al.: Fast neutron and mixed (neutron/photon) beam teletherapy for grades III and IV astrocytomas. Cancer **42** (1978) 96–103.
[45] Lassmann, L. P., G. W. Rearce, J. Gang: Sensitivity of intracranial gliomas to vincristine sulphate. Lancet **1** (1965) 296–298.
[46] Lerner, H. J., B. L. Beckloff, M. C. Godwin: Treatment of astrocytoma with hydroxyurea and irradiation – A report of six patients with 18 months follow up. Am. Surg. **36** (1970) 401–402.
[47] Levin, V. A., C. B. Wilson, P. Gutin, et al.: Brain tumor research center clinical trial 1979–1981. The U.S.-Japanese Conf. On Brain Tumor Therapy, Nikko, Japan (metting abstract) 1981.
[48] Malaker, K.: Treatment of glioblastoma with radiotherapy and BCNU and radiosensitizer. 2nd Int. Conf. on the Adjuvant Therapy of Cancer, Tucson 1979.
[49] Markulin-Grgic, L., S. Pavicic, B. Jelicica: Radiotherapy in the treatment of brain tumors. Int. Symposium on multidisciplinary aspects of brain tumor therapy, Brescia, Italy (meeting abstract) 1979.
[50] Marsa, G. W., J. C. Probert, L. J. Rubinstein, et al.: Megavoltage irradiation in the treatment of gliomas of the brain and spinal cord. Cancer **36** (1975) 1681–1689.
[51] Matsutani, M., K. Takakura: Experience with radiation and radiation-drug combinations for glioblastoma. The U.S.-Japanese Conf. On Brain Tumor Therapy, Nikko, Japan (meeting abstract) 1981.
[52] Monfardine, S., C. Brambilla, C. L. Solero, et al.: Controlled study with BCNU versus CCNU as adjuvant chemotherapy following surgery in glioblastoma multiforme. Int. Symposium On Multidisciplinary Aspects of Brain Tumor Therapy, Brescia 1979.
[53] Monfardini, S., A. Brambilla, C. L. Solero, et al.: Adjuvant chemotherapy with nitrosourea compounds following surgery plus radiotherapy in glioblastoma multiforme. Recent Results Cancer Res. **68** (1978) 393–398.
[54] Mori, T., J. Suzuki: Experimental and clinical study of ACNU and its combined therapy for malignant brain tumor. The U.S.-Japanese Conf. In Brain Tumor Therapy, Nikko, Japan (meeting abstract) 1981.
[55] Muller, H., W. Roggendorf, M. Brock: Malignant brain glioma: The possible role of preoperative radiotherapy. UICC conference on Clinical Oncology, Lausanne, Switzerland 1981.
[56] Paoletti, P., R. Knerich, G. Butti, et al.: Italian Cooperative Study on Malignant Glial Tumor Therapy. In: Therapie maligner Neoplasien des Gehirns (P. Krauseneck, H. G. Martens, eds.), pp. 46–49. Perimed Verlag, Erlangen 1983.
[57] Paoletti, P., D. Schiffer, R. Knerich, et al: Experimental and clinical studies on malignant brain tumors in Italy. The U.S.-Japanese Conf. On Brain Tumor Thterapy, Nikko, Japan (meeting abstract) 1981.
[58] Parker, R. G., H. C. Berry, A. J. Gerdes, et al.: Fast neutron beam radiotherapy of glioblastoma multiforme. Am. J. Roentgenol. Radium Ther. Nucl. Med. **127** (1976) 331–335.
[59] Payne, D. G., W. J. Simpson, C. Keen, et al.: Malignant glioma: Hyperfractionated and standard radiotherapy and chemo therapy in an radomized prospective clinical trial. Int. J. Radiat. Oncol. Biol. Phys. **7** (1981) 1217 (meeting abstract).
[60] Payne, D. G., W. J. Simpson, C. Keen, et al.: Malignant Astrocytoma. Hyperfractionated and standard radiotherapy with chemotherapy in a randomized prospective trial. Cancer **50** (1982) 2301–2306.
[61] Pouillard, O., G. Mathe, Th. Thy, et al.: Treatment of malignant gliomas and brain metastasis in adults with a combination of adriamycin, VM 26 and CCNU. Cancer **38** (1976) 1909–1912.
[62] Reagan, T. J., H. F. Bisel, D. S. Childs, et al.: Controlled study of CCNU and radiation therapy in malignant astrocytomas. J. Neurosurg. **44** (1976) 186–188.
[63] Rutten, E. H. J. M., I. Kazem, J. L. Sloof, et al.: Post-operative radiation therapy in the manage-

ment of brain astrocytoma: A retrospective study of 142 patients. Int. J. Radiat. Oncol. Biol. Phys. 7 (1981) 191–195.

[64] Sack, H., A. Calcanis, E. Godehardt, et al.: Die postoperative Strahlenbehandlung von Astrozytomen Grad 3 und 4 mit dem Strahlensensibilisator Misonidazol. Strahlentherapie **158** (1982) 466–469.

[65] Salazar, O. M., P. Rubin, M. L. Feldstein, et al.: High dose radiation therapy in the treatment of malignant gliomas: final report. Int. J. Radiat. Oncol. Biol. Phys. **5** (1979) 1733–1740.

[66] Salcman, M., F. M. Samanas, H. Mena, et al.: Whole-body hyperthermia: Potential hazards in its application to glioblastoma. In: Multidisciplinary Aspects of Brain Tumor Therapy (P. Paoletti, M. D. Walker, G. Butti, R. Knerich, eds.), pp. 197–208. Elsevier/North Holland, Biomedical Press, Amsterdam – New York – Oxford 1979.

[67] Sano, K.: Chemo-radiotherapy of malignant brain tumors. Excerpta Med. Int. Congr. Ser. **433** (1978) 79–87.

[68] Sano, K., T. Hoshino, M. Nagai: Radiosensitization of brain tumor cells with a thymidine analogue bromouridine. J. Neurosurg. **28** (1968) 530–538.

[69] Sato, K., A. Ishizawa, F. Takahura, et al.: Therapeutic effects of adjuvant immunotherapy to radiotherapy of glioblastoma. Combined use of nonspecific immunopotentiator and infusion of autologous lymphocytes. The U.S.-Japanese Conf. On Brain Tumor Therapy, Nikko, Japan (meeting abstract) 1981.

[70] Seiler, R. W., R. H. Greiner, A. Zimmermann, et al.: Radiotherapy combined with procarbazine, bleomycin and CCNU in the treatment of high-grade supratentorial astrocytomas. J. Neurosurg. **48** (1978) 861–865.

[71] Seiler, R. W., A. Zimmermann, E. A. Bleher, et al.: Preoperative radiotherapy and chemotherapy in hypervascular high-grade supratentorial astrocytomas. Surg. Neurol. **12** (1979) 131–133.

[72] Seiler, R. W., A. Zimmermann, H. Markwalder: Adjuvant chemotherapy with VM 26 and CCNU after operation and radiotherapy of high-grade supratentorial astrocytomas. Surg. Neurol. **13** (1980) 65–68.

[73] Selker, R. G., S. Jacobs, R. Stoller, et al.: Total body hyperthermia possible use in a variety of primary malignant intracranial and extracranial diseases. The U.S.-Japanese Conf. On Brain Tumor Therapy, Nikko, Japan (meeting abstract) 1981.

[74] Shapiro, W. R., D. F. Young: Treatment of malignant glioma. Arch. Neurol. **33** (1976) 494–498.

[75] Shehata, W. M., et al.: Rapid fractionation technique and re-treatment of cerebral metastases by irradiation. Cancer **34** (1974) 257–261.

[76] Sheline, G. E.: Radiation therapy of brain tumors. Cancer **39** (1977) 873–881.

[77] Simpson, W. J., M. E. Platts: Fractionation study in the treatment of glioblastoma multiforme. Int. J. Radiat. Oncol. Biol. Phys. (1976) 639–644.

[78] Slansky, B. D., R. S. Manu-Kaplan, A. F. Reynolds, et al.: PTG in the treatment of malignant intracranial neoplasmas. Cancer **33** (1974) 460–463.

[79] Solero, C. L., et al.: Controlles study with BCNU versus CCNU as adjuvant chemotherapy following surgery plus radiotherapy for glioblastoma multiforme. Cancer Clin. Trials **2** (1979) 43–48.

[80] Sweet, D. L., F. J. Hendler, K. Hanlon, et al.: Treatment of grade III and IV astrocytomas with BCNU alone and in combination with VM 26 following surgery and radiation therapy. Cancer Treat. Rep. **63** (1979) 1707–1713.

[81] Takakura, K., K. Sano: Role of immunopotentiators in brain tumor therapy. In: Multidisciplinary Aspects of Brain Tumor Therapy (P. Paoletti, M. D. Walker, G. Butti, R. Knerich, eds), pp. 223–234. Elsevier/North Holland, Biomedical Press, Amsterdam – New York – Oxford 1979.

[82] Takeuchi, K., K. Hoshino: Statistical analysis of factors affecting survival after glioblastoma multiforme. Acta Neurochir. (Wien) **37** (1977) 57–61.

[83] Tamulevicius, P., M. Bamberg, E. Scherer, et al.: Misonidazole as a radiosensitizer in the radiotherapy of glioblastomas and oesophageal cancer. Pharmakokinetic and clinical studies. Br. J. Radiol. **54** (1981) 318–324.

[84] Tamura, M. H. Yamasaki, H. Inoue, et al.: Evaluation of high dose radiotherapy (500 rad two times weekly) in glioblastoma. The U.S.-Japanese Conf. On Brain Tumor Therapy, Nikko, Japan (meeting abstract) 1981.

[85] Tator, C. H., W. Wassernaar, A. Day, et al.: Therapy of an experimental glioma with systemic or intraneoplastic methotrexate or radiation. J. Neurosurg. **46** (1977) 175–178.
[86] Taveras, J. A., H. G. Thompson, J. L. Pool: Should we treat glioblastoma multiforme? Am. J. Roentgenol. 87 (1962) 473–479.
[87] Taylor, S. G., L. Nelson, D. Baxter, et al.: Treatment of grade III and IV astrocytoma with dimethyl triazeno imidazole carboxamide (DTIC, NSC-45388) alone and in combination with CCNU (NSC 79 037) or methyl-CCNU (MeCCNU NSC 95 441). Cancer **36** (1975) 1269–1276.
[88] Uihlein, A., et al.: Comparison of surgery and surgery plus irradiation in the treatment of supratentorial gliomas. Acta Radiologica **5** (1966) 67–78.
[89] Urtasun, R. C., J. D. Miller, V. Frunchak, et al.: Radiotherapy pilot trials with sensitizers of hypoxic cells: Metronidazole in supratentorial glioblastomas. Br. J. Radiol. **50** (1977) 602–603.
[90] Urtasun, R. C., P. R. Band, D. Chapman, et al.: Clinical phase I study of the hypoxic cell radiosensitizer RO-07-0582, a 2-nitroimidazolederivative. Radiology **122** (1977) 801–804.
[91] Ushio, Y., T. Hayakawa, H. Mogami: Combination Chemotherapy with methyl-CCNU and bleomycin in the treatment of malignant gliomas, a prospective randomized study. The U.S.-Japanese Conf. On Brain Tumor Therapy, Nikko, Japan (meeting abstract) 1981.
[92] Walker, M. D., BTSG: An evaluation of methyl-CCNU, BCNU and radiotherapy in treatment of malignant gliomas. Proc. Amer. Assoc. Cancer Res. **17** (1976) 652–657.
[93] Walker, M. D., BTSG: Evaluation of mithramycin in the treatment of anaplastic gliomas. J. Neurosurg. **44** (1976) 655–658.
[94] Walker, M. D., BTSG: Evaluation of BCNU and/or radiotherapy in the treatment of anaplastic gliomas. A cooperative clinical trial. J. Neurosurg. **49** (1978) 337–343.
[95] Walker, M. D., T. A. Strike: A phase II evaluation of misonidazole in the treatment of malignant glioma. Proc. Assoc. Cancer Res. **20** (1979) 433.
[96] Walker, M. D., BTSG: Randomized comparisons of radiotherapy and nitrosoureas for the treatment of malignant glioma after surgery. N. Engl. J. Med. **303** (1980) 1323–1329.
[97] Weir, B., P. R. Band, R. C. Urtasun, et al.: Radiotherapy and CCNU in the treatment of high-grade supratentorial astrocytomas. J. Neurosurg. **45** (1976) 129–134.
[98] Wikstrand, C. J., D. D. Bigner: Immunobiologic aspects of the brain and human brain gliomas. A review. Am. J. Pathol. **98** (1980) 517–526.
[99] Wilson, C. B.: Single-agent chemotherapy of brain tumors. Arch. Neurol. **33** (1976) 739–743.
[100] Yamamoto, H., K. Takakura, K. Sano: Combined chemo-radiotherapy with VM 26 (NSC 122 819) and ACNU (NSC D 24 532) for glioblastoma. The Japanese Cancer Association **170** (1980) 367.
[101] Young, D. F., et al.: Rapid Course Radiation Therapy of Cerebral Metastases, Results and Complications. Cancer **34** (1974) 1069–1076.
[102] Yung, W., E. Steward, J. E. Marks, et al.: Glioblastoma multiforme: treatment with radiation and triiodothyronine. Int. J. Radiat. Oncol. Biol. Phys. **1** (1976) 645–650.
[103] Zülch, K. J.: Histological typing of tumors of the central nervous system. International histological classification of tumors No. 21, WHO, Geneva 1979.

CT-stereotactic interstitial irradiation therapy of non resectable and recurrant intracranial tumour in children and adolescents

F. Mundinger, K. Weigel

The possibilities of active treatment in dealing with tumours of the central nervous system in children are limited, because of their location and nature. Some of these tumours either cannot be removed surgically or can be operated on only at the risk of causing severe functional damage. This particularly holds true for brain tumours in the midline, i. e., of the diencephalon, of the mesencephalon and its neighbouring structures (corpus callosum, medio-temporal, etc.), as well as for tumours of the brain stem and pons [14]. The surgical indications and techniques are listed in another volume of these series [32].

Up to the present the treatment of such inoperable tumours which occur relatively frequently in children, has been limited to putting in a ventriculo-atrial shunt (if there is an obstructive hydrocephalus) and to percutaneous irradiation. The latter is only appropriate however, for the more malignant tumours. In our experience the more benign gliomas which have been histologically verified after a CT-stereotactic biopsy, show in most cases no evidence of regression after a focal dose of 6500–7000 Gy has been given. Any changes seen are confined to the surroundings, in the form of a diffuse gliosis or small cystic necroses. A kind of internal decompression then brings on relief, which can lead to temporary clinical improvement [9].

We therefore pointed out in our report on CT stereotactic biopsy [18] that percutaneous irradiation or conservative therapy should only be carried out if the diagnosis has been histologically confirmed. This is the only way to prevent results being published in the literature on successfully radiated non-resectable tumours, which were diagnosed solely on the basis of their neurological state and the neuroradiological results, but not on confirmation by biopsy. Underlying such "tumours" could be benign non-tumorous lesions (cysts, necroses, etc.). To demonstrate this point, we can give numerous examples from our own experiences of such lesions which we later confirmed by biopsy (cf. the list of references, tab. 1).

These examples show in how few cases there is a histological diagnosis of the tumour. This can partially be explained by the fact that the technique of biopsy used to be very complicated and unsafe. The integration of computers and computed tomo-

Table 1 Summary of literatur

Author	no. of cases	histolog. confirmed	therapy	survival rate
Marsa et al. (1973)	9	5	Betatron (4875–6675 cGy 33–54 d)	75.0%
Bataini et al. (1975)	45	20	Telekob., Betatron (5000–6500 cGy 30–45 d)	50.0%
Lütolf et al. (1978)	27	??	??	61.9%
Greenberger et al. (1977)	14	4	Telekob., Betatron (4900–5600 cGy)	58.0%
Mundinger	69	69	Ir-192 permanent implant	59.0%

graphy into the stereotactic localization and biopsy technique has greatly reduced the risk associated with biopsy [1–4, 14, 19, 28]. Histological confirmation must therefore again be called for before any conservative treatment of tumours is started – whether it be percutaneous irradiation or cortison- and chemo-cytostatic therapy [18].

For about the last 25 years, interstitial or intracavitary (local) Curie therapy, i.e., the implantation or insertion of radioactive nuclides with an appropriate physical characteristic, has been considered an alternative radio-therapeutic method of treatment for tumours that have been located and delineated using neuroradiological methods, particularly computed-tomography, and which are non-resectable or recurrent tumours. This method of treatment can also be used in combination with other methods.

Depending on the nature and the location of the tumour, two types of application are used:

1. The nuclides are implanted *permanently*. The dose is administered within a few weeks, as for example, with yttrium-90, rhenium-186, or gold-198. For protracted long-term irradiation – a method developed by Mundinger – [12, 15, 17] the tumour surface dose is accumulated over a period of moths. Permanent implantation is known as *Curie therapy* [22]. It is indicated only for slow-growing, low-grade (I and II) intracranial tumours, or for tumours in grades II–III [23, 27]. Here Curie therapy can be employed, for example, in combination with percutaneous irradition procedures [31]. The radionuclides suitable for Curie therapy are iridium-192 in the form of tiny wires* (which, however, for reasons of radiation

* Irium-192 wires: Isotopentechnik Dr. Sauerwein GmbH, Bergische Straße 16, D-5657 Haan

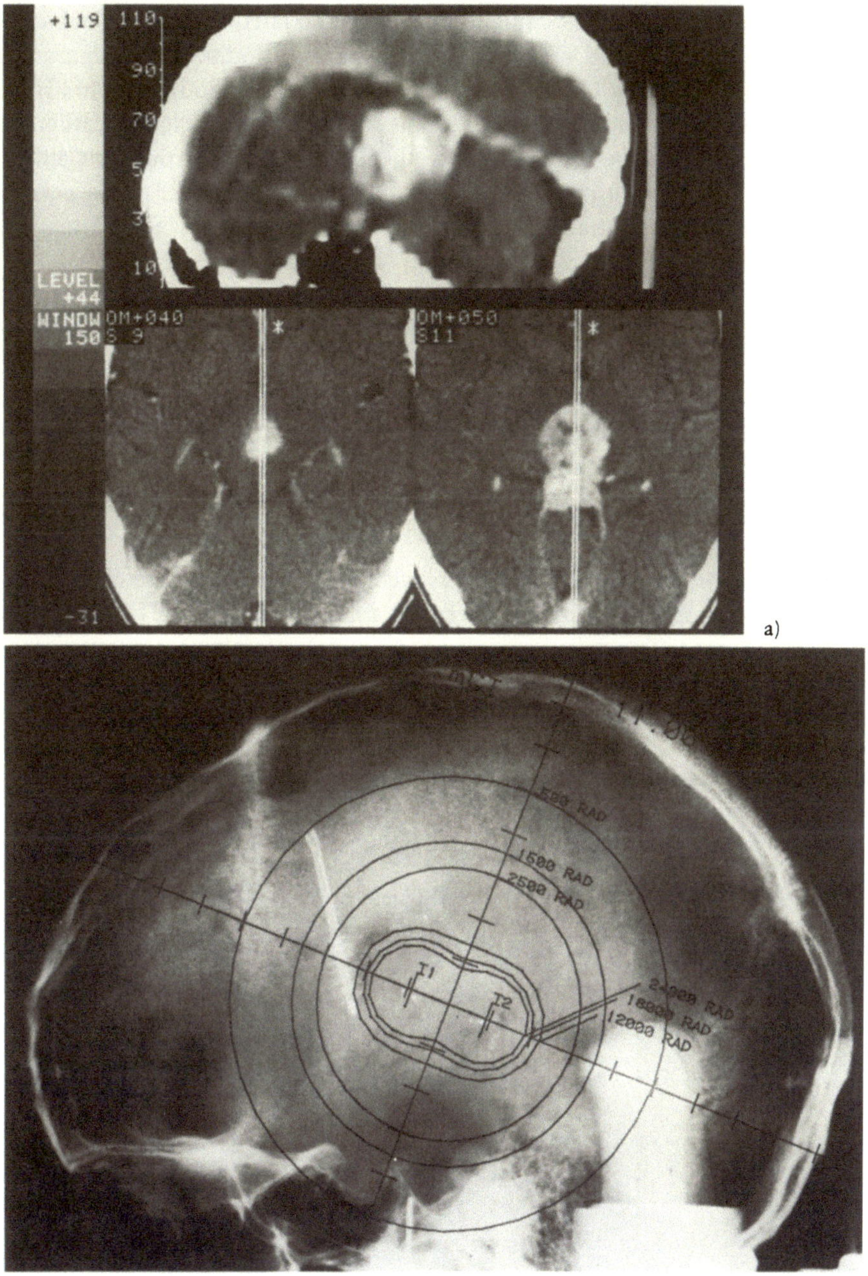

a)

b)

Fig. 1 N., C., 15 y. Estensive histologically confirmed germinoma of the quadrigeminal region and of the upper mesencephalon,

a) sagittal reconstruction of 5 mm CT-slices;

b) position of the stereotactically implanted iodine seeds (I1 and I2). The diagram projected into the X-ray shows isodose distribution which is approcimate to the configuration of the tumour (12000 cGy).

protection is used today only for smaller tumours) and lately iodine-125, which is filled in titanium seeds and absorbed on Dowex. The iodine-125 preparation method was developed by Hilaris [7] and he has used it for body tumours since 1975. Using the after-loading method, iodine-125 seeds* are filled in catheters, which are led through the tumours. Since then it has found further use. In February 1979, we in Freiburg were the first to implant iodine-125 seeds permanently into intracranial extracerebral and cerebral tumours [16]. Since then this has been the method we have favoured (figs. 1, a, b; 2 a, b).

2. The radionuclides are implanted *temporarily*. In malignant tumours of the central nervous system (III and IV), in which cases the dose should be rapidly accumulated, iridium-192 or iodine-125 are temporarily implanted or inserted according to the after-loading technique [29, 30]. The dose was delivered with a contact radiation device having a high dose rate either intraoperatively within minutes or the radionuclides filled in a catheter are implanted into the tumour, also according to the after loading method, for a few days and are then removed. We refer to this radiation techniques as *brachy-Curie therapy* [13] (figs. 3 a, b).

The determination of the tumour volume as well as the dosimetry are carried out using computed-tomography with enhancement immediately after CT-stereotactic biopsy. The dosimetry is worked out using a special interactive computer programme which was developed together with Birg [1, 2, 3, 4, 5]. The distribution of

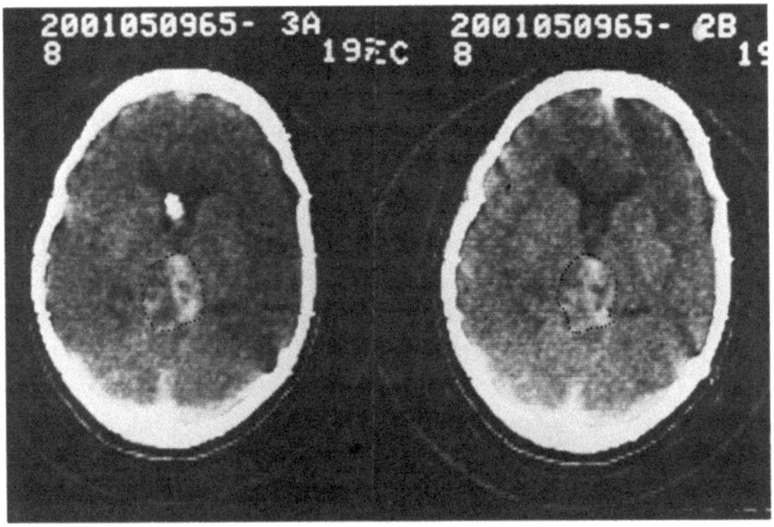

Fig. 2 K., K., 13 y.
a) Histologically confirmed germinoma in the quadrigeminal region;

* Iodine-125 seeds: 3M Deutschland GmbH, Postfach 642, D-4040 Neuss 1

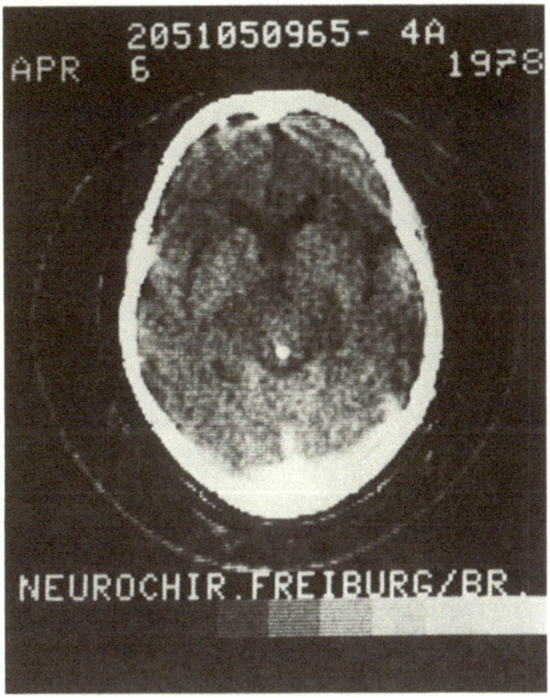

Fig. 2 b) five months after iodine-125 permanent implantion.
The tumour can no longer be seen, only the artefact left by the nuclide.

the isodoses on the tumour surface is given, as well as the location and the level of activity of the one or more radionuclide seeds to be implanted. With our CT-stereotactic technique [1], it is possible to hit these sites with better than 1 mm precision.

Depending on the tumour volume, the tumor surface dose for Curie therapy is 9000–12000 cGy iridium-192 or iodine-125. It is reduced depending on the dose distribution in the entire brain and on whether or not percutaneous radiation therapy had been carried out previously [6].

For intraoperative brachy-Curietherapy, 3500–4500 cGy are delivered in one operation to the tumour surface within a few minutes. This is done using the contact-radiation-device* iridium-192 GammaMed® [24, 11, 10], which was developed by Mundinger and Sauerwein (fig. 4). With the after-loading method, the isodose distribution can be adjusted to stereometrically complicated tumours by altering the radionuclide and the radiation time (figs. 5 a–d).

* Manufacturer of the Irium-192-Contact Radiation Device: Isotopentechnik Dr. Sauerwein GmbH, Bergische Straße 16, D-5657 Haan

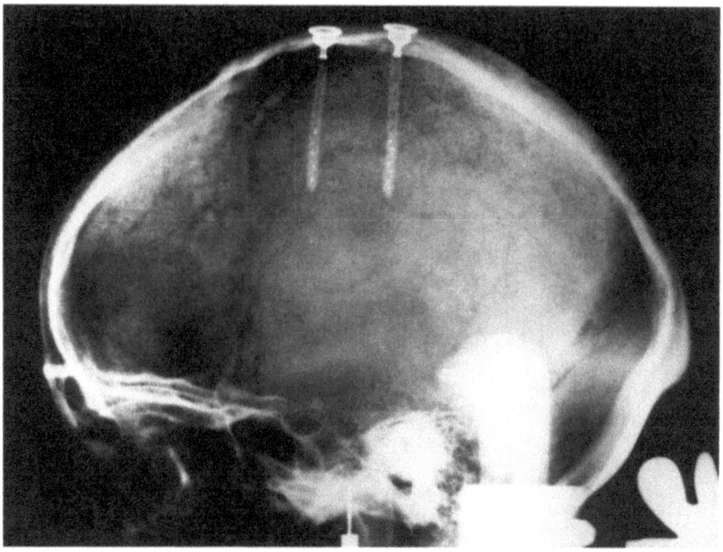

a)

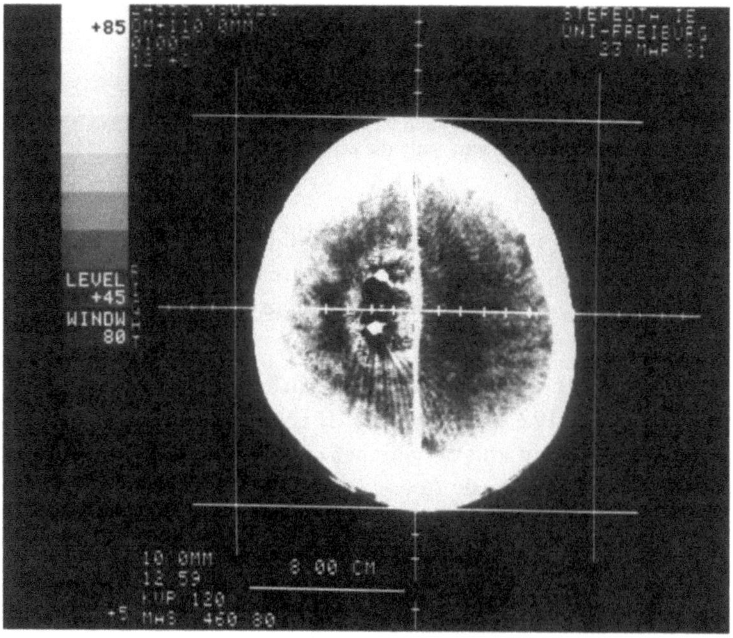

b)

Fig. 3 K., M. Extensive parasagittal glioblastoma in the right central region.
a) The lateral X-ray shows the two catheters filled with iodine-125 seeds;
b) the computer tomographic control establishes the position of the catheter in the anterior and posterior third of the tumour. This assures a sufficient dose of radiation for the tumour.

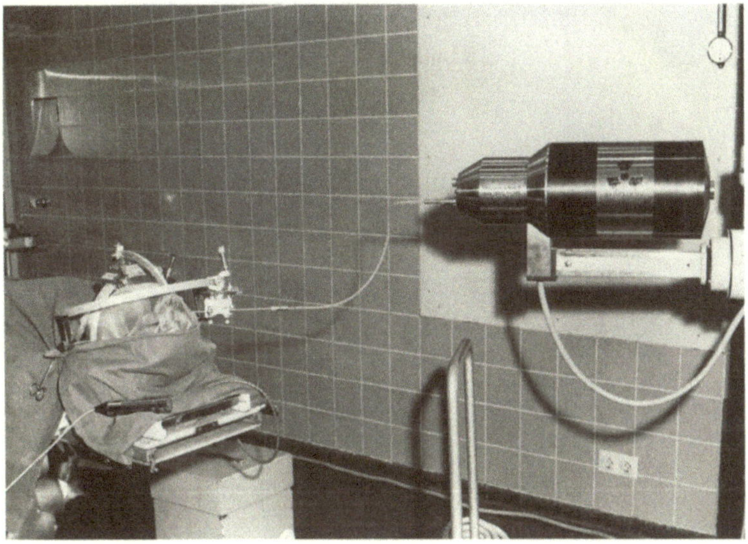

Fig. 4 Iridium-192-contact radiation device GammaMed®.
The connecting tube is attached to the stereotactically introduced application cannula at one end and to the exit channel of the shielding container at the other. With the aid of remote automatic control the emitter is introduced into the application cannula which has been inserted into the tumour and it is automatically withdrawn into the shielding container after the calculated exposure has been completed.

For temporary implantation of iodine-125 seeds – also following the after-loading method – 4000–4500 cGy are absorbed within a few days. The focal dose, which in these cases is additionally applied percutaneously, should then be 4500 cGy. For malignant tumours with a tendency to metastasise (over the CSF space for instance), radiation of the neuroaxis with 3500–4000 cGy is indicated. In order to prevent spreading in the CSF space, we have recently resumed instilling radiogold-198 colloid (3–5 mCi) into the open ventricular system [26]. This is done intraoperatively.

Curie-/brachy-Curietherapy is subject to the conditions of small volume irradiation. In the medio-temporal direction, the diameter of the tumour should not exceed 4 cm; in the rostro-caudal or the dorso-ventral direction, the tumour diameter should not exceed 5 cm, at the most, 5.5 cm. The maximum volume is 150 ml. The advantages of Curie-/brachy-Curietherapy are listed in table 2. An additional psychological advantage is that the patient is only required to stay in the hospital for a few days.

The permanent implantation technique, the after-loading method, and the dosimetry program are described in detail elsewhere [10–17].

As we have already mentioned, *complications* are mainly brought on intraoperatively by the biopsies (tab. 3 shows the morbidity rates) and less by the subsequent

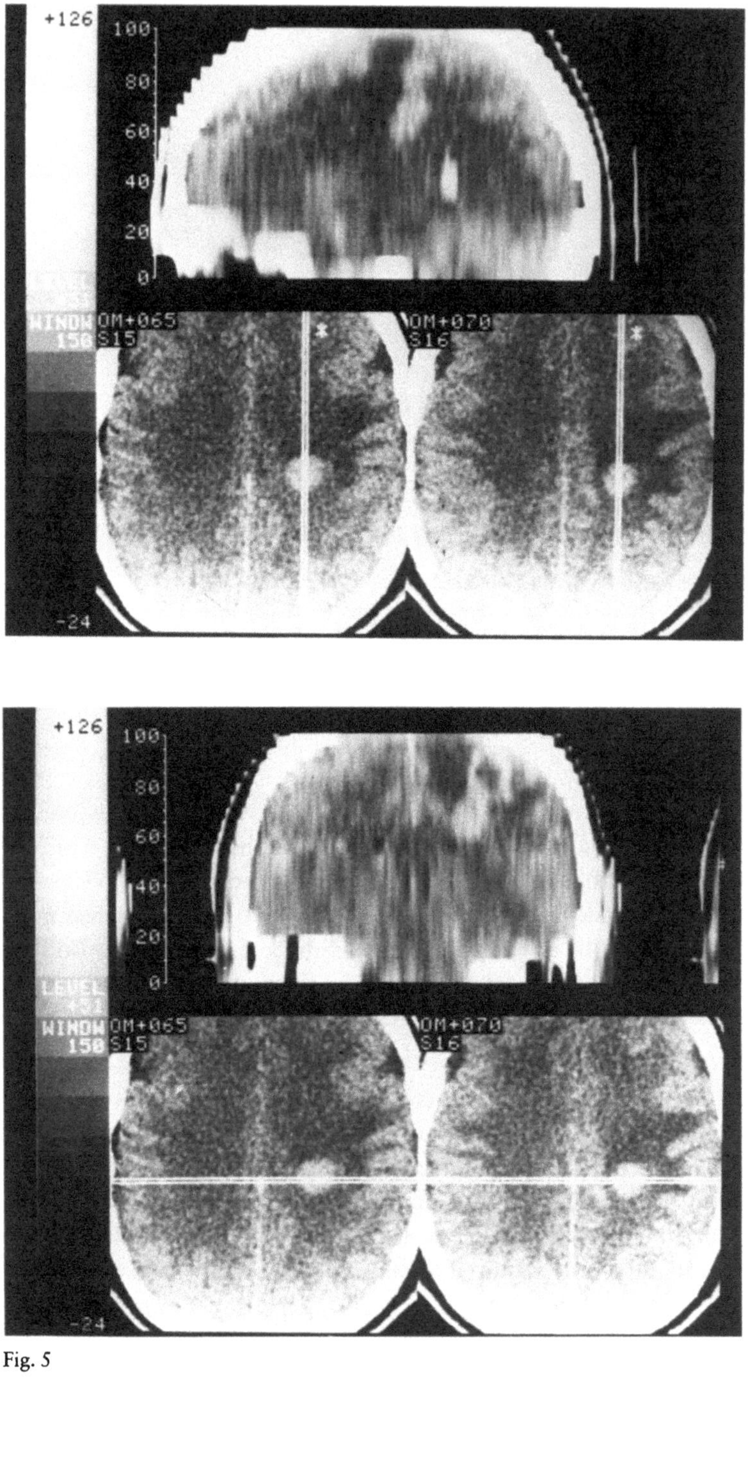
+126
100
80
60
40
20
0
WINDOW
150
OM+065
S15
OM+070
S16
-24
+126
100
80
60
40
20
0
LEVEL
WINDOW
150
OM+065
S15
OM+070
S16
-24

a)

b)

Fig. 5

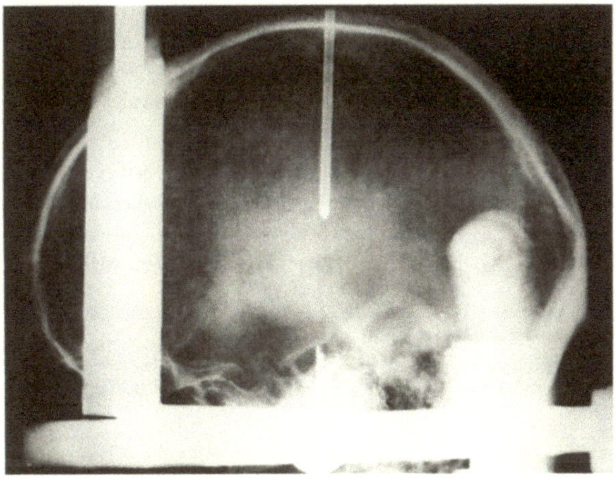

c)

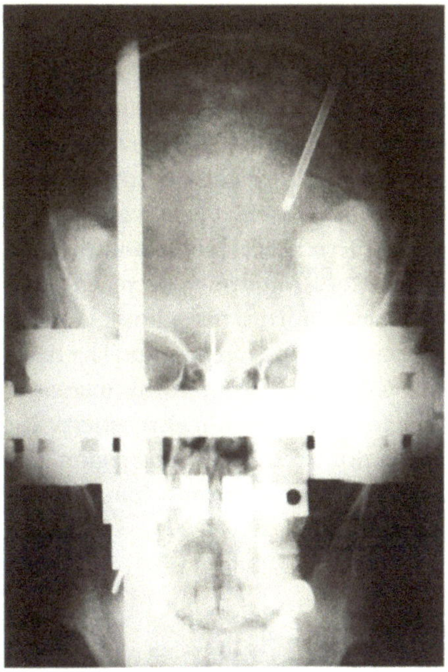

d)

Fig. 5 Sch., B. Astrocytoma III–IV.
This malignant tumour confirmed by stereotactic biopsy lies in the central region and is therefore without severe functional deficit, but it is not resectable by open operation.
The a) sagittal, b) coronal reconstruction shows the cylindrical extension of the tumour (4 cm long 2 cm in diameter), c) lateral and d) a.p. X-ray with the GammaMed® cannula placed in the axis of the tumour. The isodose distribution of the short-term irradiation (37.5 min., 2500 cGy, isodose 1 cm = tumour surface) is superimposed.

Table 2

Brachy-Curie therapy (short-term irradiation for minutes or hours)	→	quickly and highly concentrated "active centres" (direct ionization, chemically short-term intermediate products)
Permanent Curie therapy (protracted long-term irradiation for months)	→	vascular component, increase in cell cycle time by continous irradiation, higher differentiation between recovery rates and normal tissue, less oxygen-dependent effect with reduced OER in hypoxic cells

Table 3 Transient complications of stereotactically treated children (1–15 y) with intracranial tumours (1965–1982) n = 187

	no. of cases	%
haemorrhage	1	0.5
pareses	3	1.6
seizures	4	2.1

local irradiation treatment. Our series with adult patients, however, yielded several significant aspects of the iodine-125 application, which indicate that the soft, more dense ionizing X-ray of iodine-125, as opposed to the harder gamma spectrum of iridium-192, clearly shows a greater focal and perifocal effect on the vessels with subsequent occlusions [16, 20]. This in part leads to cystic necrotic foci in the distribution area of the thrombosed vessels. Also the local intratumoral reaction as necrosis, as well as the perifocal reaction as oedema and reactive gliosis is more pronounced. This holds true particularly for tumours of the white matter. The reactive changes manifest themselves as hypodense CT areas. Temporarily increased intracranial pressure symptoms caused by these local and perifocal reactions are observed and need to be treated. Particularly in the brain stem and pons region, the perifocal irritation of pathways and centres can cause such symptoms, for example, an increase in eye muscle disturbances or pareses.

Results

Out of a total number of 7664 stereotactic operations (tab. 4), the histological classification from and the nuclides used in 1494 curietherapeutic operations are listed (tabs. 5, 6). The order of the nuclides indicates a certain historical development in their use. Special attention is paid in the following to the Curie- and brachy-Curie-therapeutic stereotactic operations with iridium-192 and iodine-125 on children. The results from the total series are reported elsewhere.

Table 4 Stereotactic operations (1950–19. 9. 1983) (Stereotactic biopsies only are not included)

Parkinsonism	3778
Hyperkinesia	1217
Curie therapy	1473
Intractable pain	353
Psychosurgery	172
Epilepsy	99
Angiomas	17
Combined stereotact./ open pituitary operation	107
Others	448
total	7664

Table 5 Radionuclides and number of stereotactic interstitial irradiation procedures (1952–30. 11. 1983)

P-32	6
Co-60	179
Y-90	44
Ta-182	21
Au-198	129
I-125	257
I-125 Brachy Curie	29
Ir-192 Gamma Med	270
Ir-192	559
total	1494

Table 6 Biopsy diagnosis and number of stereotactic interstitial irradiation procedures (1952–30. 9. 1983)

Glioblastoma	211
Astrocytoma	546
Oligodendroglioma	105
Ependymoma	34
PNET	31
Meningioma	18
Metastasis	39
Sarcoma	11
Pituitary adenoma	253
Craniopharyngioma	34
Other lesions	75
Hypophysectomy	57
Pallidotomy	21
total	1435

Tables 7 and 8 give the age distribution, sex and therapeutic procedures of the 187 cases we have treated since 1965. Table 9 shows the method of treatment, whereby in eight cases post-resection of the tumour was indicated on the basis of the biopsy findings and in a further 21 cases symptomatic treatment only.

Table 10 gives the location distribution of these cases and shows that the majority of tumours were in the midline region. Table 11 gives the previously obtained biopsy confirmation of the cerebral gliomas and the non-glial tumours. The majority of glial tumours were pilocytic and fibrillary astrocytomas. Most of the non-glial tumours were germinomas. The survival time up till now under long-term treatment is three years – too short for an assessment, especially of the low-grade gliomas. Table 12 shows how many of the glial and non-glial tumour patients are still alive.

For pilocytic astrocytomas that are permanently implanted with iridium-192, the probability of survival taken from a 12-year follow-up period is more than 60% (5 years) and for fibrillary astrocytomas (grade II) 50-% after three years. However, for the more recent series of cases, which were implanted permanently with iodine-125,

Table 7 Distribution of age of children (1–15 y) 1965–1982

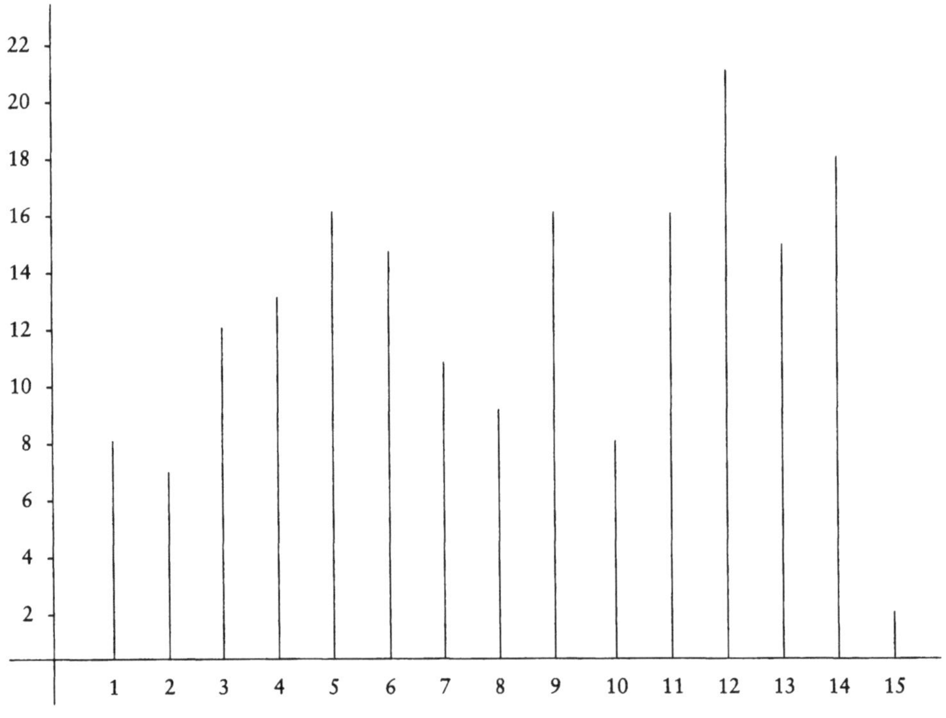

Table 8 Number of children (1–15 y) treated from 1965–1982

male		93
female		94
only punctured	92	
implanted with Ir^{192}	54	
implanted with J^{125}	41	
total		187

Table 9 Treatment of intracranial lesions in children (1–15 y) 1965–1982

treatment	number	%
interstitial therapy	95	50.8
external irradiation	23	12.3
cyst drainage	23	12.3
tumour resection	11	5.9
only punctured	35	18.7
total	187	100.0

Table 10 Treatment of intracranial tumours in children (1–15 y) 1965–1982

location	number	%
cerebral hemisphere	19	10.2
basal ganglia	49	26.2
brain stem, pons	70	37.4
hypothalamic region and chiasm	49	26.2
total	187	100.0

Table 11 Number of children (1–15 y) treated from 1965–1982

type of tumour	number
Astrocytoma Grade I	77
Astrocytoma Grade II	31
Astrocytoma Grade III	14
Oligodendroglioma	3
Glioblastoma	8
Ependymoma	4
Germinoma	11
Teratoma	7
Craniopharyngioma	10
Metastasis	2
Gliosis	6
Other	24
total	187

Table 12 Stereotactically treated children (1–15 y) n = 187 (1965–1982)

	number of patients	still alive
Astrocytoma Grade I	77	49
Astrocytoma Grade II	31	22
Astrocytoma Grade III	16	6
Oligodendroglioma	3	1
Glioblastoma	5	3
Ependymoma	4	2
Germinoma	11	5
Teratoma	6	3
Craniopharyngioma	10	7
Other	24	17
total	187	115

the follow-up period is still too short. The 39% survival probability for astrocytoma I, which is given in table 13 classified according to location and surface dose can be explained by the fact that tumours in the hypothalamus and brain stem-pons area have a lower chance of survival because of their effect on vital structures (tabs. 14 a, b; 15 a, b) [25].

Because of the steeper dose fall-off of iodine-125 (half-life layer thickness 2 cm), tumours of this location have been treated in the last three years with Curie therapy to an increasing degree [33]. Further observations are necessary to decide on the use of iodine-125 permanent implantation for tumours of the hypothalamus and the brain stem and pons region.

Indications for Curie-brachy-Curietherapy

Based on our experience of 25 years [28], we have established the following pre-

Table 13 Survival rates among children (1–15 y) 1970–1982

	only punctured	Ir^{192}–impl.	J^{125}–impl.
Astrocytoma Grade I			
number	26	27	24
3 years	51%	80%	39%
5 years	49%	56%	–
Astrocytoma Grade II			
number	15	9	5
2 years	28%	50%	–
3 years	–	50%	–
Astrocytoma Grade III			
number	8	3	3
1 year	35%	31%	29%

Table 14 Results of Curie therapy in children (1–15 y) with intracranial tumours related to location and surface-dosage of the tumour (1965–1982)

	Frontal region				Temporal region				Basal ganglia					
	Ir^{192}		I^{125}		Ir^{192}		I^{125}		Ir^{192}		I^{125}		total	
cGy	impl.	dead	impl.	dead	impl.	dead	impl.	dead	impl.	dead	impl.	dead	punctured	dead
7000	–	–	–	–	–	–	–	–	–	–	–	–	–	–
9000	–	–	–	–	–	–	–	–	1	1	1	–	2	1
10000	–	–	–	–	–	–	1	1	5	3	4	–	10	4
11000	–	–	–	–	–	–	–	–	–	–	–	–	–	–
12000	1	1	–	–	1	–	2	–	10	2	8	2	22	5
14000	–	–	–	–	–	–	–	–	2	1	–	–	2	1
16000	–	–	–	–	–	–	–	–	–	–	–	–	–	–
total	1	1	–	–	1	–	3	1	18	7	13	2	36	11

alive 25 = 69%
dead 11 = 31%

requisites for CT-stereotactic Curie therapy for inoperable tumours or recurrences of tumours of the central nervous system in children:

1. The tumour must have been histologically confirmed.
2. The tumour must be demarcated from the surrounding structures, particularly in the hypothalamus, the brain stem and the pons. This assures reliable calculation of the tumour surface dosage taking the surrounding structures into consideration.

Table 14 b Results of Curie therapy in children (1–15 y) with intracranial tumours related to location and surface-dosage of the tumour (1965–1982)

	Location									
cGy	Brainstem – pons				Hypothalamus-Chiasm					
	Ir^{192}		I^{125}		Ir^{192}		I^{125}		total	
cGy	impl.	dead	impl.	dead	impl.	dead	impl.	dead	punctured	dead
7000	–	–	2	–	–	–	1	–	3	–
9000	1	1	3	2	–	–	1	–	5	3
10000	5	3	4	2	6	4	3	1	18	10
11000	1	–	–	–	–	1	–	–	1	–
12000	10	6	5	2	8	4	6	4	29	16
14000	1	1	–	–	–	–	–	–	1	1
16000	1	1	–	–	1	–	–	–	2	1
total	19	12	14	6	15	8	11	5	59	31

alive 28 = 47%
dead 31 = 53%

Table 15 a Results of Curie therapy in children (1–15 y) with astrocytoma grade I related to location and surface-dosage of the tumour (1965–1982)

	Location									
	Temporal region				Basal ganglia					
	Ir^{192}		J^{125}		Ir^{192}		J^{125}		total	
cGy	impl.	dead	impl.	dead	impl.	dead	impl.	dead	punctured	dead
9000	–	–	–	–	–	–	1	–	1	–
10000	–	–	–	–	3	1	2	–	5	1
12000	1	–	–	–	6	1	6	1	13	2
14000	–	–	–	–	1	–	–	–	1	–
total	1	–	–	–	10	2	9	1	20	3

alive 17 = 85%
dead 3 = 15%

3. The pre-requisites for small volume irradiation (maximum tumour volume 150 ml) must be present.
4. The clinical picture has to be taken into special account.

Curie therapy is indicated for low-grad (I. II) glial and non-glial cerebral and extracerebral tumours. Depending on the size and the configuration of the tumour, one or more active nuclides are distributed in the centre or over more sites which have been previously determined using special computer programs. These are left there *permanently*. The preferred radionuclides are iridium-192 and iodine-125 seeds [8, 16].

Table 15 b Results of Curie therapy in children (1–15 y) with astrocytoma grade I related to location and surface-dosage of the tumour (1965–1982)

	Location									
	Brain stem – pons				Hypothalamus-Chiasm					
	Ir^{192}		J^{125}		Ir^{192}		J^{125}		total	
cGy	impl.	dead	impl.	dead	impl.	dead	impl.	dead	punctured	dead
7000	–	–	2	–	–	–	–	–	2	–
9000	1	1	–	–	–	–	1	–	2	1
10000	2	2	1	–	2	2	2	–	7	4
12000	5	2	4	2	6	3	5	3	20	10
14000	–	–	–	–	–	–	–	–	–	–
total	8	5	7	2	8	5	8	3	31	15

alive 16 = 51%
dead 15 = 49%

Should the biopsy confirm a higher grade tumour (II–III, III), the combination of interstitial Curie therapy with percutaneous irradiation is indicated for smaller volumes (up to 40 ml). *Brachy-Curietherapy* following the after-loading method with the iridium-192 contact radiation device GammaMed® is indicated intraoperatively for larger inoperable tumour masses of grade III and IV located in the corpus callosum, in the medio-temporal, anterior frontal or rostro-occipital cerebral regions.

Depending on the course of the further CT controls, the therapy must be repeated either alone or in combination with subsequent percutaneous irradiation treatment. Iodine-125 brachy-Curietherapy is indicated if the neighbouring structures demand a steeper dose-fall off towards the midline (basal ganglia). The therapy usually consists of a transiently central implantation of one or two catheters which match the contours of the tumour and which are filled with iodine-125 seeds of varying strength. Percutaneous irradiation therapy may still be indicated if appears necessary. With more malignant tumours, the treatment described above can be carried out in combination with cystostatics and corticosteroid therapy – if the corresponding oncological requirements are met.

If the tumour cannot be outlined with certainty and if it has reached a certain size (more than 150 ml), the CT-stereotactic operation is restricted to a biopsy. Depending on the nature, the combination of percutaneous irradiation therapy and cytochemotherapy is subsequently used in the more malignant tumours. We do not recommend any further irradiation for low-grade, in particular, pilocytic astrocytomas, as low-grade gliomas do not react to percutaneous irradiation because of their radioresistance [25]. At most, low-dose dexamethasone therapy would be worth considering as symptomatic treatment.

If there are cysts or developing cysts, stereotactic puncture and drainage of these cysts is indicated to relieve the pressure. A beta emitter such as rhenium-186 or yttrium-90 colloid could be applied for wall radiation, if necessary. In addition to this any other supporting measures required such as atrio-ventricular or peritoneal shunt should be taken.

After open operation, Curietherapeutic irradiation is indicated for recurrent tumours and for the non-resectable parts of tumours. Brachy-Curietherapy is also indicated in the case of locally recurrent tumours that occur after percutaneous radiation therapy, if they are malignant gliomas or solitary metastases. The additional radiation stress for the brain is minimal. If these tumours are more benign, Curie therapy is indicated [20]. Again the pre-requisite is that they are small. CT controls today make it possible to detect recurrent tumours in their early stages and, to confirm them with little risk by means of stereotactic biopsy if there is uncertainty about the differential diagnosis, and then to treat them agean [21].

With Curie- and brachy-Curietherapy, as an alternative and as a combined treatment for tumours of the central nervous system in children higher probability of survival is attained if the treatment is used for the appropriate indications and according to the nature of the tumour. The highly technical precision of the CT-stereotactic Curie-brachy-Curietherapy is the first essential technical requirement.

References

[1] Birg, W., F. Mundinger: Computer calculations of target parameters for a stereotactic apparatus. Acta Neurochir. **29** (1973) 123–129.

[2] W. Birg, F. Mundinger: Direct target point determination for stereotactic brain operations from CT data and the calculation of seeting parameters for polar-coordinate stereotactic devices. Proc. 8th meeting World Soc. Stereotactic and Functional Neurosurgery, Part III, Zürich 1981. Apl. Neurophysiol. **45** (1982) 387–395.

[3] Birg, W., F. Mundinger, M. Klar: A computer programme system for stereotactic neurosurgery. Acta Neurochir. Suppl. **24** (1977) 99–108.

[4] Birg, W., F. Mundinger, M. Klar: Computer assistance for stereotactic brain operations. Advances in Neurosurgery **4** (1977) 287–291.

[5] Birg, W., J. Schneider, S. Bauer, et al.: An interactive program system for the stereotactic interstitial implantation of radionuclids in brain tumors. In: Stereotactic Cerebral Irradiation, INSERM Symposium Nr. 12, (G. Szikla, ed.), pp. 77–80. Elsevier/North Holland, Biomedical Press, Amsterdam – New York – Oxford 1979.

[6] Brown, B., J. R. Thompson, T. B. Barkley, et al.: Theoretical considerations of dose rate factors influencing radiation strategy. Radiology **110** (1975) 197–202.

[7] Hilaris, B. S.: Handbook of interstitial Brachy-Therapy. Memorial Sloan-Kettering, Cancer-Center, New York, N.Y. Publishing Sciences Group, Inc. Acton, Massachusetts 1975.

[8] M. Kiessling, J. Anagnostopoulos, G. Lombeck, et al.: Diagnostic Potential of Stereotactic Biopsy of Brain Tumours. A Report of 400 Cases. In: Tumours of the Central Nervous System in Infancy and Childhood. (D. Voth, P. Gutjahr, C. Langmaid, eds.), pp. 247–256. Springer-Verlag, Berlin–Heidelberg–New York 1982.

[9] Kuhlendahl, H., H. Miltz, R. Wüllenweber: Die Astrocytome des Großhirns. Acta Neurochirurg. **29** (1973) 151–162.

[10] Mundinger, F.: Iridium-192-"GammaMed" a new Irradiation of Localized Brachytherapy of Tumors. III. European Congress of Neurosurgery, Madrid, April 23.–26., 1967. Experta Med. Int. Congr. Series, 139, 1967.

[11] Mundinger, F.: Erfahrungen mit der stereotaktischen interstitiellen Brachytherapie mit Ir^{192}-"GammaMed" bei infiltrierenden Hirntumoren. Fortschr. Röntgenstr. **110** (1969) 254–261.

[12] Mundinger, F.: The Treatment of Brain Tumors With Interstitially Applied Radioactive Isotopes. In: Radionuclide Applications In Neurology And Neurosurgery (Yen Wang, P. Paoletti, eds.), pp. 199–265. Charles C. Thomas, Springfield, Ill., 1970.

[13] Mundinger, F.: Brachy-Curie-Therapy Combined with Radiosensitizers in Treating Malignant Tumors of the Brain Hemispheres. Fifth International Congress of Neurological Surgery, Tokyo, 7.–12. 10. 1973. Excerpta Medica Int. Congr. Series No. **293** (1973) 36.

[14] Mundinger, F.: Stereotaktische Operationen am Gehirn. Grundlagen – Indikationen – Resultate. Hippokrates-Verlag, Stuttgart 1975.

[15] Mundinger, F.: Rationale and Methods of Interstitia Iridium-192-Brachy-Curie-Therapy and Iridium-192 or Iodine-125 Protracted Long Term Irradiation. In: Stereotactic Cerebral Irradiation, INSERM Symposium Nr. 12 (G. Szikla, ed.), pp. 101–116. Elsevier/North Holland, Biomedical Press, Amsterdam–New York–Oxford 1979.

[16] Mundinger, F.: Die stereotaktische interstitielle Therapie nicht resezierbarer intracranieller Tumoren mit Ir-192 und Jod-12. In: Kombinierte chirurgische und radiologische Behandlung maligner Tumoren (M. Wannenmacher, H. W. Schreiber, F. Gauwerky, eds.), pp. 90–112. Urban & Schwarzenberg, München 1981.

[17] Mundinger, F.: Implantation of Radioisotopes (Curietherapy). In: Textbook of Stereotaxy of the Human Brain. (Schaltenbrand/Walker, eds.). Thieme, Stuttgart 1982.

[18] Mundinger, F.: CT-Stereotactic Biopsy of Brain Tumours. In: Tumors of the central nervous system in infancy and childhood. (D. Voth, B. Gutjahr, C. Langmaid, eds.). Springer-Verlag, Berlin–Heidelberg–New York 1982.

[19] Mundinger, F., W. Birg: CT-Aided Stereotaxy for Functional Neurosurgery and Deep Brain Implants. Advances in Neurosurgery **10** (1981).

[20] Mundinger, F., Ch. B. Ostertag, W. Birg, et al.: Stereotactic Treatment of Brain Lesions: Biopsy, Interstitial Radiotherapy (Iridium-192 and Iodine-125) and Drainage Procedures. Proceedings of the Meeting of the American Society for Stereotactic and Functional Neurosurgery (P. L. Gildenberg, ed.), (Appl. Neurophysiol. **43** (1980) 198–204.

[21] Mundinger, F., B. Busam, W. Birg, et al.: Results of Interstitial Iridium-192-Brachy-Curie Therapy and Iridium-192 Protracted Long Term Irradiation. In: Stereotactic Cerebral Irradiation, INSERM Symposium Nr. 12 (G. Szikla, ed.), pp. 303–320. Elsevier/North Holland, Biomedical Press, Amsterdam–New York–Oxford 1979.

[22] Mundinger, F., T. Hoefer: Protracted long-term irradiation of inoperable midbrain tumors by stereotactic Curie-Therapy using Iridium-192. Acta Neurochirurg. **21** (1974) 93–100.

[23] Mundinger, F., E. Metzel: Interstitial Radioisotope Therapy of Intractable Diencephalic Tumors by the Stereotaxic Permanent Implantation of Iridium-192, Including Bioptic Control. Confin. neurol. **32** (1970) 195–202.

[24] Mundinger, F., K. Sauerwein: "GammaMed", ein neues Gerät zur interstitiellen, nur einige Minuten dauernden Bestrahlung von Hirngeschwülsten mit Radioisotopen, auch intraoperativ anwendbar. Acta radiol. (Stockh.) **5** (1966) 48–52.

[25] Mundinger, F., K. Weigel: Indication and Results of Stereotactic Curietherapy with Iridium-192 and Iodine-125 for non-resectable Tumors of the Hypothalamic Region. Acta Neurochir., suppl. **33** (in press).

[26] Imm, W., O. Fürste, Ch. Ostertag, et al.: Intralumbale Radiogoldapplikation (^{198}Au) zur Prophylaxe zentral nervöser Leukämie-Rezidive. Dtsch. Hämatologenkongreß, Göttingen, 8.–10. 10. 1978.

[27] Poblete, M., R. Zamboni: Stereotactic Implant of Iridium-192 in Brain Tumors. In: Stereotactic Cerebral Irradiation, INSERM Symposium Nr. 12 (G. Szikla, ed.), pp. 321–328. Elsevier/North Holland, Biomedical Press, Amsterdam–New York–Oxford 1979.

[28] Riechert, T., F. Mundinger: Beschreibung und Anwendung eines Zielgerätes für stereotaktische Hirnoperationen (2. Modell). Acta Neurochir. (Wien) **III** (1956) 308–337.

[29] Scott, W P.: Interstitial therapy using non-absorbable (Ir-192 Nylon Ribbon) and absorbable J-125 Vicryl suturing techniques. Am. J. Roent. Rad. Ther. **124** (197 a) 560–564.

[30] Szikla, G., J. C. Peragut: Irradiation interstitielle des Gliomes. In: Radiothérapie des tumeurs du systéme nerveux central de l'adul (J. P. Constans, M. Schlienger, (ed.). Neurochirurgie **21**, suppl. 2, (1975) 187–228.

[31] Szikla, G., et al.: Combined interstitial and external irradiation of gliomas. In: Stereotactic Cerebral Irradiation, INSERM Symposium Nr. 12 (G. Szikla, ed.), pp 329–338. Elsevier/North Holland, Biomedical Press, Amsterdam–New York–Oxford 1979.

[32] Voth, D.: Standard Techniques and Microsurgical Procedures in the Removal of Supratentorial and Infratentorial Tumours. In: Tumours of the Central Nervous system in Infancy and Childhood. (D. Voth, P. Gutjahr, C. Langmaid, eds.), pp. 199–213. Springer-Verlag, Berlin–Heidelberg–New York 1982.

[33] Weigel, K., Ch. B. Ostertag, F. Mundinger: Interstitial Long Term Irradiation of Tumors in the Pineal Region. In: Stereotactic Cerebral Irradiation. INSERM Symposium Nr. 1 (G. Szikla, ed.) pp. 283–292. Elsevier/North Holland, Biomedical Press, Amsterdam–New York–Oxford 1979.

Treatment of astrocymatomas grade III and IV with high-dose irradiation and misonidazole: preliminary report

B. Stadler, K. H. Kärcher, T. Szepesi, H. D. Kogelnik, P. Wessely

Introduction

The prognosis for malignant cerebral astrocytomas is extremely grave. The high failure rate in the treatment of these tumours is related to our current inability to controll the disease locally, with local failure being the major cause of death in at least 95% of the patients [11]. Though postoperative radiation therapy, with or without adjuvant chemotherapy, has resulted in a statistically significant improvement of survival [15, 16], virtually no long-term cures are reported.

The relative radioresistance of grade III and IV astrocytomas to conventional fractionated radiotherapy is believed to be associated with the presence of hypoxic tumour cells and their ability to accumulate sublethal damage. In an attempt to overcome the radioresistance of this astrocytomas, a randomized trial was initiated at the University Clinic for Radiotherapy and Radiobiology of Vienna using unconventional fractionated radiotherapy and the hypoxic-cell sensitizer misonidazole, a 2-nitromidazole.

Materials and methods

Until February 1982, 40 patients with histologically confirmed grade III and IV astrocytomas referred to the University Clinic for Radiotherapy and Radiobiology of Vienna for postoperative irradiation entered the study: Patients with recurrent astrocytoma or those who received chemotherapy were excluded. A reasonable functional ability was required and patients with a modified Karnofsky performance status of less than 20 were not elegible for the study. Patients with adrenal steroid incompatibility and significant coexisting diseases were excluded.

All patients were in hospital for most of the treatment time. Routine neurological and ophthalmologic examinations and pre- and postoperative brain scans and electroencephalograms were performed. Repeated examinations of CBC, sedimentation rate, urine analysis, electrolytes and hepatic and renal functions were obtained. The patients were randomized in two treatment schedules. Radiotherapy was identical for both groups. A tumour dose (TD) of 66.5 Gy was given in 31 fractions over 7$^1/_2$ weeks using 43 MeV photons. In the first, second and eight week 4 Gy TD were given on Monday and Thursday. From the third until the seventh week, daily tumor doses of 1,7 Gy were administered from Monday through Friday. The whole brain was treated with parallel opposing fields until 45 Gy TD has been given. Then the field size was reduced to cover the tumour area with a small margin of safety. By randomization 23 patients received radiation alone; in 17 patients misonidazole was administered orally 4–5 hours before irradiation on those six treatment days, when fractional radiation doses of 4 Gy TD were used. The cumulative dose of misonidazole was 27 g (range 12.6–16.4 g/m^2), corresponding to 4–4.5 g (2.1–2.7 g/m^2) per treatment day. Steroids and diuretics were used in conjunction with the high fractional doses of 4 Gy. Antiemetic drugs were used when necessary. Only patients at risk obtained antiepileptic medication.

Results

In general, the treatment was well-tolerated with no untoward side effects related to radiation doses used. Survival curves for both treatment groups are illustrated in figure 1. Median survival for the group receiving irradiation alone was 8.7 months compared with 15.5 months for the misonidazole group. The superiority of the misonidazole group survival is significant at the 0.0025 level (Wilcoxon test statistic for independent samples). The corresponding 1-year survival rates are 13.0% and 58.8% respectively.

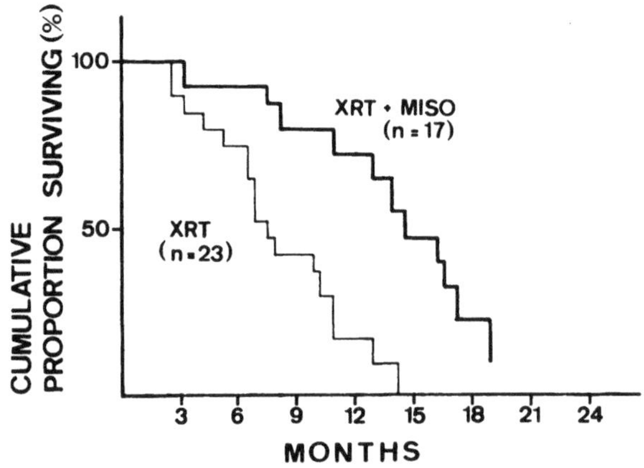

Fig. 1 Survival plots for patients receiving radiation alone (XRT) or irradiation plus misonidazole. Survival is statistically significantly better in the misonidazole group ($p < 0.0025$).

Figure 2 shows the survival curves according to the type of operation (complete or subtotal). There is no significant difference between the two groups. Also the histological grade did not influence survival either.

The mean age for the patients is 51 years in the sensitizer group and 56 years for patients who only received irradiation. The age distribution between the two groups shows no statistically significant difference ($p > 0,4$).

With the use of antinausea medication 30 minutes before misonidazole administration the drug was tolerated well. Repeated controls of the blood counts, renal and hepatic functions were all within normal limits. A significant sensitizer enhacement ratio [1, 7] may be expected (1.6 with a mean serum level at 4 hours after the administration of 4.5 g of misonidazole (2.1–2.7 g/m^2) [9, 10]. Although 12.6–16.4 g/m^2 (mean 14.2 g/m^2) of midonidazole were given, neurotoxic side effects were minimal. Three patients experienced mild paraesthesiae of the lower extremities, lasting a few weeks, in five patients a transient tinnitus occurred in the second week of treatment. No other significant side effects could be observed and no enhanced normal tissue reactions were found due to the interaction of misonidazole with irradiation.

Discussion

The results of our study demonstrate a significant advantage in survival for patients with astrocytomas grade III–IV treated with irradiation and misonidazole. This finding is in contradiction to most other reports [5, 7, 8, 12], whereas Urtasun et al. also found a benificial effect of a radiosensitizer in a glioblastoma study using metronidazole [13]. In addition encouraging results are reported in an EORTC pilot study, using misonidazole and multiple daily radiation fractions [2]. The type of operation

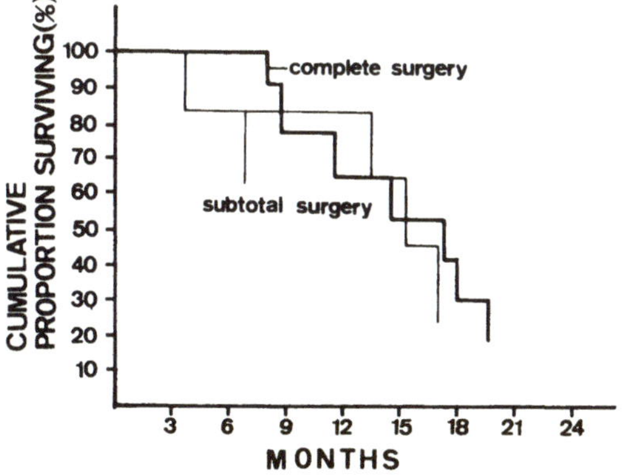

Fig. 2 Survival plots for patients with complete or subtotal operation ($p>0.4$).

(radical or subtotal) did not influence survival in our study as opposed to the finding of the Cambridge glioma trial [3, 5]. There was an even patient distribution concerning age, histological grade and initial performance status between our two treatment groups. With cumulative misonidazole doses of 27 g (12.6–16.4 g/m^2), the neurotoxic side effects like peripheral neuropathy and tinnitus were minimal in combination with steroid administration [14]. Other investigators [4, 5] also came to similar conclusions, although lesser cumulative doses of misonidazole were employed. One of the difficulties in comparing the different studies in progress is related to major differences in treatment schedules. The rationale for our fractionation scheme was to decrease quickly the number of hypoxic cells at the beginning of treatment and then to let reoxygenation take place with the daily fractionation scheme from the third to the seventh week of treatment. In the last week of treatment further high-dose fractionation and sensitizer administration possibly helps to destroy remaining hypoxic tumour cells.

In conclusion at the present time, we can therefore only speculate about the reasons for the better outcome of patients treated with misonidazole in our study. The results should not lead to premature conclusions about the efficacy of radiation sensitizers of hypoxic cells but they point out the possibility of obtaining an improvement in survival in patients with grade III–IV astrocytomas, when unconventional fractionation schemes are used in combination with the hypoxic cell sinsitizer misonidazole.*

Summary

In a randomized study, investigating the hypoxic cell sensitizer misonidazole, 40 patients with high-grade astrocytomas were referred for postoperative radiotherapy to the University Clinic for Radiotherapy and Radiobiology of Vienna. The improved survival of the misonidazole group is significant at the 0.0025 level. Side effects of treatment were minimal. Radiosensitizers for hypoxic cells might play a role in the future management of high-grade astrocytomas, expecially when combined with altered radiation fractionation schedules.

References

[1] Adams, G. E., K. Dawson, I. J. Stratford: Electron-affinic radiation sensitizers for hypoxic cells: Prospects and limitations with present and future drugs. In: Progress in Radio-Oncology (Proc. Int. Symp. Baden, Austria, 1978. K. H. Kärcher, H. D. Kogelnik, H. J. Meyer, eds.), pp. 84–95. Georg Thieme Verlag, Stuttgart, and Thieme- Stratton Inc., New York 1980.

* We are indepted to Hoffmann-La Roche A.G., Basle, for making misonidazole available to us for this study.

[2] Ang, K. K., E. van der Scueren, et al.: Split Course Multiple Daily Fractional Radiotherapy Schedule combined with Misonidazole for the Management of Grade III and IV Gliomas: A pilot feasibility study of the Radiotherapy Group of the EORTC. Int. J. Radiat. Oncol. Biol. Phys. **10** (1982) 1657–1664.

[3] Bleehen, N. M.: The Cambridge Glioma Trial of Misonidazole and Radiation Therapy with associated Pharmacocinetic Studies. Cancer Clin. Trials **3** (1980) 267–273.

[4[Bleehen, N. M.: Misonidazole, MRC Trials-Glioblastoma. Proceedings I. Meeting of ESTRO, London, UK (1982) 26.

[5] Bleehen, N. M.: MRC Study of Misonidazole and Radiotherapy for High Grade Astrozytomas. Proceedings II. Meeting of ESTRO, Bordeaux, France (1983) 21.

[6] Dische, S.: Hypoxic cell sensitizers. In: Proceedings of 2nd International Symposium on Biological Bases and Clinical Implications of Tumour Resistance, Rome 1980. Masson Publishing USA Inc. (in press).

[7] Gonzalez-Gonzalez, D.: Randomized double blind Study in Patients operated for Malignant Brain Glioma, using Radiotherapy in Proceedings I. Meeting of ESTRO, London, UK (1982) 32.

[8] Hagen, S.: A Randomized Study of Radiotherapy, Misonidazole and CCNU in operated Patients with Astrozytomas Grade 3/4. Proceedings II. Meeting of ESTRO, Bordeaux, France (1983) 41.

[9] Kogelnik, H. D.: Clinical experience with Misonidazole – High dose Fractions versus daily low Doses. Cancer Clin. Trials **3** (1980) 179–186.

[10] Kogelnik, H. D., H. J. Meyer, K. Jentzsch: Hypoxic cell Sensitizers in Radiobiology and Radiotherapy (Proc. 8th L. H. Gray Conf., Cambridge, UK, 1977). Br. J. Cancer **37**, suppl. III (1978) 281–285.

[11] Maire, J. Ph.: The Spread of Supratentorial malignant Gliomas: A Follow-up Study with Computerized Tomography after Treatment. Proceedings II. Meeting of the ESTRO, Bordeaux, France (1983) 35.

[12] Sack, H.: Postoperative Radiotherapy of Astrozytomas Grade III and IV with the Radiosensitizer Misonidazole – End Results of a Multicentric controlled German Study. Proceedings II. Meeting of ESTRO, Bordeaux, France (1983) 7.

[13] Urtasun, R. C., P. Band, J. D. Chapman, et al.: Radiation and high-dose Metronidazole in supratentorial glioblastomas. N. Engl. J. Med. **294** (1976) 1364–1367.

[14] Urtasun, R. C., H. Tanasichuk, D. Fulton, et al.: High dose Misonidazole with Dexamethasone Rescue: A possible Approach to circumvent Neurotoxicity. Int. J. Rad. Oncol. Biol. Phys. **8** (1982) 365–369.

[15] Walker, M. D., E. Alexander Jr., W. E. Hunt: Evaluation of BCNU and/or Radiotherapy in the Treatment of Gliomas. A cooperative clinical Trial. J. Neurosurg. **49** (1978) 333–343.

[16] Walker, M. D., S. B. Green, D. P. Byar: Randomized Comparisons of Radiotherapy and Nitrosureas for the Treatment of malignant anaplastic Glioma after Surgery. New Engl. J. Med. 303 (1980) 1323–1329.

Reflections on the radiation treatment of gliomas

J. Halama, W. Falk

For the neurosurgeon it may be said that it is only the site of a tumour which is the limiting factor in any operative procedure, and here, as a rule the motor areas, brain stem, midbrain, pons, thalamus and medulla are areas to be spared. However, for the radiotherapist it is desirable in every case to try to obtain a histological or cytological classification of the lesion. Apart from the histology and the site and size of the tumour he must also consider the tolerance of the tissues to radiation in relation to the total dosage and the time [1, 2, 9, 13, 16, 17, 21] particularly in the brain stem, and also in children the increased biological sensitivity to radiation of the brain [4], as well as the different types and grades of tumour. Thus, astrocytomas in children favour the cerebellum and brain stem, while in juveniles they occur predominantly in the cerebral hemispheres. Only recently the old concept of 'site specifity' in brain tumours has been rivived, whereby tumours of the same type and grade are influenced quite differently in their prognosis according to their location in the different parts of the brain [2]. This is not only a matter of the varying sensitivity of the different parts of the brain. For example, it is well-known that neoplasms in the cerebello-pontine angle can lead, through vascular effects, to brain stem dysfunction and to a significantly less favourable outcome [6]. Burger [2] has found with supratentorial astrocytomas that as one moves towards the occipital region there is an increase in the mean survival time, which varied from a minimum of 29 weeks in the temporal region to the highest figure of 53 weeks in the occipital region. With glioblastoma multiforme this amounted to 16 weeks with operation alone, 42.2 weeks with operation and radiation, but with the combination of operation and BCNU it was lower at 23.9 weeks, than the combination with radiotherapy.

Apart from the two factors, dose and time, the size of the radiation field used has gained great significance [10] in the biological assessment of brain tolerance of the Nominal Standard Dose (NSD) in ret (roentgen equivalent therapy). With a total brain radiation using 18 cm^2 fields and 5 × weekly administration of 200 cGy, a total tumour dose of 60 Gy* leads to the value of brain tolerance: 1600 ret and tumour-NSD of 1867 ret. The limit of brain tolerance is definitely transgressed and hence, in over 5 per cent of cases, the risk of damaging normal tissue is increased. For midline structures it amounts to 1500 ret [5].

---

* 1 Gy (Gray) = 100 rad

An 8 × 8 cm field covers only 40 per cent of the brain volume and with a similar type of radiation produces a tolerance of 1849 ret and NSD 1727 ret. The possible incidence of injury is definitely under 5 per cent! Outpatient small field radiation over the stated field size, three times weekly with 250 cGy, gives similarly favourable ret values at 1849:1783.

Raising the tumour dose to 65 Gy, but otherwise with the same method of radiation, rapidly changes the relationship – 1849:1934 ret. A half total brain and half small field series given one after the other with 200 cGy five times weekly produces 1724:1798 ret. With the total target dose 200 cGy five times weekly large field, and 250 cGy three times weekly with a small field technique there are similarly favourable relationships at 1724:1833.

Thus it is, that with the requirements of a partial large field radiation such as we have to employ with undifferentiated astrocytomas, glioblastoma and ependymomas, with high total doses of up to 60 Gy, side effects on the healthy brain may be expected in 5–10 per cent of the cases. It may then be, for example, that one can fall short of the calculated tumour dose of 60 Gy after an extensive radical operation. Thus a combination of large field and small field radiation, 200 cGy five times weekly and a total dosage of 50 Gy, gives a tolerance dose of 1742 ret and NSD tumour dose of 1500 ret. Side effects are therefore eliminated. On the other hand Salazar [14] has stated that taking the ependymoma as an example, only those patients had a chance of cure whose field size was over 150 cm^2 and whose ret dose was more than 1350, even going as high as 1600.

In this way, by taking note of the limiting factors such as the site of the tumour and the age of the patients, in many cases the necessary high radiation dose and the ret-dose for the destruction of the tumour can be given for the most part using small fields only, into the actual area of the tumour. In this way the tolerance of the healthy brain tissue becomes raised. Without consideration of the field size, the danger of a radiogenic brain lesion starts [9], in up to 5 per cent of the cases with a fractionation giving about 50 Gy in 60 days, 40 Gy in 30 days and 30 Gy in just 10 days. The risk rises considerably in the case of total target doses of 70, 60 and 42 Gy for the same administration times of 60, 30 and about 10 days, from which the limit of an efficient second radiation for a recurrence becomes evident. The indications for radiating a recurrence would be markedly reduced in cases who have had preceding small field radiation and fresh evidence of a tumour in regions other than the original site.

The radiotherapist moves along a very narrow line in giving his treatment, where on the one side he must consider the destruction of the tumour and, on the other, the possibility of a worthwhile existence for the patient. It has been increasingly referred to in the literature [6] that a clinical cure of the tumour must occasionally be accepted with neurological deficits, impairment of intelligence and retardation. It is thus particularly important to record the clinical and social state before treatment, in order to have adequate information for comparison. The limiting values mentioned at the beginning, for the appearance of radiogenic brain changes apply to radiotherapy on its own. The dose must clearly be reduced by including chemotherapy in the scheme of management, as for example in the treatment of leukaemia or MXT-therapy. This means a primarily determined interdisciplinary programme of radiotherapy.

The multiaxial small field rotational radiation favoured in Offenbach requires – according to the radical nature of the operative intervention and the respective histological grades of the tumour – target doses between 45 and 65 Gy related to the limits of the tumour, plus a safety margin of at least 2 cm.

In the case of markedly anaplastic gliomas (Stages III and IV) and glioblastoma multiforme, as well as medulloblastomas, we give first of all whole brain radiation with parallel opposing fields, up to a dose of about 30 Gy in adults and 20 Gy in children. "Saturation" of the tumour is then achieved with small fields – according to the mobility of the patient – with static fields, but for preference by rotational radiation with filting head given over the forehead, the vertex and the occiput. By using this small field technique we rarely see permanent epilation and if there should be small areas of hair loss, these can be easily dealt with by the hairdresser. We believe that in this way we are able, after curing the tumour, to make a psychologically important contribution to the well-being of the patient who will not feel branded as an outcast, either at home with the family or even after return to work. In tumours which are less radiosensitive and where a radical operation has not been performed, we give the patient radiation 2–3 times daily with a total daily dose of up to 300 cGy, five times weekly, with a reduced total tumour dose of 50 Gy, in two separate courses.

The technique of radiotherapy of the spinal cord ist well-known. Tumour doses of between 20 and 25 Gy are given. While medulloblastomas are given this prophylaxis more or less routinely, with infratentorial ependymomas it is only used for the more malignant grades [17].

The indications for radiotherapy are familiar. While appreciating the necessity for caution in giving radiation, there is a tendency to set rather more ambitious targets. As Walker [7, 19] has shown, in a so-called total resection one gram of tumour still remains and after a subtotal resection of a malignant glioma 10 g of residual tumour remain, so that in practice a total tumour extirpation is impossible. According to his view, this demands further though on the subject of efficient radiotherapy or chemotherapy.

Sheline [18], in a group of 108 incompletely resected cerebral astrocytomas (I–II) was able to report a very definitely improved chance of cure after 5, 10 and 20 years, when additional radiotherapy was given, as compared with those treated by operation alone (18%:46%; 11%:25%; 0%:23%). If the grade of malignancy is considered the five-year survival in grade I amounts to 25% (58%); grade II 0% (25%). Scanlon and Taylor [15] have seen an astonishingly high percentage of cures in 417 radiated intracranial astrocytomas: I (76%), II (58%), III (6%), IV (4%), in which 68 per cent of the cases were in grades III and IV.

In the case of ependymomas inoperability or partial operability is always supposed to exist, so that radiotherapy as an additional measure must be given. Thus Sheline as well as Mørk and Løken [11] were able to improve the five-year results of postoperative radiotherapy from 24% to 60%, in cases where the supratentorial lesions were definitely worse than the infratentorial.

The slow growth of oligodendrogliomas really contraindicates any postoperative radiation if a radical operation has been done. On the other hand Sheline, using supplementary radiation in these cases, has been able to improve the results of operation alone from 23–37% to 53–85%, and increase the ten-year cure from 25% to 55%, so that even with this tumour, which is somewhat less than radiosensitive, something can be done with target doses of 60 Gy. After purely surgical treatment 50% of oligodendrogliomas recur [6].

From 1976 to 1982, 147 brain tumours, including eight non-intrinsic neoplasms were treated in Offenbach by the recommended small field rotating therapy. At the present time we see something over 30 cases per year. The operation or other diagnostic procedure takes place in the University Clinics of Frankfurt, Mainz, Giessen and in the accident clinic in Frankfurt (Herr Hübner) and the neurosurgical clinics at Offenbach (Fromm). The Curie therapy implantations were, as a rule, undertaken by Dr. Mundinger in Freiburg (tab. 1).

The mean period of survival in the astrocytomas (I–II) who have died was 24–29 months, in grades III–IV 12.5–24.8 months and in the survivors grade I–II 19.5–84 months and in grades III–IV 14.5–26 months.

In combination with chemotherapy using BCNU, VCR and PCB, when there was evidence of a recurrence, no significant improvement in the survival time was recorded in four cases, compared with ten deaths in those who had not received chemotherapy, with a survival time of between 14 and 15.8 months. However, in the ten glioblastoma patients who had died, the mean survival time was raised to 12.5 months compared with 6.8 months in 44 who were not treated with chemotherapy. The mean survival time of all who had died was between 2.0 and 13.2 months, depending on the radicality of the operation. Thirty-three neoplasms not histologically verified were assigned mainly to the group of the astrocytomas and glioblastomas as described, according to the clinical and neuroradiological evidence and were removed from the data in the table, as well as a further eight non-intrinsic intracranial tumours (tab. 2).

Table 1 Radiotherapy of the cranial cavity in 147 brain tumours

a/n	D/age	Histology	Median survival time. Radical oper'n		Subtotal Op'n		No operation		No report about radicality	
3/10	*34.6*	*Astrocytoma I-II*		–	3/6	d: 26.5	2/2	d: 24.0	1/2	d: 29.0
				–	2/6	a: 19.5		–	1/2	a: 84.0
9/22	*49.3*	*Astrocytoma III-IV*	2/5	d: 12.5	7/11	d: 14.4	2/4	d: 16.8	2/2	d: 24.8
			3/5	a: 14.5	4/11	a: 26.6	2/4	a: 11.0		
1/54	*52.8*	*Gliobl. (2 × sarcomatous)*	11/2	d: 8.6	34/34	d: 7.3	3/3	d: 2.0	4/5	d: 13.2
			1/12	a: 20.5		–		–		–
4	19.8	Medulloblastoma	1/1	a: 39.0	2/2	a: 33.5		–	1/1	d: 17.5
5	48.5	Oligodendroglioma	2/2	a: 26.5	1/3	a: 45.5		–		–
					1/3	b: 64.5				
1	54	Oligodendrospongiobl. glioma		–		d: 4.0		–		–
1	37.0	Oligodendroastrocytomatous Gl.		–		d: 6.5		–		–
1	31	Spongioblastoma		–		–		d: 8.0		–
1	35	Pinealoma		–		d: 54.5		–		–
1	52	Malignant meningioma		–		d: 75.0		–		–
4	33.5	Pituitary adenoma		d: 22.0		–		d: 23.0		–
						a: 52.0		a: 38.5		
2	67.5	Unclassified malignant tumour		–		–		d: 9.0		–
33		*Neoplasms without histology*								
20	54	Glioblastoma					1/20	a: 12.0		
							18/20	d: 7.4		
2	46	Astrocytoma					2/2	d: 15.5		
1	32	Oligodendroglioma						a: 10.0		
1	56	Craniopharyngioma						d: 12.0		
9	46	Unclassified					1/9	a: 21.0		
							8/9	d: 7.2		
8		5 malignant lymphomas, one each haemangioblastoma, giant-cell sarcoma, (periadventitial) sarcoma								

Radiation therapy of the skull cavity (Radio-oncology Clinic, Offenbach 1976–1982) 147 brain tumours, including 8 non-intrinsic and 62 metastases treated with chemotherapy (30 breast + 18 bronchus) (a = alive d = dead)

In summary it must now be stated that a mainly small-field rotation radiation given routinely to intrinsic brain tumours in Offenbach, has not led to any worth-while improvement in the well-known results of radiotherapy. However the incidence of side-effects was extremely small and this carefully administered radiation treatment has been well tolerated by the patients.

According to our experience it was only in patients with glioblastomas that chemotherapy seemed able to improve the chances of survival. However, in Offenbach it has for a long time only been used in significant recurrences, in accordance with the statements of Levin et al. [7] and of Eagan and Scott [3] who, apart from the important treatment with corticosteroids, have only seen positive results with the use of Procarbacin and BCNU, either alone or in combination.

The significance of the blood-brain barrier in the treatment of brain metastases has recently been called into question by general oncologists [12] as they secured good results in brain metastases, using the customary schema for carcinoma of the breast.

Up to the present time 66 brain metastases that have been treated by radiation and chemotherapy are being investigated. Of these, 30 were from the breast and 18 from

Table 2 Combined radiotherapy and chemotherapy in 18 brain tumours and 62 intracranial metastases

Tpye of tumour	Median survival time in months		Courses
Astrocytoma III-IV	Chemotherapy	4 d : 14.0	4.2
	No Chemotherapy	10 d : 15.8	
Glioblastoma	Chemotherapy	10 d : 12.5	4.9
	No Chemotherapy	44 d : 6.8	
Medulloblastoma	Chemotherapy	1 d : 3.0	3.0
Oligodendroglioma	Chemotherapy	1 a : 45.5	5.0
Spongioblastoma	Chemotherapy	1 d : 8.0	3.0
No histology / Corpus callosum	Chemotherapy	1 d : 7.5	1.0

Brain tumours			Cerebral metastases (Ca. breast)				Cerebral metastases (bronchial carc.)			
Day 1	BCNU	75 mg/m²	Day 1	ADB	40 mg/m²	i. v.	Day 1	ADB	40 mg/m²	i. v.
Day 1 + 8	VCR	1–2 mg²	Day 3–6	CTX	200 mg/m²	p. o.		CTX	600 mg/m²	i. v.
Day 1–14	PCB	100 mg/m²	Days 3–10	PCB	100 mg/m²	p. o.		BCNU	65 mg/m²	i. v.
							Day 2	VCR	1–2 mg	i. v.
								BLEO	15 mg	i. m.

Combined radiotherapy and chemotherapy in 18 brain tumours and 62 cerebral metastases (a = alive, d = dead)

the bronchus. In the case of the breast carcinomas they were treated by a combination of Adriablastin, Endoxana (cyclophosphamide) and Natulan (procarbazine), while for the bronchial carcinomas the well-known BACON-schema was preferred on account of its extension of the use of BCNU. With brain metastases small field radiation, which is otherwise to be recommended, cannot be used, but opposing field radiation with a dose of 25–30 Gy is necessary. This includes the whole cranial cavity, in which case larger solitary metastases in individual cases can be saturated by additional small fields with 15 Gy. The CT follow-up occasionally shows almost complete regression of the metastases.

Summary

In the radiotherapy department in Offenbach between 1976 and 1982 we have treated 147 brain tumours, by careful dose planning and small fields of about 8 × 8 cm, by three-axial rotating radiotherapy. The importance of the Nominal Standard Dose in roentgen equivalent therapy (rets) for brain tolerance, is demonstrated.

References

[1] Berg, N. O., M. Lindgren: Relation between field size and tolerance of rabbit's brain to roentgen irradiation (200 KV). Acta Radiol. 1 (1963) 147–168.

[2] Burger, P. C., R. T. Vollmer: Histologic factors of prognostic significance in the glioblastoma multiforme. Cancer 46 (1980) 1179–1186.

[3] Eagan, R. T., M. Scott: Evaluation of prognostic factors in chemotherapy of recurrent brain tumors. J. Clin. Oncol. 1 (1983) 38–44.
[4] Halama, J.: Die Hirntumoren aus strahlenklinischer Sicht. Med. Welt 18 (1967) 810–818.
[5] Holdorff, B.: Der Unterschied zwischen zerebralen Hemisphären- und Mittellinien-Strahlenspätnekrosen und seine Bedeutung für die Strahlentherapie. Strahlentherapie 156 (1980) 530–536.
[6] Kornblith, P. L., M. D. Walker, J. R. Cassady: Neoplasms of the central nervous system. In: Cancer, pp. 1181–1253. Principles and practice of oncology (V. T. De Vita, S. Hellmann, St. A. Rosenberg, eds.). Lippincott, Philadelphia – Toronto 1982.
[7] Levin, V. A., Ph. H. Gutin, Ch. B. Wilson: Brain tumors. In: Clinical interpretation and practice of cancer chemotherapy (E. M. Greenspan, ed.), pp. 393–408. Raven Press, New York 1982.
[8] Leibel, St. A., G. E. Sheline, W. M. Wara, et al.: The role of radiation therapy in the treatment of astrocytomas. Cancer 35 (1975) 1551–1557.
[9] Lindgren, M.: On tolerance of brain tissue and sensitivity of brain tumors to irradiation. Acta Radiol., Suppl. 170 (1958) 1–73.
[10] Marquardt, B., A.-C. Voss, A. Markewitz: Ergebnisse der Strahlentherapie bei 214 primären Hirntumoren und 27 Hirnmetastasen (1969–1978). Strahlentherapie 156 (1980) 371–381.
[11] Mørks, S. J., A. C. Løken: Ependymoma. Cancer 40 (1977) 907–915.
[12] Rosner, D.: Annual ASCO Meeting San Diego 1983.
[13] Rubin, Ph., G. W. Casarett: Clinical radiation pathology. Vol. II. Saunders Comp., Philadelphia – London – Toronto 1968.
[14] Salazar, O. M., Ph. Rubin, D. Bassano, et al.: Improved survival of patients with intracranial ependymomas by irradiation. Cancer 35 (1975) 1563–1573.
[15] Scanlon, P. W., W. F. Taylor: Radiotherapy of intracranial astrocytomas: Analysis of 417 cases treated from 1960 through 1969. Neurosurg. 5 (1979) 301–308.
[16] Schmitt, H. P.: Akute und intercelläre Strahlenschäden des Zentralnervensystems. Springer-Verlag, Berlin – Heidelberg – New York 1979.
[17] Schnepper, E.: Tumoren des Nervensystems. In: Strahlentherapie (E. Scherer, ed.), pp. 831–862. Springer-Verlag, Berlin – Heidelberg – New York 1980 (II).
[18] Sheline, G. E.: The importance of distinguished tumor grade in malignant glioma: Treatment and prognosis. Int. J. Radiat. Oncol. Biol. Phys. 1 (1976) 781–786.
[19] Walker, M. D., E. Alexander, W. E. Hunt, et al.: Evaluation of BCNU and/or radiotherapy in the treatment of anaplastic gliomas. A cooperative clinical trial. J. Neurosurg. 49, (1978) 333–343.
[20] Walker, M. D., S. B. Green, D. P. Byar: Randomized comparison of radiotherapy and nitrosoureas for the treatment of malignant glioma after surgery. N. Engl. J. Med. 303 (1980) 1323–1329.
[21] Wendhausen, H.: Untersuchungen zur biophysikalischen Dosisplanung bei der Strahlentherapie maligner Tumoren. Habil. Schr. Kiel 1980.

Therapeutic results in malignant gliomas with special respect to radiotherapy

H. Keim, P. C. Potthoff, A. Neiss

Introduction

In 1980, we reported on the results of operation and radiotherapy in 49 glioblastomas and astrocytomas grade III–IV [10]. At that time, we were able to show a considerably better survival time for younger patients than for older ones.

We now present a group of 161 patients of malignant, irradiated, and in most cases primarily operated brain tumours whose treatment started in 1972 and had been terminated by June 30, 1983.

This group of 161 comprises

- 111 patients that had been operated and whose tumours were histologically classified according to the WHO-classification and whose post-operative condition permitted post-operative irradiation,
  and
- 50 patients with primary brain tumours that appeared inoperable because of size and location and that received radiotherapy alone. In these cases the diagnosis was based on the CT-findings and mostly involved extensive space-occupying lesions encroaching upon the midline or in both cerebral hemispheres. Biopsies were not used because of their uncertainty in histological classification.

It was the intention of this retrospective study to evaluate our treatment results, to elucidate correlations between patient groups and results, to find differences between operable and non-operable patients, between sex groups, between age groups, and possibly between different dosage techniques of radiotherapy, and possibly to find indications for an improved strategy in radiotherapy.

Patient groups

Sex: Among 111 operated patients there were 68 male and 43 female, among 50 non-operated patients were 28 male and 22 female patients.

Age distribution: The peak of male as well as female patients was in the sixth decade, secondly in the seventh decade, in which women were represented by 50% and not, as usual, by only 30%.

Site: Only one case – a glioblastoma – showed multifocal distribution in its phase of recurrence, in all other cases, operated as well as non-operated patients, the tumour was solitary and the later recurrence within the region of operation and/or radiation remained solitary.

Histology: Most cases were classified as glioblastoma multiforme. In three cases the histological variant of a gliosarcoma was diagnosed. In one other case the histological diagnosis was "gigantocellular glioblastoma"; this 26-year-old patient died after an unusually long survival time of 111 months not from his cerebral recurrence, but from a generalized neurofibromatosis manifesting itself one year before the patient's death (this case has not been included in the following survival time calculations).

Irradiation technique: Radiation was begun postoperatively after the wound was healed, usually between the 12th and 14th postoperative day. A longer interval between operation and irradiation, sometimes caused by the necessity of a prolonged intensive care treatment or prolonged local wound complications, usually also included a worse prognosis, while on the other side a neurological deficit and the initial necessity of intravenous nutrition presented no obstacle for starting radiotherapy.

With inoperable tumours irradiation was started immediately after diagnosis and transfer of patients for radiotherapy.

Methods of irradiation

Irradiation was given with a cobalt 60 unit and with opposed fields. The irradiation volume was whole brain irradiation for large inoperable tumours. In operated cases – as far as possible – the irradiation was confined to the region of tumour-resection including a 2 cm margin of safety.

In the past 12 years *three different dosage variants* have been used:

1. Until February 1979 and in the last quarter of 1981: 50 Gy in five weeks, corresponding to 1572 ret NSD.
2. From March 1979 till October 1980 40 Gy in four weeks whole brain irradiation, and, after a break of two weeks, 20 Gy booster dose on the tumour area in two weeks, corresponding to 1698 ret NSD.
3. Since 1982 60 Gy in 18 days, corresponding to 1825 ret NSD on the tumour area (mostly partial brain irradiation) including larger daily dosages in three sections every 4 hours and with administration of irradiation also during holidays and Saturdays (HDMDF = high dose multiple day fractionation).

Accessory treatment

This included anticonvulsive prophylaxis by Luminal (100 mg twice daily) or Zentropil® 3 times daily; treatment of cerebral oedema, if necessary, with 4.5 milligrams Dexamethason orally 3 times per day, in cases with marked signs of brain oedema increase of Dexamethason medication and osmotherapy. In 14 cases tumour sensitization for irradiation was induced by the administration of Misonidazol® 400 mg/cm^2/day in a randomized study. All patients received physiotherapeutic rehabilitation to an intensive degree during their hospital stay. All patients received oxygen-inhalations of 4 l oxygen/per minute for 3 hours daily.

Results

For a comparison of results the *median survival time* was calculated, starting with the day of operation in operated patients and starting with the first day of irradiation in non-operated patients. *Quality of survival* was expressed in three simplified categories in accordance to the Karnofski-scale:

K I = 75 – 100%
K II = 50 – 75%
K III = Karnofski below 50%.

The calculation of survival curves was accomplished by the method of Kaplan-Meyer.

Corresponding to other authors [1, 9, 19] all those patients were included in the evaluation whose general condition at the end of irradiation corresponded to groups K I or K II, whose general status therefore was better than 50% of the Karnofski-scale.

Under these conditions, 86 patients remained within the group of operated and irradiated patients, while within the group of non-operated patients 30 patients remained for survival calculations.

Median survival times were as follows in both groups:

	n	average age	months
After operation and radiotherapy	86	52.2	*10.8*
Radiotherapy alone	30	52.2	*7.6*

Median survival times for male and female patients in both groups were

		n	average age	months
After operation and	male	56	51.9	*10.8*
radiotherapy	female	30	52.8	*10.9*
Radiotherapy alone	male	20	51.8	*6.2*
	female	10	53.0	*9.3*

Median survival times in relation to dosage of radiotherapy were

	n	average age	months
Operation + 50 Gy corr. 1572 ret	36	45.0	*12.8*
Operation + 60 Gy corr. 1698 ret	23	55.6	*8.9*
Operation + 60 Gy corr. 1825 ret (HDMDF)	27	53.4	*10.3*
Radiotherapy alone			
50 Gy corr. 1572 ret	16	56.1	*6.3*
60 Gy corr. 1825 ret (HDMDF)	14	47.9	*12.6*

Median survival times in relation to age in patients with survival quality Karnofski over 50%, irradiation dosage over 1572 ret.

	n	average age	months
Operation + irradiation			
up to 40 years	13	31.2	*20.0*
41 to 60 years	53	52.3	*9.7*
over 61 years	20	65.7	*10.4*
Radiotherapy alone (inoperable)			
up to 40 years	4	23.2	*30.0*
41 to 60 years	17	50.5	*6.4*
over 61 years	9	68.3	*7.1*

Discussion

In spite of all efforts for a radical tumour cure, results so far have mostly been modest and must be improved. This aspect is not altered by the fact that our survival times take one of the better ranges among those authors cited by Jellinger [9], and that our operated patients were classified entirely among the most malignant gliomas and that in our material anaplastic astrocytomas are excluded [compare 2, 3, 5, 6, 17, 19]. This study shows in the first range that survival chances of operated patients are significantly better with an median survival time of 10.8 months compared with only 7.5 months of non-operated patients.

There was no significant difference between male and female patients. Also the difference between 6.2 months for male and 9.3 months for female patients in the non-operated patient group was not significant.

Concerning dosage of radiotherapy, the hope of achieving a better tumour-static effect with higher irradiation dosage inducing better survival times, was not confirmed by the calculation of median survival times in the three different dosage variants. This does agree with the results as published by Salazar et al. [18]. Surprisingly, the median survival times in the group of operated patients were *shorter* with the higher dosages of 1698 and 1825 ret than with the formerly used dosage of 1572 ret.

In the group of non-operated patients with primary radiotherapy – on the other hand – a median survival time of 6.3 months after the administration of 1572 ret was improved to 12.6 months after the administration of 1825 ret.

It have to keep in mind that our results are obtained by an retrospective study and not by a controlled clinical trial. That means comparing different dosages of irradiation, the compared groups not only differ by dosage but also by other factors. One of such factors is the age of patient.

In the age group up to the 40th year of life the median survival time was 20 to 30 months, in the age group above 40 years of life only 6 to 10 months. These differences are significant. The drop after the 40th year of life is confirmed exactly by the results of Salazar [18] who described the same trend after the 45th year of life in his patients [also compare 4].

This age effect is confirmed by the survival times as observed in all different dosage variants of radiotherapy: The group of patients operated before 1979 had an average age of 45 years and a median survival time of 12.8 months. Among these are several patients with survival times above 20 months. The patient groups irradiated after 1979 had an average age of 53 to 55 years and the median survival times dropped to 9 to 10 months, among these the maximal survival time was only 15 months.

In the non-operable patient group the average age was 56.1 years before 1981 and 47.9 years since 1982, and in a reciprocal relation the median survival time increased in the second patient group irradiated after 1982.

The factor for better or decreased survival chances may therefore *not* be the dosage of postoperative radiotherapy, but the age of the patient. The hypothesis that this effect of age is also caused by a decreased irradiation tolerance of the older brain above the 50th year of life can be discussed and is in accordance to reports of different authors [7, 8, 15] who have used only partial brain irradiation instead of whole brain irradiation because of a possibly irradiation-induced encephalopathy [16], as well as in accordance with recommendations to use very high dosages in spite of a good patient tolerance only in younger patients and only with gliomas of lower grades of malignancy [18]. So far, we cannot definitely accept these consequences from our present study, but it is our intention in the future to confine higher dosages according to the HDMDF-method only to younger patients and to those of younger biological status.

It has to be discussed if, in the second group, patients were excluded and transferred into a group of operable patients by improvements in neurosurgery, patients that under earlier indications might have been considered as inoperable. As is well known, neurosurgical operation techniques and intensive care therapy have made important advances [12, 13, 14] during the time we have used our different variants of dosage of radiotherapy, and this may have had an effect on the indication for operation.

Summary

The results of treatment of 111 operated and irradiated patients with glioblastoma multiforme and astrocytoma grade III–IV (WHO-classification) and of 50 patients with primary radiotherapy of extensive inoperable brain tumours were compared in a retrospective study and examined as to their correlations with age and irradiation dosages. Median survival times in the operated group were 10.8 months, in the non-operated group 7.6 months, with an individual maximum survival time of up to 111 months in the operated and irradiated patient group.

The dosage corresponded in the consecutive phases of radiotherapy to 1572 ret NSD up to 1979, then 1698 ret NSD until October 1980, and finally 1825 ret NSD in high dose multiple day fractionation (= HDMDF-method) since 1982.

Age had a definite effect on the results with significantly better median survival times for younger patients. An increase of dosages in radiotherapy from 1572 to 1825 ret NSD did *not* show an improvement of results in the group of operated and irradiated patients. In the inoperable tumour patient group, we found a doubling of survival times under the higher dosage, however with lower age. Therefore the influence of age of a patient with a malignant brain tumour appears to be more important for survival time than any increase of radiotherapy dosages above the so far generally accepted dosage of about 1550 ret NSD. The cause for this effect of age could be the reduced tolerance of the older brain towards the traumatizing influence of irradiation. This suggests an innovation of irradiation-protective medical or physical methods in the radiotherapy of older patients over 50 or until, strategies of therapy are invented that allow for a reduction of irradiation dosages.

Acknowledgement

We are indebted to E. Kunz for doing the calculations on the CDC-Cyber-Computer of the Leibnitz-Rechenzentrum, Munich.

References

[1] Andersen, H. P.: Postoperative irradiation of glioblastomas. Acta Radiologica Oncology **17** fasc. 6 (1978) 475.

[2] Ang, K. K., E. von der Schueren, G. Notter, et al.: Split course multiple daily fractioned radiotherapy schedule combined with misonidazole for the management of grade III and IV gliomas. Int. J. Radiation Oncology Biol. Phys. Vol. 8, 1982.

[3] Ang, K. K., E. van der Schueren, G. Notter, et al.: High-dose multiple daily fractionation radiotherapy in combination with misoinidazole as a treatment of high-grade malignant gliomas. In: Progress in Radio-Oncology II (K. H. Kärcher, et al., ed.), pp. 197–201. Raven Press, New York 1982.

[4] Gehan, E. A., M. D. Walker: Prognostic factors for patients with brain tumors. Modern concepts in brain tumor therapy: Laboratory and Clinical Investigation. National Cancer Institute Monograph 46, Dept. of Health, Education and Welfare, 1977, pp. 189–196.

[5] Glanzmann, Ch., W. Horst, H. Seigert: Radiotherapie in der Behandlung primärer Hirntumoren. Fortschritte Röntgenstrahlen **121** (1974) 644.

[6] Haferkamp, G., P. Gutjahr, H. J. Reulen: Derzeitige Therapie maligner Tumoren des ZNS. Acta neurol. **5** (1978) 105–113.

[7] Hochberg, F. H., B. Slotnick: Neuropsychologic impairment in astrocytoma survivors. Neurology **30** (1980) 172–177.

[8] Hochberg, F. H., A. Pruitt: Assumptions in the radiotherapy of glioblastoma. Neurology **30** (1980) 907–911.

[9] Jellinger, K., D. Volc, I. Podreka, et al.: Ergebnisse der Kombinationsbehandlung maligner Gliome. Vergleich postoperativer Strahlen-, Polychemo- sowie kombinierter Strahlen- und Polychemotherapie. Nervenarzt **52** (1981) 41–50.

[10] Keim, H.: Zur Strahlenbehandlung maligner Hirntumoren: Methodische Aspekte und eigene Erfahrungen. In: Maligne Hirntumoren. Aktuelle Probleme in Chirurgie und Orthopädie (P. C. Potthoff, W. Schreml, eds.), Vol. 18, pp. 46–47. H. Huber, Bern–Stuttgart–Wien 1981.

[11] Marquart, B., A. C. Voss, A. Markewitz: Ergebnisse der Strahlentherapie bei 214 Hirntumoren und 27 Metastasen. Strahlentherapie **156** (1980) 371–381.

[12] Potthoff, P. C.: Neurochirurgische Eingriffe bei malignen Hirntumoren. In: Maligne Hirntumoren. Aktuelle Probleme in Chirurgie und Orthopädie (P. C. Potthoff, W. Schreml, eds.), Vol. 18, pp. 37–45. H. Huber, Bern–Stuttgart–Wien 1981.

[13] Potthoff, P. C.: Ergebnisse der Therapie maligner Hirntumoren. In: Maligne Hirntumoren. Aktuelle Probleme in Chirurgie und Orthopädie (P. C. Potthoff, W. Schreml, eds.), Vol. 18, pp. 78–86. H. Huber, Bern–Stuttgart–Wien 1981.

[14] Potthoff, P. C., W. Schreml: Therapiestandard und Therapieziel bei malignen Hirntumoren. In: Maligne Hirntumoren. Aktuelle Probleme in Chirurgie und Orthopädie (P. C. Potthoff, W. Schreml, eds.), Vol. 18, pp. 91–93. H. Huber, Bern–Stuttgart–Wien 1981.
[15] Ramsey, R. G., W. N. Brand: Radiotherapy of glioblastoma multiforme. J. Neurosurgery 39 (1973) 197–202.
[16] Schmitt, H. P.: Akute und intervalläre Strahlenschäden des Zentralnervensystems. Sitzungsberichte der Heidelberger Akademie der Wissenschaften. Mathem.-naturwissenschaftl. Klasse, Jg. 1979, 1. Abhandlung. Springer, Berlin–Heidelberg–New York.
[17] Trott, K. R.: Strahlenbiologische Probleme bei der Strahlentherapie von Hirngeschwülsten. Röntgenbl. 31 (1978) 282–288.
[18] Salazar, O. M., P. Rubin, M. L. Feldstein, et al.: High dose radiation therapy in the treatment of malignant gliomas. Final report. Int. J. Radiation Oncology Biol. Phys. 5 (1979) 1733–1740.
[19] Walker, M. D., Th. A. Strike, G. E. Sheline: An analysis of dose-effect relationsship in the radiotherapy of malignant gliomas. Int. J. Radiation Oncology Biol. Phys. 5 (1979) 1725–1731.

Pseudo-recurrence in malignant brain tumours

P. Krauseneck, D. Seybold, H. G. Mertens

Deciding about the onset of a recurrence in malignant brain tumours has become more and more important in recent years because, with the expansion of the cytostatic spectrum and the more active attitude to a second operation, essential decisions must be made about further treatments. The exact measurement of the free interval is of great importance for improving the chronological sequence of the various steps of treatment. In studies by the EORTC the moment of recurrence and not the death of the patient was chosen as the terminal point for each study section. In the multicentred study on malignant glioma which began in Germany and Austria in 1983 chemotherapy can be altered following a safety period after the clinical onset of recurrence. We have, therefore, in recent years particularly tried to determine the onset of recurrence exactly. Earlier on, an obvious deterioration of the neurological state of a patient with malignant brain tumour was always accepted as proof of recurrence. Only in rare cases were other causes for the deterioration successfully found. With the increased efficiency of multimodal, more active and aggressive treatment, we have encountered in recent years longer periods of freedom and also to some extent new complications which can simulate a relapse. Diagnosis substantially improved mainly by investigations computer tomography, exposes, however, a long list of other possible causes for the clinical deterioration. Examples of this and some misinterpretations of the diagnostic findings seem to be worth reporting. Table 1 shows these findings.

Table 1 Causes of pseudo-recurrences

Endocrine disorders – Hypothyroidism – Adrenal gland insufficiency	Ischaemic stroke
Vitamin deficiency – Wernicke encephalopathy	Radiation necrosis
Cerebral hypoxia – chronic purulent pneumonia – toxic interstitial pneumonia (espec. Bleomycine, BCNU)	Growing pseudo-cysts
	Acute increase of cerebral oedema – epileptic seizures – local infection
	Disorders of CSF circulation – Hydrocephalus aresorptivus – Low pressure syndrome

Case 1:
This 37-year old female patient with a centrally located histologically unclassified malignant growth showed a very good response to combined radio-chemo-therapy during February and March 1978 (fig. 1), but fell ill again at the beginning of April with a left-sided hemiparesis and was again disoriented so that an early relapse was supposed. The control CT surprisingly showed an ischaemic partial block of the right middle cerebral artery. Corresponding to the frequent appearance of thrombo-embolic complications in patients with malignant growths we have also repeatedly seen additional ischaemic strokes in patients with brain tumours.

Case 2:
A well-known complication hardly diagnosable during life-time, and rare in spite of aggressive radio-therapy, is radiation necrosis. With this patient, however, the sus-

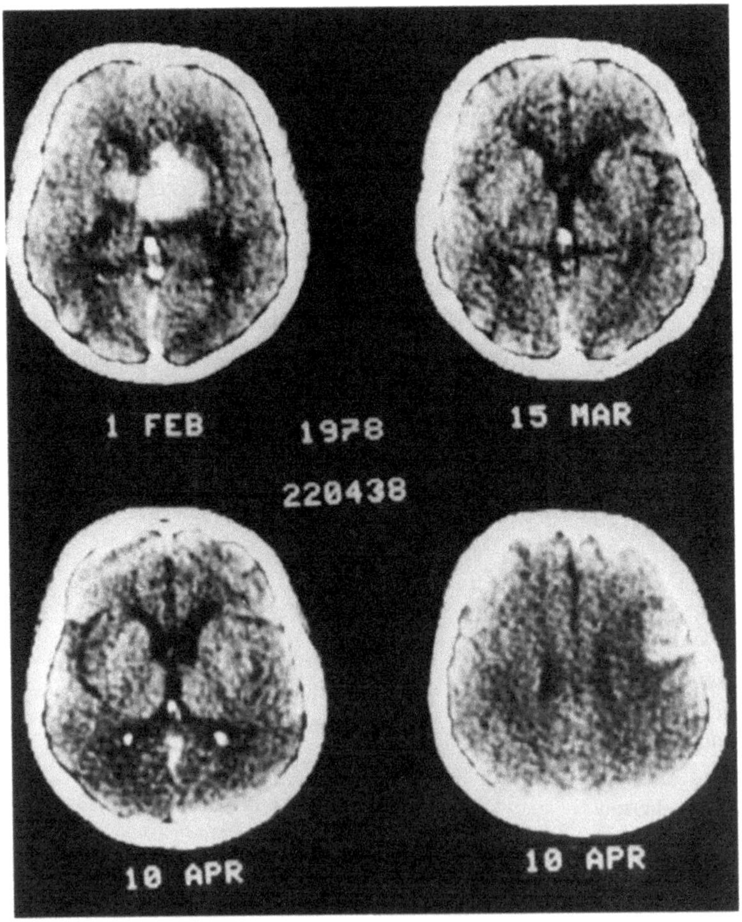

Fig. 1 Complete response of the tumour of the basal ganglia after six weeks of combined therapy (upper row). Clinical relapse in April is explained by a right temporal ischaemic stroke (lower row).

picion of radiation necrosis was fairly obvious as he had been given irradiation up to a total of 100 Gray to the seat of the tumour while being well aware of the risk of a possible radiation necrosis. The "tumour progression" from August 1979 until February 1980 (fig. 2) also turned out to be histological radiation necrosis. The appearance of growing pseudo-cysts after combined therapy must also be mentioned in this connection [1].

Case 3:
Not until the introduction of computer tomography was there any success in differentiating between a tumour relapse and an acute increase of oedema following, for example, a minor injury of the skull or slight insolation. In this patient an epileptic seizure in January 1983 led to a serious hemiparesis and mental slowing from which he rapidly recovered after anti-oedema treatment and remained in a stable condition for five further months. Not until July 1983 did a genuine recurrence develop.

Case 4:
A change in chemotherapy was planned for this female patient as fresh neurological signs were discovered. The CT showed stronger contrast enhancement of the tumour and thus recurrence seemed certain. A further X-ray check, however, showed that a superficial wound infection had developed into a massive osteomyelitis of the bone-flap (fig. 3). The removal of the bone-flap resulted in abolition of her complaints and in an improvement of the CT for the last four months that she remained under observation.

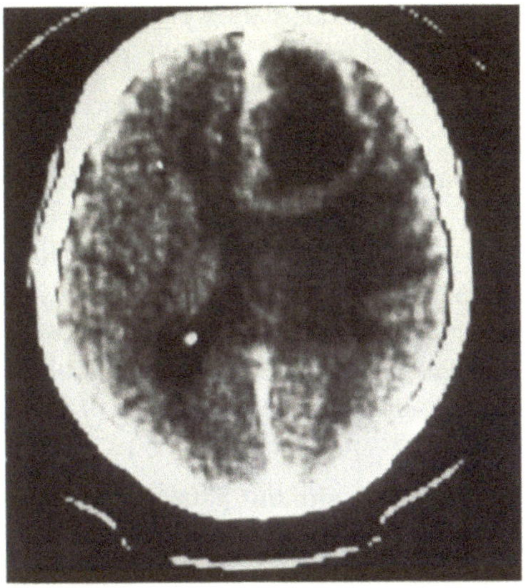

Fig. 2 This right frontal "re-growth" of a glioblastoma after a long stable period was verified at autopsy as radiation necrosis.

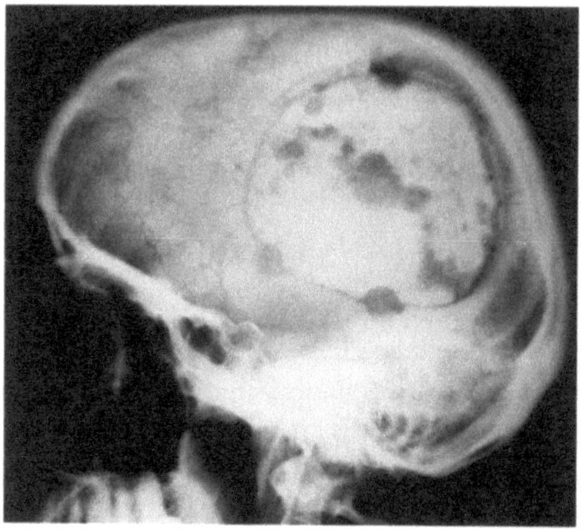

Fig. 3 Osteomyelitis of the bone flap causing intracerebral oedema with slight hemiparesis in a patient with a malignant oligodendroglioma.

Case 5:

The cranial nerve disorder and the abasia of this patient were reversed after an operation on the highly malignant right cerebral immunocytoma in July 1979 and subsequent radio-therapy. Until April 1980 the patient was in good condition. Renewed abasia and ataxia as well as intellectual impairment suggested a recurrence although no new growth of the tumour was found in CT. Further deterioration of his condition led to further admission in 1982 when the CT again showed no hint of recurrence but indicated a marked internal hydrocephalus. A spinal infusion test, a cerebral-pressure probe measurement and RISA-examination proved clearly an aresorptive hydrocephalus which was confirmed as the cause of the neurological symptoms.

Case 6:

This young patient suffered from a pinealoblastoma, grade IV, confirmed by stereotactic biopsy. This had responded very well to radiotherapy and was no longer identifiable in CT. The patient, however, vomited several times daily, had severe headaches and was not able to stand up. Repeated CSF checks revealed single atypical cells so that a meningeal dissemination of the tumour was considered. The CT findings indicated a low pressure syndrome. Six months after removal of the shunt system the patient is free from complaints and there is no evidence of tumour.

Case 7:

A misinterpretation of the CT findings occurred with this patient. He was on long-term combined treatment for Hodgkin's disease stage IV b and was in full remission when he fell ill with apathy, temporary loss of memory and uncharacteristic abasia. As the CT seemed to show the rare event of a cerebral manifestation of Hodgkin's disease (fig. 4) it was decided to irradiate this cerebral focus. The clinical symptoms,

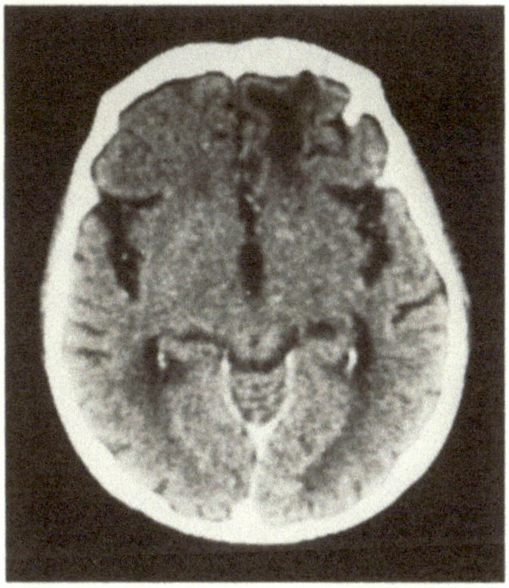

Fig. 4 Right frontal hypodense area in Hodgkin's disease, stage IV b, suggesting cerebral infiltration by the lymphoma. Relief of symptoms after substitution therapy for hypothyroidism.

however, remained as much unchanged as did the right frontal CT focus. Not until a marked hypothyroidism was diagnosed and treated did the patient's condition clearly improve. The CT findings may possibly be related to an old cerebral contusion.

Case 8:

After long-term doses of cortisone an adrenal cortical insufficiency simulated a progression of tumour in this patient. After the operation on a right frontal glioblastoma multiforme in November 1981 the recurrence of April 1982 was well stabilized by November 1982 by treatment with VM 26. However, the patient slept all day and was completely apathetic although he had neither neurological disorders nor did he need anti-oedema treatment. Further treatment was out of the question because of the patient's poor condition. A check on the adrenal cortical function then led to substitution of hydro-cortisone which resulted in almost entirely eliminating the hypersomnia and apathy of the patient, so that therapy could be successfully continued.

Case 9:

In this patient multiple cerebral metastases from a breast carcinoma had responded very well to a combined therapy when she fell ill five months later of severe ataxia, double vision and rapidly progressive conjugate paralysis so that recurrence especially of the cerebellar metastasis was suspected. Surprisingly though, neither in the CT nor in the CSF was pathological proof to be found (fig. 5). The idea of Wernicke encephalopathy and substitution with vitamin B 1 finally brought about a speedy alleviation and early relief for the patient.

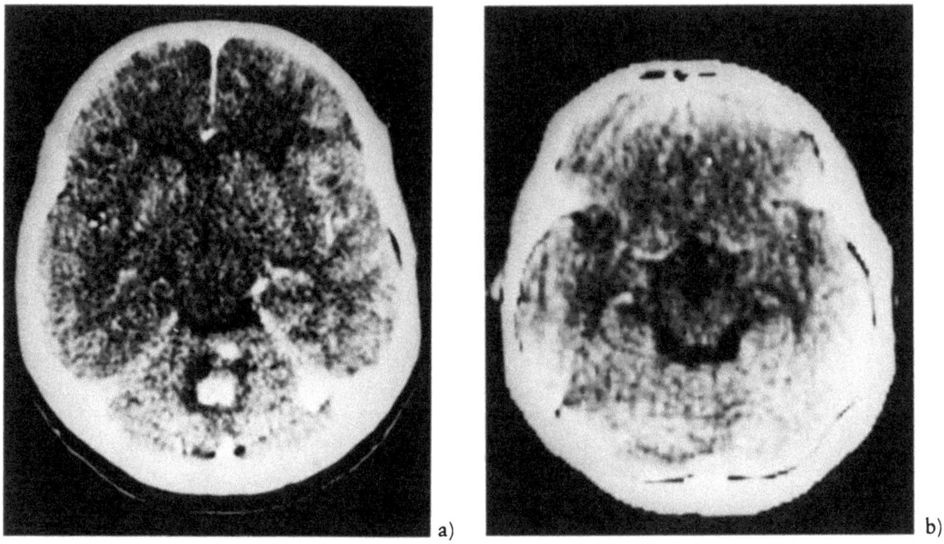

Fig. 5 This cerebellar metastasis from a carcinoma of the breast (a) had disappeared completely (b) when the patient presented with ataxia, diplopia and psychic disturbances which responded to parenteral vitamin B_1-therapy.

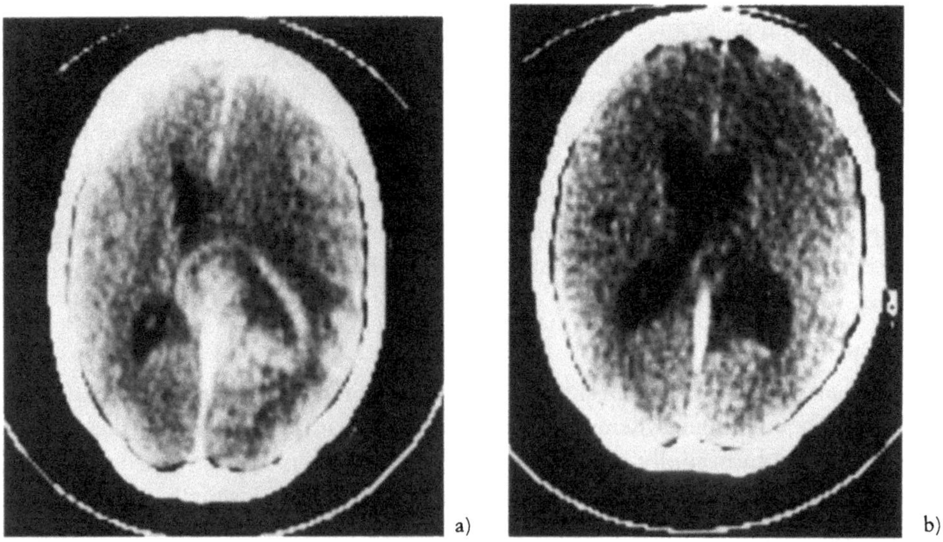

Fig. 6 Good response of the glioblastoma (a) within eight weeks (b), but bad clinical shape caused by chronic purulent pneumonia.

Case 10:
General malaise, apathy, alternating orientation can be both the expression of a central or frontal tumour as well as of a serious secondary illness as, for example, chronic pneumonia with central hypoxia. Therefore, it was possible to improve the condition of this patient only temporarily although over the months the tumour growth was reversed to a great extent (fig. 6). She died of chronic purulent pneumonia.

In complete contrast, a pseudo-remission finally demonstrate a further possibility of misinterpretation of a CT finding:

Case 11:
In September 1982 this patient was operated on for a right occipital glioblastoma (fig. 7 a) which recurred in January 1983 (fig. 7 b). In Figure 7 b the corpus callosum also appears to be affected. A week of maximum anti-oedema therapy with 96 mg Dexamethason and 600 ml 40% Sorbitd daily and the tumour was hardly recognisable in the CT (fig. 7 c). Only in the high-resolution CT-scan two weeks later under reduced oedema therapy can the tumour again be outlined (fig. 7 d). This also showed that the corpus callosum had, at the most, been only marginally infiltrated. This case demonstrated impressively that high doses of steroids can mask a tumour and the CT findings can simulate a far greater extent of tumour and the involvement of central structures, as the extent of mass displacement by the tumour and the surrounding oedema cannot with certainty be adequately assessed. In critical cases, therefore, a short-term CT check is to be recommended before the final decision about any surgical intervention.

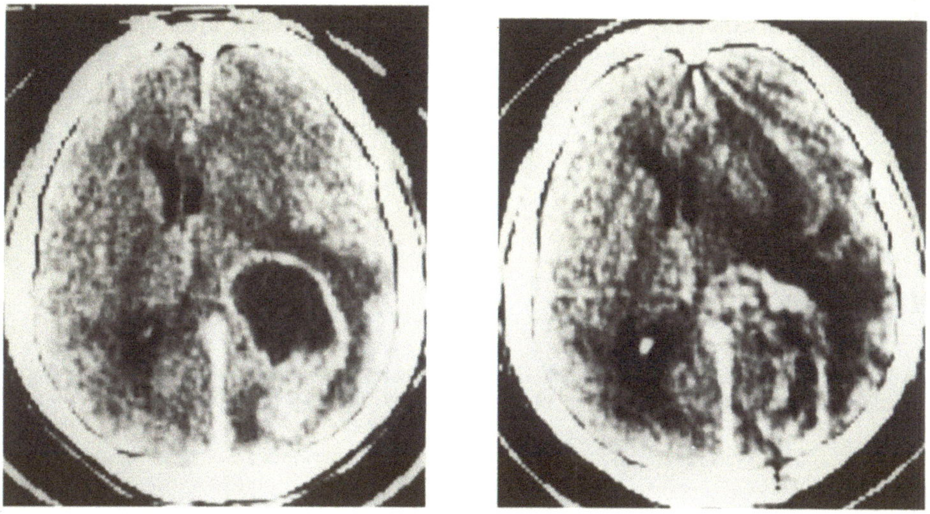

Fig. 7 a) b)

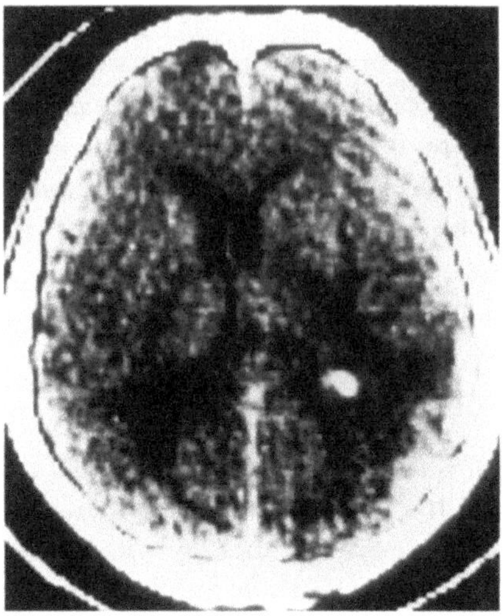

c)

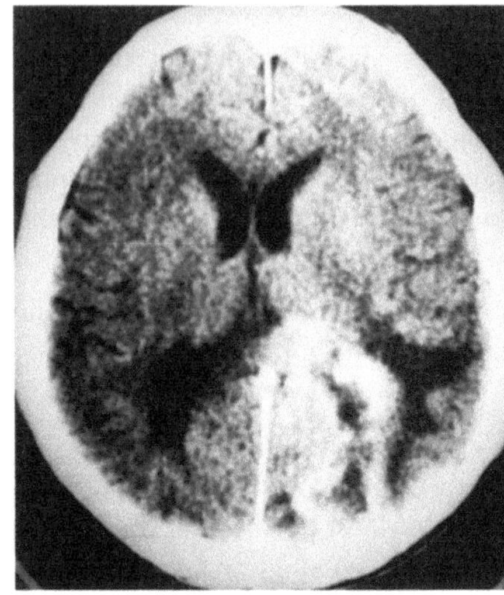

d)

Fig. 7 a) Right occipital glioblastoma in Sept 1982,
b) recurrence (4. 1. 83) suggesting infiltration of the basal ganglia/corpus callosum,
c) tumour hardly visible after one week of intensive anti-oedema therapy,
d) high-resolution scan two weeks later: infiltration of the basal ganglia/corpus callosum is doubtful.

The problems encountered in determining the onset of recurrence in malignant brain tumours are reflected in this collection of cases. In spite of the great accuracy of the CT diagnosis critical cases often need a detailed case control as to the surgical indication and determination of the onset of recurrence in order to make exact decisions. Here especially the amount of any cortisone dosage must also be taken into consideration. Within the range of aggressive combined therapy of malignant brain tumours longer survival times and rare complications such as hormone deficiency, cerebral ischaemia, infections, CSF circulation disorders occur, so that extensive efforts at diagnosis are justified and necessary when there is clinical deterioration in these patients.

References

[1] Poisson, M., J. Philippon, R. van Effenterre et al.: Cerebral pseudocysts following chemotherapy of glioblastomas. Acta Neurochirurgica 39 (1977) 143–149.

Histological-cytological study of the effects of misonidazole and some related substances on the nervous system

P. Glees, K. B. Dawson

Introduction

Tumour cells situated centrally and cut off from oxygen supply resist radiotherapy, but preserve their ability to proliferate. To give the radiation a chance of attacking these cells a biochemical-biophysical approach has been made to sensitize these malignant cells by the application of nitromidazoles [1, 2, 3]. However this preparatory treatment has caused a peripheral neuropathy in 55% of the patients [10].

This neurotoxicity initiated a research project between the Dept. of Biophysics (Royal Marsden Cancer Hospital, Sutton, head Professor G. E. Adams) and the Anatomy Dept., Cambridge with partial support of the Cancer Research Campaign. It was hoped that the special experimental techniques developed in earlier research on neurotoxicity [5, 6] could be employed in this clinically orientated study, which lasted for over five years.

This research project had the following aims:

1. The development of a reliable biological model for assessing neurotoxic threshold, similar to vinca alkaloid studies [12].
2. To investigate whether the neurotoxic damage was morphologically diffuse or whether definite target areas were detectable.
3. Were the signs of neurotoxic damage in animals comparable to those seen in patients.
4. Which neurohistological and ultrastructural changes could be attributed to neurotoxicity directly or whether they were secondary sequels.
5. Special attention was paid to ultrastructural investigations of spinal ganglion cells in view of the clinical picture of neuropathy.

Materials and methods

The animals examined included chickens, rats, cats and primates, whose behaviour especially motor performance was closely observed. Specialised histological techniques are a necessity in any detail study of this type on the central nervous system. For this reason a very careful tissue preparation and fixation and the employment of a battery of neuro-histological and histochemical stains for fatty degeneration were employed, e.g. modified Marchi, for degenerating myelinated nerve tracts, Glees silver method for degenerating neurones and fragmented non-myelinated fibres and their terminations, Hortega's method for revealing microglia reactions and the Cresyl Violet method for demonstrating neuronal chromatolysis. In addition after Glutaraldehyde fixation and suitable embedding selected neuronal areas have been examined for ultrastructural changes, looking first at semi-thin sections at high power in the light microscope and then using ultra-thin sections in the electron microscope.

The investigations very soon showed important species differences in the neural changes caused by misonidazole. Due to the use of specialised techniques in particular, fixation and perfusion, in the detection of some of these changes the amount of information obtainable from human p. m. material was very limited and we had to rely on animal experiments for almost all our data. Our standard substance was misonidazole and we compared other drugs with this. Animals were dosed daily by a suitable route for one, two or three weeks, and were sacrificed two or three weeks after the last dose. This gave time for any lesions to become histologically established.

Observations

Chickens were the first animals to be used as previous experimental work with toxic substances such as tricresyl phosphate. The clear results obtained suggested these birds could also be suitable animals for the present study. Unfortunately, they were relatively resistant to misonidazole given orally and long periods of survival were necessary to see neurological signs such as ataxia, when climbing the ladder and general malaise. Changes were then found in the Purkinje cells of the cerebellum and particularly in the deep cerebellar nuclei (fig. 1) some degeneration of long fibre tracts in the cord occurred, but no evidence of damage to spinal ganglia as seen later in the monkey could be detected. The chick's spinal ganglia are much smaller than those of mammals differently organised and possibly a feathered animal with spiny legs and wings is less prone to show signs of sensory neuropathy. We continued our observations on mammals, using rats, cats and monkeys. Because larger numbers of animals might be needed, if it was necessary to obtain any statistical verification, or

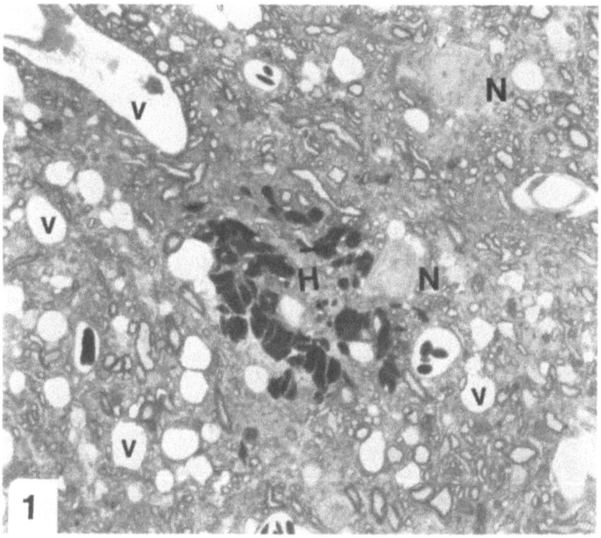

Fig. 1 Misonidazole hen, fixation by perfusion. Haemorrhage (H) in deep cerebellar nuclei. N = neuron, v = vessel. Semithin section. Osmium, toluidin blue × 400.

to examine any of the many variables such as sex or the animal's age, a number of experiments have been done on rats. Some experiments have also been performed on cats. However their histological examination was secondary to a physiological orientated series of experiments and the animals were killed very shortly after the final dose or drug, when definite neurological changes have had no time to fully develop and a more complete comparison could not be made with other species.

It is however from the trials with *primates* that the significant results have been obtained in baboons. We have had the chance to examine selected material of some of these animals, but as the material could not especially be fixed for some of our special histological techniques, it has not been possible to make a complete analysis of the lesions and fibre degeneration observed at higher brain levels. A further opportunity arose to examine primate material (Cynomologus monkeys). Some animals were killed by perfusion with special fixatives and brain, cord and spinal ganglia removed for detailed histological and ultrastructural examination. Two animals had been dosed daily until they showed severe neurological and general symptoms, in others the dosing lasted for a shorter period and the animals were left for two weeks before sacrifice.

In these animals neural lesions were found at lumbar levels of spinal cord, at medullary pontine and midbrain levels (figs. 2–7). These were of *symmetrical size* in both halves of the brain and cord. The focal destruction of neural tissue was of equal extent on both sides. The neural damage consisted of an intense loss of neuropil (terminating axons and branching dendrites) and neuronal cell body loss. The focal

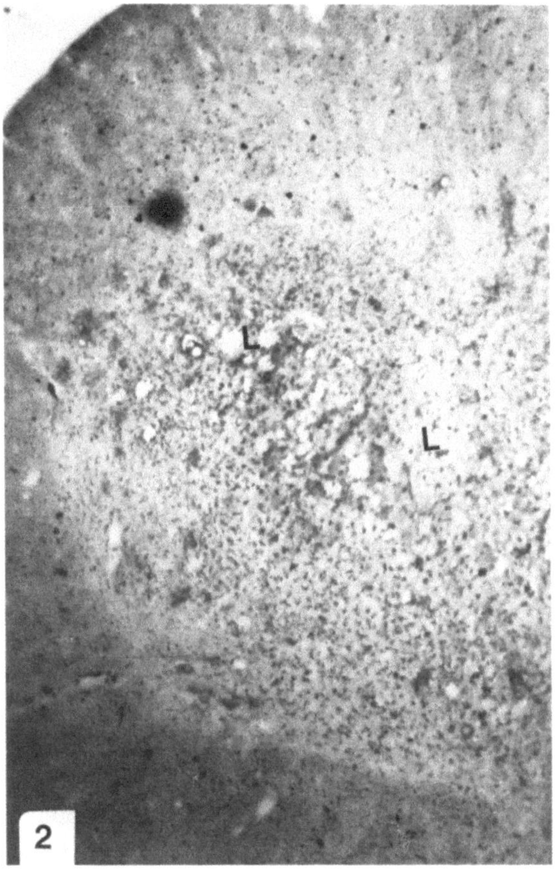

Fig. 2 Misonidazole monkey. Focal destruction (L) of cuneate nucleus in medulla (symmetrical), Marchi stain, low power.

lesions were very circumscribed and sharply delienated from normal tissue. Areas of focal destruction were invaded by microglia or phagocytes which could be followed entering capillary walls. Study of semi-thin Marchi sections counter-stained with Cresyl Violet showed the behaviour of microglia in great detail. These cells break down homogeneously stained neurones which have lost all intracellular organelles. Under high power, some neurones exhibited a vacuolated pattern whilst surrounding microglia cells were laden with fatty debris. Examination of spinal ganglia showed vacuolated neurons due to lipid degeneration of ultrastructure (figs. 8–11). A great number of cells were still normal showing centrally placed nucleus, well ordered granulated endoplasmic reticulum, clusters of ribosomes with normally spaced mitochondria. The toxic neurons seen in semi-thin sections and in electron microscopic pictures, however show all these organelles at varying stages of degeneration. In the cord, apart from some myelinated fibre degeneration in the posterior columns, no significant degeneration of long ascending or descending tracts was seen.

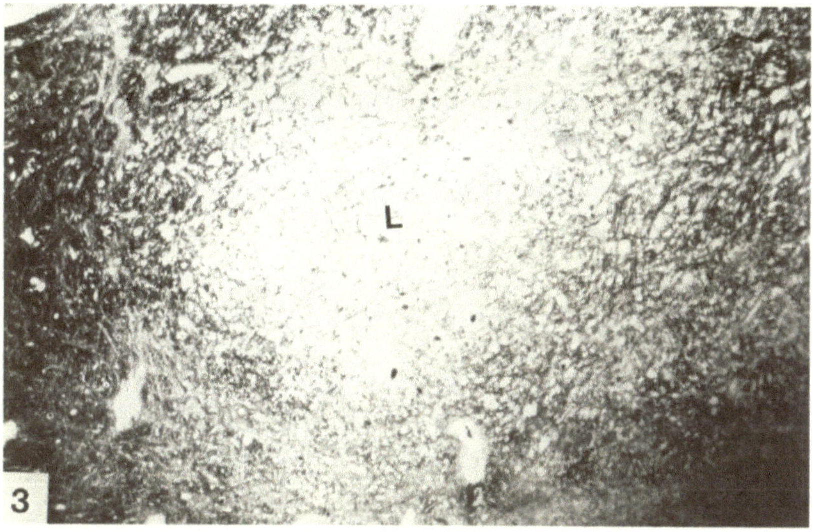

Fig. 3 Misonidazole monkey. Focal lesion (L) at medullary level (symmetrical), both lateral reticular nuclei). Complete loss of nerve fibres and cells. Glees silver stain × 200.

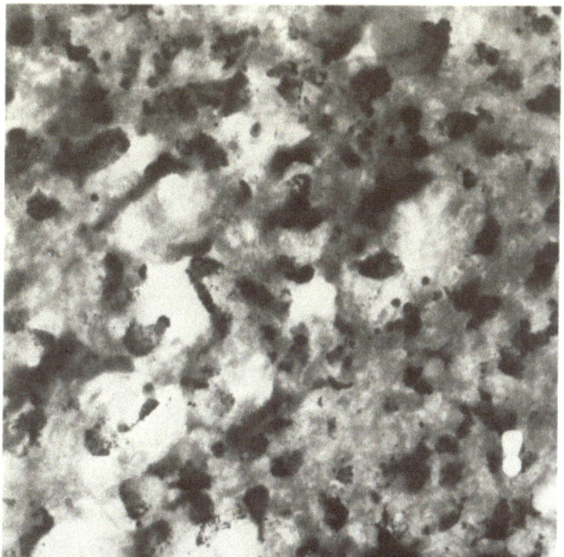

Fig. 4 Misonidazole monkey. Focal lesion in ventral horn of lumbar cord. Massive invasion of fat laden microglia cells stained black by Osmium × 200.

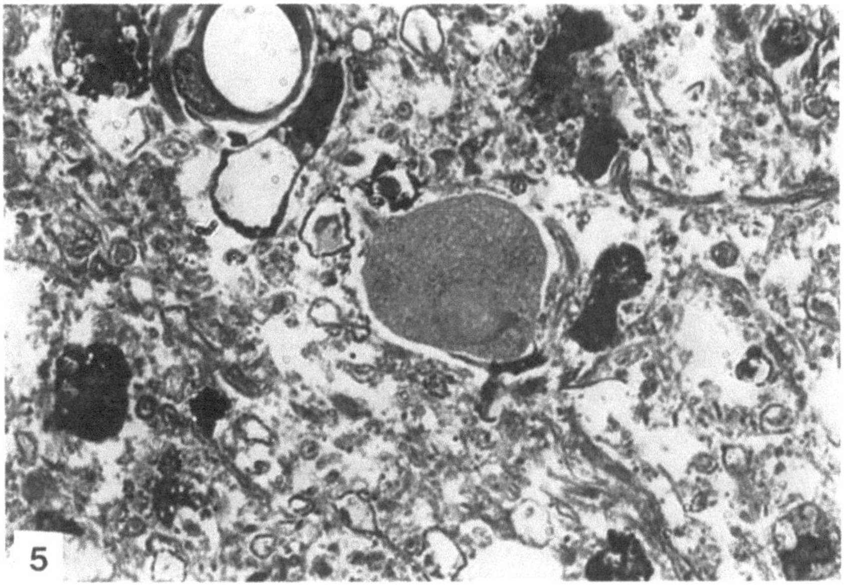

Fig. 5 Misonidazole monkey. Degenerating structureless neuron and disintegrating neurophil. Semithin section. Toluidin blue, × 1000.

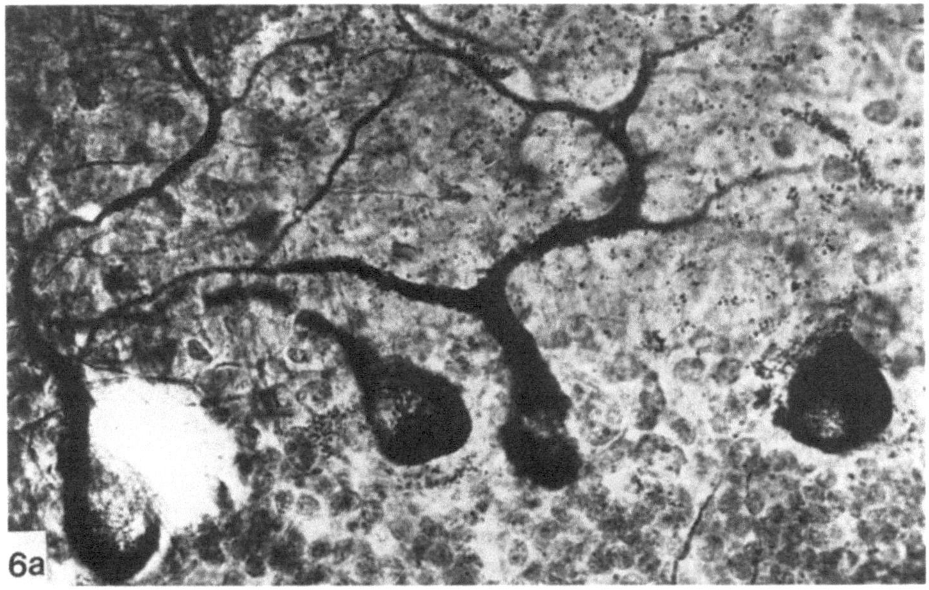

Fig. 6a Misonidazole monkey. Degeneration of Purkinje cells. Loss of climbing fibres, basket fibres and tangential fibres. The picture exhibits typical terminal degeneration in form of fine silver granules. × 600. Compare with figure 7.

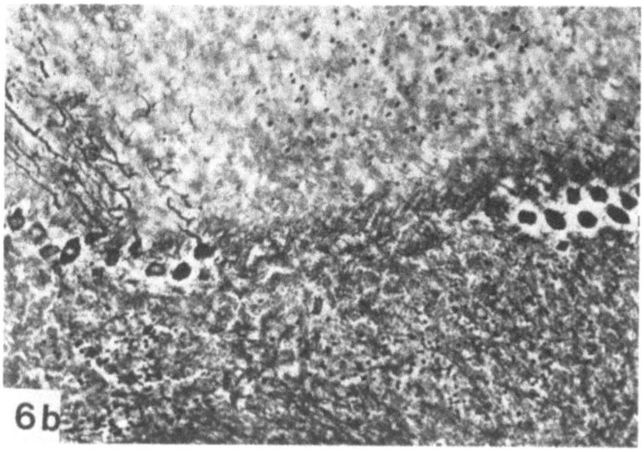

Fig. 6b Misonidazole monkey. Numerous degenerating Purkinje cells.

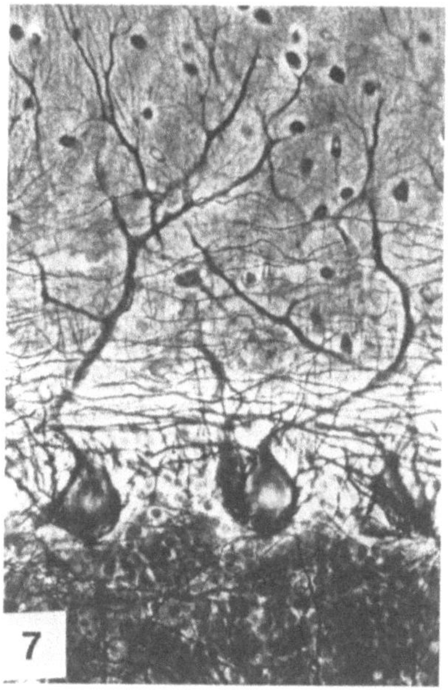

Fig. 7 Control monkey cerebellum, note normal cell bodies and fibre pattern. Glees silver × 300.

A similar but smaller study was undertaken in Cynomologus monkeys with a modified misonidazole. After a dose of this drug twice the size of that which produced very severe symptoms in the misonidazole treated monkeys, these animals appeared perfectly healthy. A detailed histological study showed the appearance of some very slight changes, but these were in the histological "grey region" in the sense that they could have been normal age variations, fixation artefacts or the beginning of toxicological changes. Because this drug was going into clinical trial the investigation was continued in rats dosed at high levels for a week and then killed at weekly

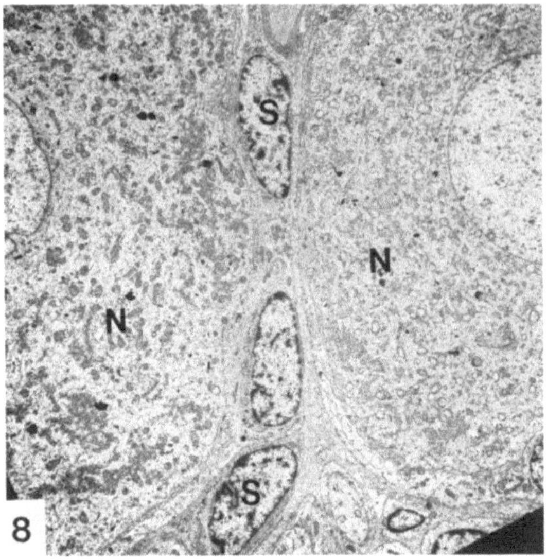

Fig. 8 Control monkey. EM picture of spinal ganglion neurons (N) showing normal distribution and appearance of ultrastructure, e. g. mitochondria and endoplasmic reticulum, only few osmiophilic granules visible. S = satellite cell nucleus.

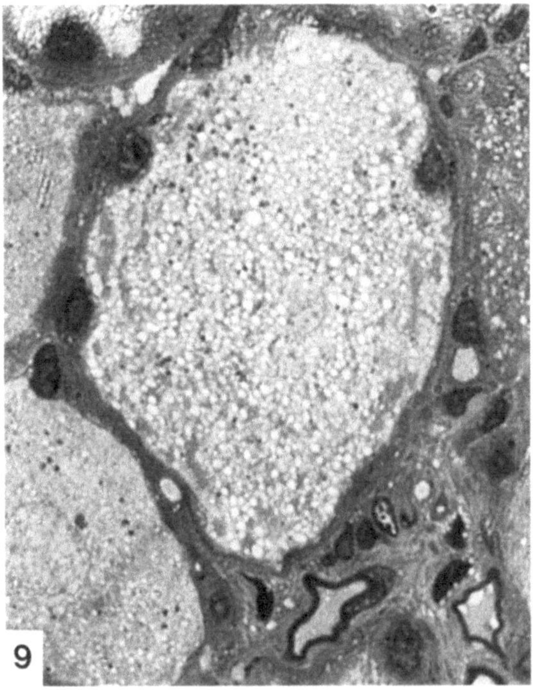

Fig. 9 Misonidazole monkey. Lipid degeneration of a spinal ganglion neuron. Semithin section, toluidin blue, × 1000.

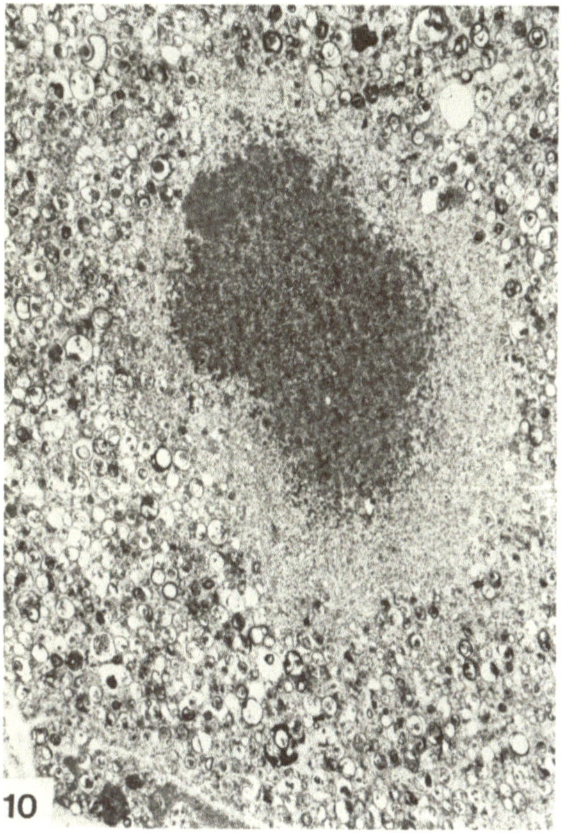

Fig. 10 Misonidazole monkey. Spinal ganglion neuron. E. M. Severe destruction of ultrastructure, × 2000.

intervals or dosed continually for three weeks. Of these animals, those dosed chronically and sacrificed two weeks after ceasing dosing showed very slight histological reactions. Nothing significant in the brain but a mild positive Marchi reaction in the anterior medial tract of the spinal cord. The neurones of these fibres are most likely vestibular and reticular spinal tract neurones which were always involved in the misonidazole experiments in chickens. It suggests this is an early sign of neurotoxicity. In summary, one can say that the drug coded '8799' RMH is not free of neurotoxicity but is considerably less toxic in equivalent amounts than misonidazole.

From the work we have done to date, we finally conclude that any investigation of this type of drug must at some stage involve the use of primates, but preliminary screening or testing should not exclude rodents.

To examine two of the promising drugs (RSU 1047 and 1069) synthesised at Sutton we have used marmosets. These are small lower primates, but have the advantage

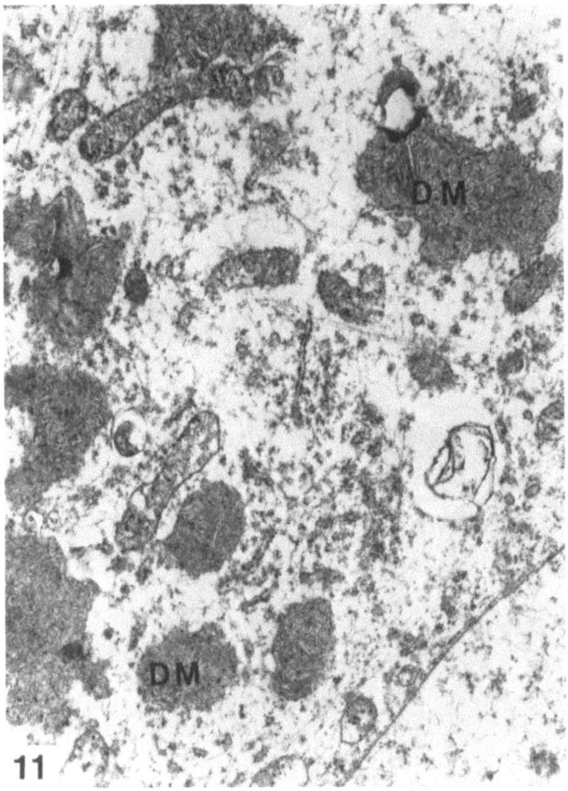

Fig. 11 Misonidazole monkey. Spinal ganglion neuron. E. M. Degenerating mitochondria (DM), × 5000.

that they have been laboratory bred for some generations, and are more easily maintained and handled than most monkeys.

To establish suitable doses of the untested drugs from the known dose of misonidazole that would cause marked neurotoxicity in a monkey and the known LD_{50} dose of misonidazole, '1047' and '1069' in rodents, we gave corresponding doses of these drugs in the marmoset experiments. Control animals and a misonidazole treated animal as standard, were examined at the same time, animals were dosed by the appropriate route (i. p. and i. v. for '1047', orally for misonidazole and '1069') for a week and then sacrificed by perfusing with fixative two weeks later.

The misonidazole treated marmoset showed just the same pattern and type of change that was seen in the Cynomologus monkey and is described above. Neither of the two animals treated with '1047' showed any evidence of neurotoxicity or any effects of the drug.

The first '1069' animal appeared perfectly normal during dosing but ten days later (i.e. four days before the projected end of the test) this normally very active animal appeared listless and very ill, and was trying to vomit and lost quite a lot of weight (13%). It was killed at this time by perfusion. No superficial changes seen at p. m. but major organs taken for histological examination as well as the brain and spinal cord. In terms of neurotoxicity, there was a lesion at midbrain level, between the superior colliculus and the lower thalamus with some microglia reaction. In the lumbar and cervical cord there was some pseudo-Marchi reaction due to the dissection which could have obscured any genuine Marchi reaction. Silver staining of the spinal cord, pons and cerebellum showed that the larger neurons and in particular the Purkinje cells of the cerebellum showed definite pathology such as altered cell bodies and gross swelling and enlarged dendritic processes. In the viscera the only change was a very small lesion in the liver, but severe changes were seen in the kidney (fig. 12). In contrast the second animal treated with this drug appeared perfectly normal throughout the experiment apart from a very small weight loss and at sacrifice showed no evidence of neurotoxicity in the CNS. The electron microscope sections of all these animals have yet to be examined but the light-microscopy is complete and from this we can conclude [1] the marmoset appears to be a perfectly suitable animal for investigation, [2] the drug 'RSU 1047' is non-neurotoxic at comparable doses producing marked neurotoxicity with misonidazole. We [3] cannot yet make any categorical statements about 'RSU 1069'.

Discussion and summary

The neurotoxicity of misonidazole (2-nitro-imidazole) originally used in protozoal infections – had been recognised in clinical trials [10] not only in cancer treatment but also in treating other conditions such as Morbus Crohn [4].

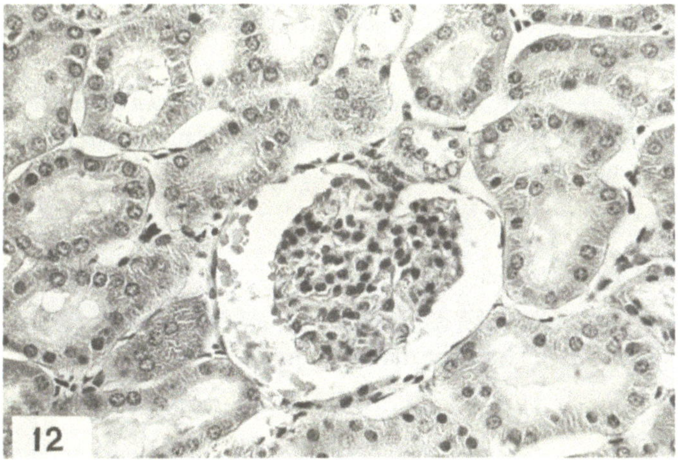

Fig. 12 Misonidazole monkey. Kidney. Shrunken glomerulus shows pycnotic nuclei and space of Bowman and renal tubules contain hyaline material.

Numerous experimental investigations have confirmed the neurotoxicity of misonidazole and drawn special attention to central lesions [7, 8]. A careful study of this kind using the conventional animal model, the rat, is from Griffin et al. [9], who review the literature as well and should be consulted. Griffin et al. believe that the CNS pathology found, resembles thiamine deficiency, but adding thiamine to the diet, did not prevent the neurotoxicity. The underlying disease process, apart from embolic or haemorrhagic lesions appears to be fundamentally different from an inflammatory infectious event. It is different also from the dying back process seen in studies of organic phosphate intoxication [6] or thiamine deficiency. Misonidazole appears to interact primarily with capillary endothelial and neuronal mitochondria, causing in the latter their complete degeneration leading to neuronal cell death and rapid removal of neuronal debris by massive microglia invasion. This direct action on neuronal ultrastructure is clearly seen in the spinal ganglia of primates. Spinal ganglia neurons apart from satellite cells have no protection from neurotoxic agents due to the absence of a blood-brain barrier in the capillary circulation. Pannese [11] has shown that invaginations of the connective tissue spaces into the spinal ganglion satellites are present which follow the outer contour of the satellite cell sheath (c. f. Pannese, fig. 20). These two factors might explain the greater vulnerability of these neurons in toxicity expressed in peripheral neuropathy as a first stage. These facts have been insufficiently considered in previous studies on toxicity. It is of interest too, that haemorrhages have never been seen in spinal ganglia of primates used in these studies which showed distinct central lesions including interstitial bleedings.

We believe therefore that overlapping causes for central nervous lesions exist, haemorrhage and toxic action on neuronal ultrastructure, but that peripherally, the spinal ganglia exhibit primary neurotoxic damage. The screening of these neurons by the satellite cell sheaths is less efficient than the glial envelopes centrally as the connective tissue space invaginations into satellite cytoplasm come close to the neuronal membranes.

Neurotoxic experiments should be extended to primates, as we have seen definite ultrastructural changes in spinal ganglia of primates. This can explain the peripheral neuropathy seen in man, the highest primate.

Acknowledgements

We wish to thank J. F. Crane, John Almond and Ann Muir for their technical assistance and the Cancer Research Campaign for funding.

Special thanks are due to Professor Enrico Pannese for his discussions on spinal ganglia ultrastructure.

References

[1] Adams, G. E.: Chemical radiosensitization of hypoxic cells. Brit. Med. Bull. **29** (1973) 48.

[2] Adams, G. E., D. L. Dewey: Hydrated electrons and radiobiological sensitization. Biochim. Biophys. Res. Commun. **12** (1963) 473.

[3] Asquith, J. C., M. E. Watts, K. Patel et al.: Electron affinic sensitization v. radiosensitization of hypoxic bacteria and mammalian cells in vitro by some nitroimidazoles and nitropyrazoles. Radiat. Res. **60** (1974) 108.

[4] Druschky, K. F., K. A. Flugel, H. Daun et al.: Zur Metronidazol-Polyneuropathie. Verhandlungen der Deutschen Gesellschaft für Neurologie **2**, pp. 580–584. Springer-Verlag, Berlin–Heidelberg–New York–Tokyo 1983.

[5] Glees, P.: Terminal degeneration within the central nervous system as studied by a new silver method. J. Neuropathol. Exp. Neurol. **5** (1946) 54–59.

[6] Glees, P.: A morphological and neurological analysis of neurotoxicity illustrated by tricrecylphosphate intoxication in the chick. Neurotox. Drugs **8** (1966) 136–148.

[7] Glees, P., J. Almond: Experimental studies of neurotoxicity in birds. J. Anat. **133** (1981) 239.

[8] Glees, P., K. Dawson: Vergleichende tierexperimentelle Untersuchungen über die Neurotoxidität von Radiosensitizers. Verhandlungen der Deutschen Gesellschaft für Neurologie **2**, pp. 725–728. Springer-Verlag, Berlin–Heidelberg–New York–Tokyo 1983.

[9] Griffin, J. W., D. L. Price, D. O. Kuethe et al.: Neurotoxicity of Misonidazole in Rats. 1. Neuropathology I. **299** (1979) 312.

[10] Moore, J. L., I. C. M. Paterson, P. J. D. K. Dawes et al.: Misonidazole in patients receiving radical radiotherapy: Pharmacokinetic effects of Phenytoin tumor response and neurotoxicity. Int. J. Radiat. Oncol. Biol. Phys. **8** (1982) 361–364.

[11] Pannese, E.: The satellite cells of the sensory ganglia. Advances in Anatomy, Embryology and Cell Biology **65**, pp. 1–111. Springer-Verlag, Berlin–Heidelberg–New York 1981.

[12] Todd, G. C., W. J. Griffin, W. R. Gibson et al.: Animal models for the comparative assessment of neurotoxicity following repeated administration of vinca alkaloids. Cancer Treatment Reports **63** (1979) 35–41.

Local, intratumoral chemotherapy of brain gliomas in the rat, using adriamycin – a preliminary report

B. Rama, H. D. Mennel, M. Altmannsberger, M. Holzgraefe

Introduction

Chemotherapy for patients with brain gliomas, as compared with their treatment by operation and radiotherapy, has not significantly lengthened the duration of survival. According to generally accepted opinion the blood-brain barrier is responsible for this. As it may be supposed that no barrier exists within a brain tumour, in contrast to the periphery, if an effective chemotherapeutic agent is introduced directly into the tumour the blood-brain barrier will be avoided.

Up to the present this concept of treatment has not succeeded either in animal experiments or clinically. The results were unsatisfactory or were not unequivocal to evaluate, as the intraneoplastic (i. n.) chemotherapy was given in combination with radiotherapy and immunotherapy or other systemically administered chemotherapy [9]. For this reason it seemed first of all necessary to carry out i. n. treatment with only one drug (Adriamycin, ADM), in order to confirm the efficacy or otherwise of such intraneoplastic chemotherapeutic agents.

Material and methods

1. Adriamycin* is an anthracyclin antiobiotic. The chemotherapeutic effect is cell-cycle specific. Apart from the well-known side effects of chemotherapeutic drugs, Adriamycin shows a characteristic cardiotoxicity [1].

ADM was injected stereotactically into the right frontal lobe of BD IX rats in concentrations of 0.5 μg to 20 μg/10 μl injection volume, or in doses of 5.5 μg/kg body weight up to 222 μg/kg body weight.

After three days and 1, 2, 3, 4, and 8 weeks the rats were perfused with formalin (one part 37% neutral formalin + nine parts distilled water).

* Kindly supplied by Farmitalia Carlo Erba.

2. The heart muscle from the animals treated with ADM was examined by light and electron microscopy.

3. The brain tumours which had originally been induced by transplacental ethyl-nitroso-urea [6] were continuously inoculated into isologous BD IX rats. The transplantation was carried out stereotactically putting 20 µl of a tumour cell suspension into the right frontal lobe. The survival time was determined. The animals were finally perfused with formalin (v. s.). The brain tumours were histologically examined after being stained with cresyl violet or H & E.

4. ADM was injected into the tumour using the same coordinates as were used for injecting the tumour cells. The dosage was 10 µg ADM/10 µl (volume) or 111 µg, 90 µg and 71 µg ADM/kg body weight and was given on the 4th, 6th, 8th and tenth day after the tumour transplantation.

Perfusion and histological examination followed as described above.

Results

1. After intracerebral ADM injection the animals showed no alterations in their behaviour up to the time of the perfusion. No obvious neurological deficits such as e. g. hemiparesis, were apparent.

The extent of the morphological changes in the brain, in the way of intracerebral and subarachnoid bleeding and necrosis were dependent on the dose and the duration of the action.

Eventually large cysts were produced by a dose of more than 100 µg/kg body weight.

2. In the heart muscle of the animals treated with ADM there was no evidence of any morphological changes.

3. In the preterminal stages all animals had a hemiparesis. The median survival time for 20 continuously transplanted rats was 12 days (fig. 1). The growth of the transplanted tumours was mainly intracerebral, but occasionally also slightly subdural. The extracerebral growth of the tumours is the result of misplacement of tumour cells caused by the injection and should be avoided by a more precise technique. Histologically the tumour resembled an undifferentiated glioma.

4. Local chemotherapy of the rats brain tumour on the tenth and the eighth days after the tumour transplant did not prolong the survival time as compared with the untreated rats. The injection of ADM on the fourth day after tumour transplantation extended the median survival time to 19 days (fig. 1). The tumour is filled with haemorrhages right up to its surface (fig. 2). The histological picture shows a marked breaking up of the tissue taking place, going on to cyst formation. Giant cells have been formed, which is typical for glial tumours treated by chemotherapy (fig. 3).

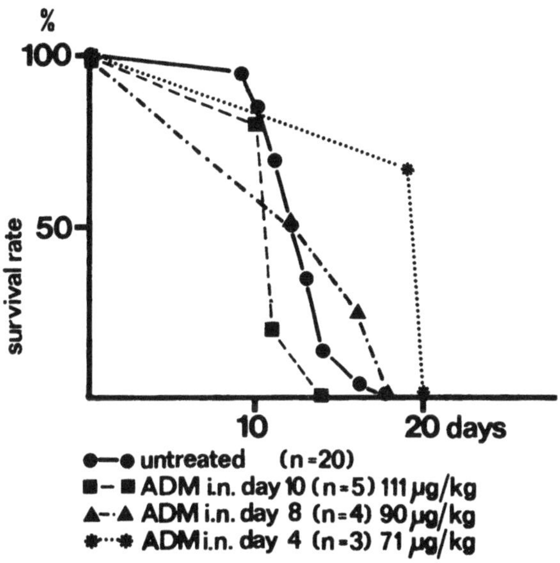

Fig. 1 Survival rates of untreated tumour-bearing rats and also of rats whose tumours were treated with intraneoplastic (i. n.) Adriamycin (ADM) on the tenth, eighth and fourth day after tumour transplantation.

Discussion

If we accept the idea that the function of the blood-brain (or blood-tumour) barrier is also effective in the opposite direction, that is in the sense of a 'tumour-blood' barrier, we have, in spite of notes of warning in the literature chosen Adriamycin for the local intraneoplastic treatment of brain tumours in rats.

After intrathecal administration of ADM [7] and after intra-arterial use with osmotic influences on the blood-brain barrier [8] severe or even fatal sequelae have been described.

ADM has been tested as systemic treatment in many malignant tumours. Its neurotoxic effect [2, 4] suggests that it may also be effective for the treatment of intrinsic brain tumours. As ADM does not pass the blood-brain barrier it seems appropriate to use it for local treatment. In this respect it can already be detected intracellularly after 12 minutes [10].

Our initial experiences with this treatment are:

1. The toxicity of the locally administered treatment is less than after treatment as described above.
2. The early intra-neoplastic injection of ADM leads to a prolongation of the median survival time of about 60%. Of course, it must be admitted that we are not dealing

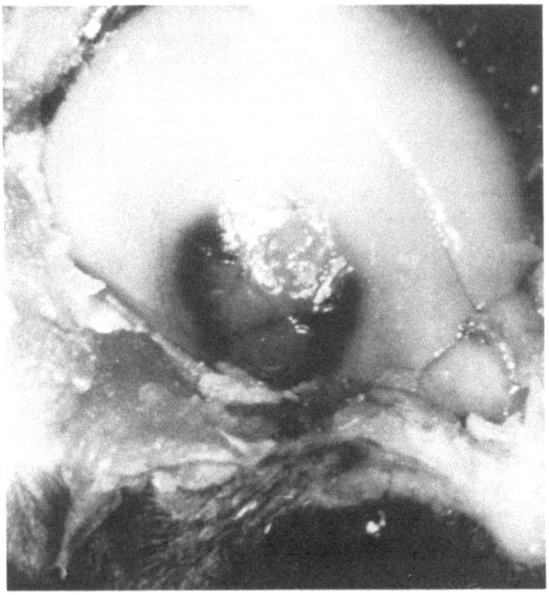

Fig. 2 Right frontal tumour in a rat, who survived 19 days. On the fourth day after the tumour inoculation 71 μg/ADM/kg were injected stereotactically into the tumour.

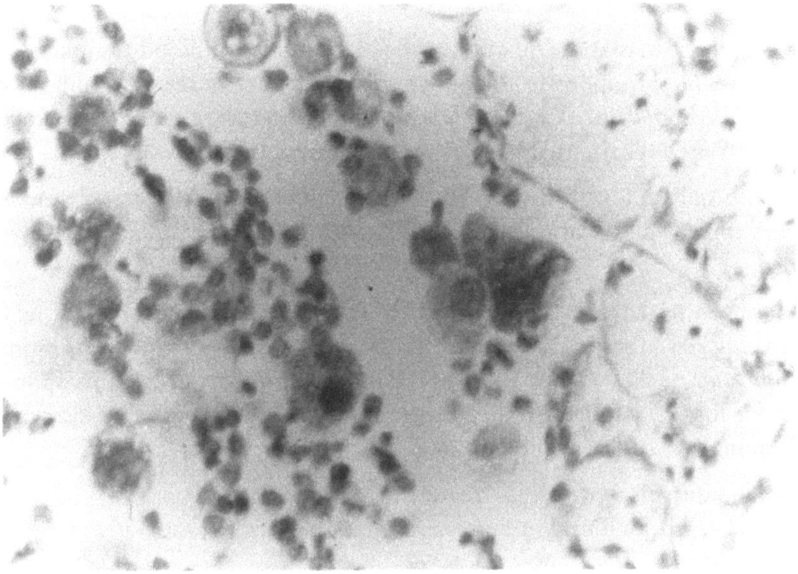

Fig. 3 Tumour after i. n. ADM injection. The appearance suggests an infarct with cavitation, oedema formation, cysts, giant cells (Cresyl violet × 77).

with a randomised series, and secondly that the results are i. n. chemotherapy with CCNU for transplanted ependymoblastomas in mice [11] were better.

3. The morphological alterations in our researches were confined to the region of the tumour. As regards this finding, further explanations must be sought.

Summary

It has been established that rats survive after an intracerebral injection of ADM (up to 200 µg/kg) and no serious deficits result. Brain tumours in the rat originally induced transplacentally with ethyl-nitroso-urea were regularly transplanted. The intraneoplastic treatment of this tumour with ADM was able to prolong the median survival time.

References

[1] Bühner, R., J. Henrichs, R. Gottschalk: Charakterisierung und Vergleich der klinischen und morphologischen Veränderungen bei der Adriamycin-Kardiomyopathie. Onkologie **2** (1979) 24–27.

[2] Cho, E. S.: Toxic effects of adriamycin on the ganglia of the peripherial nervous system: a neuropathological study. J. Neuropathol. Exp. Neurol. **36** (1977) 907–915.

[3] Füllenbach, D., G. A. Nagel, S. Seeber: Adriamycin-Symposium. S. Karger Verlag, Basel 1981.

[4] Jortner, B. S., E. S. Cho: Neurotoxicity of adriamycin in rats: a low-dose effect. Cancer Treat Rep **64** (1980) 257–261.

[5] Long, J. M.: Capillary ultrastructure and the blood-brain barrier in human malignant brain tumors. J. Neurosurg. **39** (1970) 127–144.

[6] Mennel, H. D.: Transplantation of tumors of the nervous system induced by resorptive carcinogens. I. Histological investigation of intracerebrally transplanted tumors of the central nervous system. Neurosurg. Rev. **1** (1978) 123–131.

[7] Merker, P. C., M. R. Lewis, M. D. Walker et al.: Neurotoxicity of adriamycin (doxorubicin) perfused through the cerebrospinal fluid spaces of the rhesus monkey. Toxicol. Appl. Pharmacol. **44** (1978) 191–205.

[8] Neuwelt, E. A., M. Pagel, P. Barnett et al.: Pharmacology and toxicity of intracarotid adriamycin administration following osmotic blood-brain barrier modification. Cancer Res. **41** (1981) 4466–4470.

[9] Shimura, T., S. Nakazawa: Intraneoplastic local injection of adriamycin for malignant brain tumor chemotherapy. A clinicopathological study. No Shinkei Geka **8** (1980) 35–42.

[10] Shimura, T., S. Nakazawa, K. Aihara: Intraneoplastic local injection of adriamycin for the treatment of experimental brain tumor. An autoradiographic study. J. Nippon Med. Sch. **49** (1982) 134–136.

[11] Tator, C. H.: Intraneoplastic injection of CCNU for experimental brain tumor chemotherapy. Surg. Neurol. **7** (1977) 73–77.

IV Chemotherapy: Basic principles, experiences, results and alternative procedures

Principles of cancer treatment with cytostatic agents (Brief communication)

G. Zeile

Cancer is a global problem and demands a number of different therapeutic interventions. In a generalised stage of cancer operation and irradiation offer no or little hope. Cytostatica too are incapable to fulfil a lasting hope of tumour regression or a cure. Tumour growth inhibiting substances should however be given if subjective complaints have to be reduced or some improvement in the quality of life.

In case of disseminating glioma satisfactory therapeutic results in cytostatic polychemical therapy are still exceptional.

Progress in treatment presupposes a precise knowledge of the properties of anticancer drugs. This is the only safeguard in the narrow field between growth inhibition of the tumour and the toxic side effects on the total organism. Cytostatica are classified according to their origin and action in alcaloids, anti-metabolites, mitotic inhibitors, anti-biotica and hormones. Their action is mainly the interference of nucleic acid synthesis (DNS, RNS, and protein synthesis). Future therapeutic aims must be directed to vary the combination of cytostatica and to test the efficiency in randomised, prospective studies.

Chemotherapy of malignant gliomas – present state of treatment
(Brief communication)

P. Gutjahr

Operation and radiotherapy have proved to be unsatisfactory for treating malignant glioma. Additional treatment, such as cytostatica are urgently needed [1, 2, 3, 4].

Before computertomography it was believed that the mono-therapy with some cytostatica has caused an improvement or partial remission in the condition of the patient, based on clinical and subjective impressions. Examining the relevant literature of the past eight years (tab. 1), which reports the use of lipid soluble cytostatica of the nitroso-urea substances on their own or in combination an improvement in the outcome is not apparent [4]. The present state concerning chemotherapy of primary brain tumours has been critically evaluated, in particular against the background of side effects.

Table 1 Median survival according to the method of treatment in the principal controlled studies after adjuvant nitrosoureas (BCNU, CCNU, Me-CCNU) (after [3])

Treatment	No. of evaluable cases	Median survival (months)
Surgery		3.7
BCNU	223	5.8
Radiotherapy		8.6
Radiotherapy + BCNU		9.3
Radiotherapy	22	11.5
CCNU	22	6.6
Radiotherapy + CCNU	19	12.0
Radiotherapy		8.2
Me-CCNU	332	7.1
Radiotherapy + Me-CCNU		7.1
Radiotherapy + BCNU		7.1
Radiotherapy	32	10.5
Radiotherapy + BCNU	34	12.5
Radiotherapy + CCNU	36	17.0

References

[1] EORTC Brain Tumour Group: Effect of CCNU on survival rate of objective remission and duration of free interval in patients with malignant brain glioma – Final evaluation. Europ. J. Cancer **14** (1978) 851–856.

[2] Kornblith, P. L., M. D. Walker, J. R. Cassady: Neoplasm of the Central Nervous System. In: Cancer – Principles and practice of oncology (V. T. DeVita Jr., S. Hellman, S. A. Rosenberg, eds.), pp. 1181–1253. Lippincott, Philadelphia–Toronto 1982.

[3] Monfardini, S., K. Brunner, D. Crowther, et al. (eds.): Manual of Cancer Chemotherapy (UICC Technical Reports, vol. 56), pp. 165–167. Union Internationale Contre le Cancer, Geneva 1981.

[4] Walker, M. D., S. B. Green, D. P. Byar: Randomized comparisons of radiotherapy and nitrosoureas for malignant glioma after surgery. N. Engl. J. Med. **303** (1980) 1323–1329.

Chemotherapy of malignant supratentorial gliomas in adult: a ten-year experience of the EORTC Brain Tumour Group

J. Hildebrand

Methods

Within the last ten years, the EORTC Brain Tumour Group has performed six cooperative studies. Three of them [1, 2, 3] are phase III type randomized and controlled essays. The trial 26801 is in addition a double-blind study.

The aim of these phase III type trials was to test the effect of respectively CCNU (trial 26741), VM-26 + CCNU (trial 26751) or mizonidazole, a radiosensitizer of anoxic cells (trial 26801) on *the duration of the free interval* defined as the time between the operation and a relapse of neurological signs, and *the total survival.* All the patients in the trials 26741 and 26751 were irradiated with 5500 to 6000 rads, given in 30 fractions over sex weeks. In most patients 4000 rads were delivered to the whole cranium and a 2000-rad buster to the tumour bed. The schedule of radiotherapy was modified (in order to give the radiosensitizer the best theoretical chance of being active) in the trial 26801 where patients received nine fractions of 350 rads in three weeks, four hours before each irradiation, 1.3 g/m^2 of mizonidazole were given by mouth. In addition, during the next two weeks, six fractions of 300 rads completed the treatment. The administration of CCNU or VM-26 + CCNU was started concomitantly with radiotherapy at doses indicated in table 1. In each trial the given doses of chemotherapy actually given were close to 80% of the scheduled doses, whereas the actual doses of mizonidazole given were almost 100%.

The criteria for patient's selection were the same in all studies:

a) optimal removal of histologically proven supratentorial malignant glioma,
b) over 16 years old,
c) quantitatively evaluable postoperative neurological examination, and an expected survival of eight weeks or more,
d) steroid administration had to be stopped on the tenth day after operation. All the treated patients as well as the controls were followed up every four weeks until the recurrence.

Results

The results given in table 1 show that neither CCNU nor VM-26 plus CCNU nor mizonidazole given during radiotherapy are able to prolong the free interval or the survival time. It is important to note that these two factors appeared remarkably reproducible from one study to another, and should therefore be considered as adequate criteria for the evaluation of an adjuvant chemotherapy in malignant brain tumours.

Regardless of the treatment given the same prognostic factors for the free interval and the survival emerged from every study. The most significant of these are age, performance status, and frontal location. The distribution of patients according to the main prognostic factors was comparable in the two arms of each trial.

The length and the rate of objective remissions, defined in our studies as a clear-cut clinical improvement of at least one neurological sign persisting for at least four weeks after a complete discontinuation of corticosteroids was evaluated in trials 26741 [1], 26751 [2], 26781 [4]. The results are given in table 2.

Table 1 Results of phase-III type studies

Trial	No of patients	Agent	Dose	Free interval T (weeks)	Free interval C (weeks)	Survival T (weeks)	Survival C (weeks)
26 741	81	CCNU	130 mg/m²/ 6 weeks	34.5	31.0	43	62*
26 751	116	VM-26 + CCNU	100 mg/m²/ 6 weeks + 130 mg/m²/ 6 weeks	39.0	30.7	58	61.1**
26 801	163	Mizonidazole	12 g/m² total dose	30	30	50	51

T = treated; C = controls

* received CCNU (1-(2-chloroethyl)-3-cyclohexyl-1-nitrosourea) after relapse

** received CCNU or VM-26 (4'dimethyl-epipodophyllotoxine-D-therylidene-glucoside) plus CCNU after relapse

Table 2 Results of phase-II type studies

Trial	No of patients	Drug	Doses	Objective remissions Number	Rate (%)	Length (months)
26 741	28	CCNU	130 mg/m²/ 6 weeks	8	28	3 to 18
26 751	16	CCNU		3	19	3½, 3½, 16
26 751	19	VM-26 + CCNU	130 mg/m²/ 6 weeks + 100 mg/m²/ 6 weeks	3	16	4, 19, 20
26 751	17	Procarbazine**	150–200 mg/d for 21 days	0	0	
26 781	29	DDMP*	75 mg/m²/ week × 5	2	7	3½, 18
26 811	34	AZQ***	10–20 mg/m²/ day × 5.q. 28 days	3	11	1, 2½, 20

* DDMP (2,4-Diamino-5-3′, 4′ Dichlorphenyl-6-Methylpyrimidine)

** Given to patients who relapsed while receiving VM-26 plus CCNU

*** AZQ (Diaziquone (2,5,-bis-1-aziridinyl-3,6-dioxo-1, 4-cyclohexadiene-1, 4-diyl) bis (carbamate)

Discussion

Considering the effects obtained on different clinical findings measured in our studies, apparently contradictory results have been obtained, probably because these findings do not measure exactly the same phenomenon. Therefore, the effects on different clinical signs and symptoms should be considered separately.

As with many authors [5, 6], we have found that CCNU, like other nitrosourea derivatives such as BCNU or methyl-CCNU, produces clinical improvements of the neurological status. The length of the remissions observed in our trials are comparable to those in the literature but their rate is lower.

The discrepancy is partly due to the fact that complete discontinuation of steroids and an improvement (not only a stabilisation) was required in our studies to meet the criteria of an objective remission. The activity of CCNU was not enhanced by VM-26. The activity of DDMP or AZQ appeared modest. Although the effectiveness of these agents was not compared with that of the nitrosourea derivatives in controlled or randomized studies, we feel that, when used alone, they are less active than BCNU or CCNU in malignant supratentorial brain gliomas. Procarbazine was given in our study only when nitrosoureas failed and appeared inactive, but much better results for procarbazine were reported by Wilson et al. [7].

Survival and duration of the free interval were not prolonged by CCNU nor VM-26 plus CCNU. Therefore we do not recommend the use of these agents as adjuvant chemotherapy but only after a recurrence. In contrast with our data (which are concerned with CCNU and VM-26 plus CCNU), the US Brain Tumour Study Group reported repeatedly that the percentage of long-term survivors was significantly increased by the postoperative administration of BCNU. Since chemotherapy, at least as it was used by our group, was ineffective in prolonging the free interval, we attempted to enhance the activity of radiation therapy, which is definitely effective in malignant brain gliomas, by adding mizonidazole. Unfortunately, as in other trials, this radiosensitizer appeared ineffective in the treatment of malignant brain gliomas.

References

[1] EORTC Brain Tumour Group: Effect of CCNU on survival rate, objective remission and duration of free interval in patients with malignant brain glioma. Final evaluation. Eur. J. Cancer **14** (1978) 851–856.

[2] EORTC Brain Tumour Group: Evaluation of CCNU, VM-26 plus CCNU and procarbazin in supratentorial brain gliomas. J. Neurosurg. **55** (1981) 27–31.

[3] EORTC Brain Tumour Group: Misonidazole in radiotherapy of supratentorial malignant brain gliomas in adult patients: a randomized double-blind study. Eur. J. Cancer **19** (1983) 39–42.

[4] EORTC Brain Tumour Group: Effect of DDMP (2,4-Diamino-5-3', 4'-Dichlorophenyl-6-Methyl-pyrimidine) on brain gliomas. A phase-II study. Eur. J. Cancer **16** (1980) 1639–1640.

[5] Rosenblum, M. L., A. F. Reynolds Jr., K. A. Smith, et al: Chloroethyl-cyclohexyl-nitrosourea (CCNU) in treatment of malignant brain tumours. J. Neurosurg. **39** (1973) 306–314.

[6] Wilson, C. B., P. Gutin, E. B. Boldrey, et al.: Single-agent chemotherapy of brain tumours. Arch. Neurol. **33** (1976) 739–744.

Characterization of human malignant brain tumour cells *in vitro* and comparison of three different *in vitro* assays to determine their sensitivity to BCNU*

U. Bogdahn, H. T. R. Rupniak, F. Ali-Osman, M. L. Rosenblum

Introduction

In vitro assays predicting response of individual tumours to a number of chemotherapeutic agents seem to bring new hope to oncologists and their tumour-bearing patients in improving results of clinical anti-cancer therapy. As the human tumour stem cell assay in soft agar described by Hamburger and Salmon [9] has attracted many scientists at least to give *in vitro* predictive drug assays a fair trial, results of the use of this method for a broad spectrum of tumours become available [4]. A modification of the original colony formation assay, employing lethally irradiated (44 Gy) 9L-rat gliosarcoma feeder cells and growth of individual tumour cells in a monolayer, has also been applied for human brain tumour cells [7]. This brain tumour colony formation assay has been able to predict clinical tumour resistance to BCNU (the most frequently employed single agent in brain tumour chemotherapy) correctly in 100%, however, it will correctly predict clinical sensitivity to the drug in only 42% [7].

As has been described elsewhere in the book, a non-tumour stem cell based *in vitro* assay has been developed, correctly predicting clinical response of human malignant brain tumours to BCNU in at least 85% [3], whereas clinical resistance is also predicted correctly in all cases. A third *in vitro* assay has been applied to human tumour biology increasingly frequently in the recent past: viz. the short term-precursor assay (Volm-assay [6]). Since a number of well characterized early passage human brain tumour cells were available, we compared the three different *in vitro* assays in their ability to discriminate sensitive from resistant human brain tumour cells *in vitro*.

* This work has been supported by a grant of the Deutsche Forschungsgemeinschaft and NIH-grants Ca-13525, Ca-3182, Ca-28529.

Method

Characterization of tumours: The neuropathological diagnoses of seven brain tumours and one probe of normal brain and the clinical therapy may be seen from table 1. The cells were also characterized in culture by a number of antibodies to antigenic determinants on their membranes and in their cytoplasm, as may be seen from table 2 a.

Immunofluorescence: The methods used for immunofluorescence in human brain tumour cells has been described in detail elsewhere [8]. Briefly, there were two main procedures: 1. for staining "fixed" cells FLOW tissue culture slides with brain tumour cells grown on them for 24 hours were fixed in ice-cold acetone for 1 min, then airdried for 30 min, and finally rehydrated in cold PBS for another 30 min. Then indirect immunofluorescence, as described below, was performed at room tempera-

Table 1 Clinical data on cultures used in different assays

Nr.	Age	Sex	Histology	Therapy
126	50	F	Gliobl. Mult.	Operation, Radiotherapy, BCNU
188	9	M	Gliobl. Mult.	Operation, Radiotherapy, Multidrug-Trtm.
211	57	M	Oligodendrogl.	Operation, Radiotherapy,
253	49	M	Gliobl. Mult.	Operation, Radiotherapy, Multidrug-Trtm.
344	–	F	Norm. Glia	No
354	48	F	Gliobl. Mult.	Operation, no further
358	61	M	Gliobl. Mult. (R)	Operation, no further
360	20	F	Fibrocyt. Astro.	Operation, no further

Table 2a Characterization of human brain tumour culture cells by a number of monoclonal and polyclonal antibodies

Cell culture	126	188	211	253–2	344	354	358	360	
Passage no.	20	13	11	12	3	–	3	2	
Antibody									
HLA	3+	4+	+	3+	+	ND	+	+	live cell IF
AB390	3+	4+	2+	3+	+	ND	2+	–	
UJ13A	–	–	–	+	–	ND	–	–	
GE2	+	–	–	–	–	ND	–	–	
BF7	–	–	–	–	–	ND	–	–	
α GFAP	–	–	–	3+(1.9)*	–	ND	3+(8)*	3+(.1)*	fixed cell IF
GE2	2+	2+	3+	2+	2+	ND	2+	2+	
BF7	+	+	2+	+	+	ND	2+	+	

* Percentage of +labelled cells

ture. 2. "Live" cells were stained at 4 °C without prior fixation. For the actual staining 25 μl of the appropriate dilution of each individual antibody were incubated with cells for 30 min, cells were then washed 5 × with PBS for 30 min, then the cells were again incubated for 30 min with the appropriate dilutions of either FITC-labelled anti-mouse (sheep)- or Rhodamine-labelled anti-rabbit (swine)-antibodies. Prior to observation of fluorescence pattern with a fluorescence microscope the cells were washed 5 × with PBS for 30 min and mounted in PBS-buffered glycerol (figs. 1a, 1b, 1c).

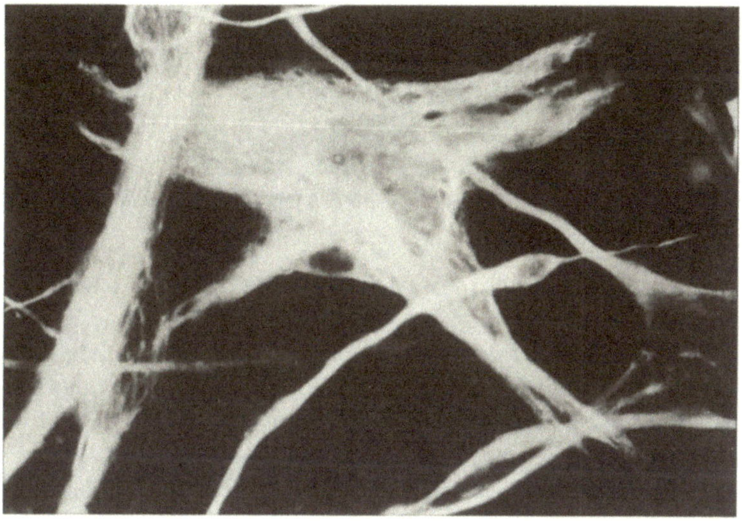

Fig. 1 a

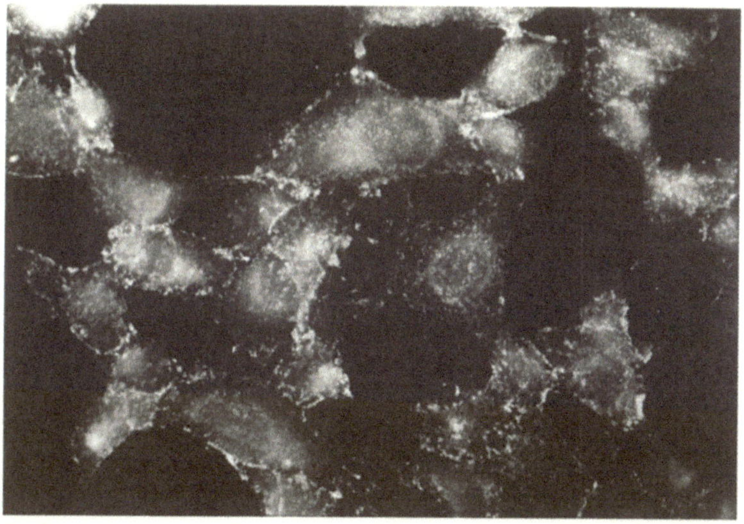

Fig. 1 b

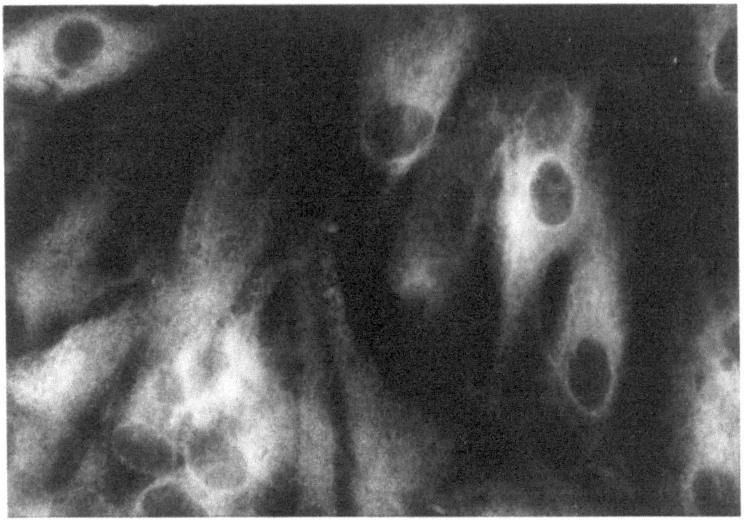

Fig. 1 c

Fig. 1 Immunofluorescent staining of human glioma cells with different antibodies: a) anti-GFAP, b) anti-THY-1, c) GE 2, "fixed cells". (320x).

In vitro assays: For the proliferation microassay (PRO) single cells were plated into 96-well micro-tissue-culture plates [3]. After 24 hours cells were treated with BCNU for one hour, then allowed to proliferate for about eight population doubling times (of untreated controls) in fresh culture medium (MEM, 20% FCS, Gentamycin). Finally (5,6-^{3}H)-uridine uptake during a six hour incubation period, determined by a liquid scintillation counting method, was employed as a measure of RNA-synthesis in surviving tumour cells. The drug effect was expressed as percent age inhibition of RNA-synthesis relative to untreated controls (fig. 2a).

The second *in vitro* assay to assess chemosensitivity was a colony forming assay (CFE) employing lethally irradiated (44 Gy) 9L-rat brain tumour cells as feeders. Single human brain tumour cells were treated for one hr with BCNU, 24 hours after plating in monolayer culture. Colony formation was assessed 2 to 4 weeks after treatment [7]. The drug effect was calculated as the ratio of the number of colonies that formed in the drug treated cultures to the number of colonies that formed in untreated controls (fig. 2b). For the short term precursor assay [6] a similar method was used as for the PRO-assay, except that ^{3}H-thymidine incorporation during a 12 hr period was measured immediately after a one hour BCNU-exposure (total BCNU-exposure 13 hrs, but $T_{1/2} = 21$ min!). The drug effect was expressed as a percentage of inhibition of DNA-synthesis relative to untreated controls (fig. 2c).

Calculation of drug effects: Drug effect on each individual tumour (assessed by the 3 different methods) was expressed in terms of a sensitivity index [2] as defined by:

$$I_s = \frac{A_{drug}}{A_{100}} = \frac{\text{area under survival curve}}{\text{area under 100\% survival curve}}$$

As the *in vitro* $T_{1/2}$ for BCNU (MEM, 20% FCS) has been found to be 21 min [5], and the achieveable *in vivo* concentration time product (cxt) has been established as 4.58 μMhr [1], for these experiments a cut-off concentration of 9.6 μM BCNU was set in order to calculate the sensitivity indices. An I_s of 1 would thus mean total drug resistance in the clinically achievable dose range (cxt), a theoretical I_s of O would mean no survival throughout the entire dose range.

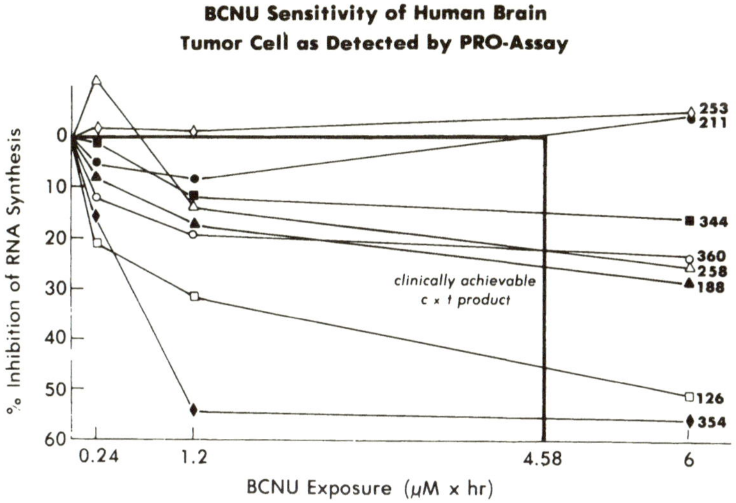

Fig. 2 a

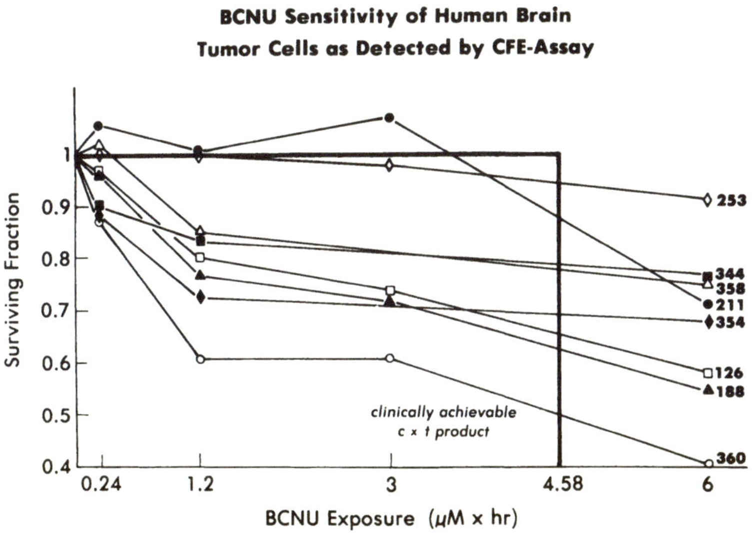

Fig. 2 b

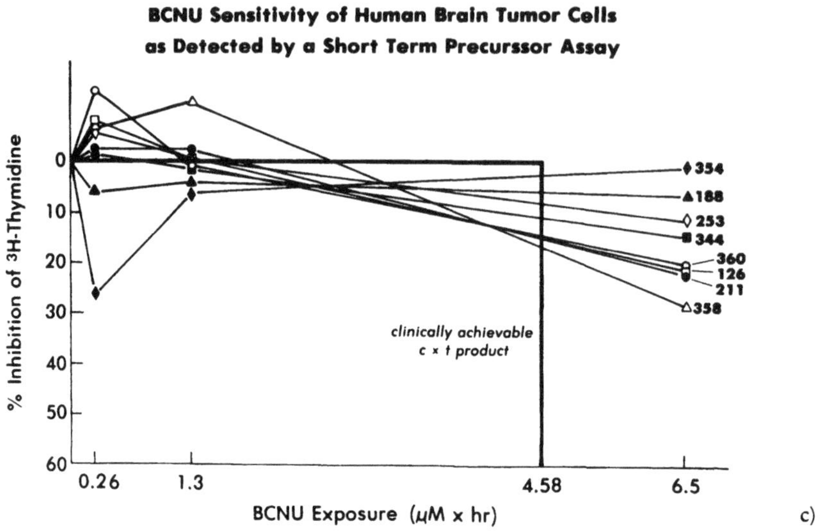

Fig. 2 BCNU-chemosensitivity of human brain tumour cells, as assayed by a) PRO-assay, b) CFE-assay, c) short term-precursor assay.

Results

The results of our characterization of human brain tumour cells *in vitro* may be seen from table 2b. All cells tested showed reactivity with glial specific antibodies GE2 and BF7.

Table 2b Adnex

Monoclonal (MAB)/ Polyclonal (PAB)	Antigen recognized/cell type	Source
HLA (mouse-MAB)	common determinant on HLA-AG of A, B, C segregant series	Cappel Laboratory Cochranville Pa. USA
AB390 (mouse-MAB)	THY-1	R. C. Seeger, Ucla, Sch. Med., Los Angeles, Ca, Ref. 7
UJ13A (mouse-MAB)	PAN-neuroectoderm marker in frozen section	J. T. Kemshead, Imp. Canc. Res. Fund, London, GB, Ref. 8
GE2 + BF7 (mouse-MAB)	2 diff. antigenic determinants on same molecule present on membranes + cytopl. preferentially of gliomas	N. De Tribolet, Centre Hospitalier Univ. Vaudois, Lausanne, CH. Ref. 9
α GFAP (rabbit-PAB)	astrocyte-ass. intracell. cytoskeletal protein	L. F. Eng, VA Hosp. Palo Alto, Ca, USA, Ref. 10

The results of the different *in vitro* test systems to detect *in vitro* BCNU chemosensitivity are summarized in table 3. It can be clearly seen that the PRO-assay detected sensitivities between $I_s = 1$ and 0.5, the CFE assay between $I_s = 1$ and 0.65, and the precursor short term assay between $I_s = 1$ and 0.95: the short term assay thus predicted tumour cell resistance to BCNU in all lines (and the normal brain) investigated, whereas both CFE and PRO were able to discriminate different degrees of chemosensitivity among the diverse lines.

Conclusion and discussion

Under standardized conditions (with slight experimental advantages for the precursor short term assay) PRO-assay and CFE-assay were both able to discriminate BCNU-sensitive from BCNU-resistant brain tumour cell cultures in our experimental set-up. However, the precursor short term assay failed to do so, but predicted only BCNU-resistance in all cell cultures investigated. As data on clinical courses of the tumours investigated were not evaluable in most cases for an *in vitro/in vivo* correlation, the differences in I_s for the individual tumours as measured by PRO- and CFE-assays could also not be correlated to *in vivo* tumour sensitivity or resistance. As the PRO-assay is semiautomated, not dependant on subjective criteria in evaluating human tumour colony formation, superior to CFE in predicting *in vivo* tumour BCNU-sensitivity (85 versus 42% correct prediction [3, 7]), and much less time and labour consuming, it may be more advantageous for *in vitro* drug screening of human malignant brain tumour cells than the CFE-assay. In contrast, the CFE-assay is based on cloning of human tumour stem cells, and therefore it may be further improved to be applicable for studies on human brain tumour biology.

Table 3

Sensitivity index for the various cell cultures assayed by			
I_s	PRO	CFE	Short term
1.00	253	253, 211	253, 358, 344
0.95	211	–	188, 126, 211, 360, 354
0.90	344, 358	–	–
0.85	188, 360	–	–
0.80	–	344, 358	–
0.75	–	126, 188, 354	–
0.70	–	–	–
0.65	126	360	–
0.60	–	–	–
0.55	–	–	–
0.50	354	–	–

Summary

Human malignant brain tumour cells were characterized by a number of antibodies reactive with antigenic determinants in their cytoplasms or cell-membranes, and by conventional neuropathological classification. Employing these cells, a proliferation microassay (PRO), a colony assay (CFE) and a precursor short term assay were compared in their ability to predict *in vitro* sensitivity or resistance of human malignant brain tumour cells to BCNU, the drug most frequently used in single agent chemotherapy of this disease. The drug effect on each individual tumour (assessed by the three different methods) was expressed in terms of a sensitivity index, as defined by I_s = area under survival curve/area under 100% survival curve. PRO-assay and CFE-assay are both able to discriminate BCNU-sensitive from BCNU-resistant brain tumour cell cultures, whereas the precursor short term assay predicted drug resistance for all tumour cell cultures investigated. As the PRO-assay has a number of advantages over the currently presented CFE-assay, especially in predicting *in vivo* tumour sensitivity to BCNU, it may be more advantageous for *in vitro* drug screening purposes.

Acknowledgement

The authors are especially grateful to R. C. Seeger, J. T. Kemshead, N. DeTribolet, and L. F. Eng, for generously providing the different antibodies.

References

[1] Albers, D. S., et al.: Tabular summary of pharmacokinetic parameters relevant to *in vitro* drug assays. In: Cloning of human tumour stem cells (S. Salmon, ed.), p. 351. Alan R. Liss, New York 1980.

[2] Ali-Osman, F., et al.: *In vitro* cytostatic drug testing in the human stem cell assay: a modified method for the determination of the sensitivity index. Tum. Diagn. Ther. **4** (1983) 1.

[3] Bogdahn, U.: Chemosensitivity of malignant human brain tumours. Preliminary results. J. Neuro-Oncol. **1** (1983) 149.

[4] Conference on predictive drug testing in human tumour cells, Zurich, July 1983.

[5] Genini, D., et al.: Determination of *in vitro* pharmacokinetics of different nitrosoureas. Unpublished results. BTRC, UCSF, San Francisco, Ca, USA.

[6] Group of KSST: *In vitro* short term test to determine the resistance of human tumours to chemotherapy. Cancer **48** (1981) 2127.

[7] Rosenblum, M. L., et al.: Stem cell studies of human malignant brain tumours. J. Neurosurg. **58** (1983) 170.

[8] Rupniak, H. T. R., et al.: Characterization of human brain tumour cells *in vitro*. Manuscript in preparation.

[9] Salmon, S.: Clinical correlation of *in vitro* drug sensitivity. In: Cloning of human tumour stem cells (S. Salmon, ed.). Alan R. Liss, New York 1980.

Combined modality treatment of operated astrocytomas grade 3–4

A prospective and randomized study of misonidazole and radiotherapy with two different radiation schedules and subsequent CCNU chemotherapy

Stage II of a prospective multicenter trial of the Scandinavian Glioblastoma Study Group:

R. Hatlevoll, K. F. Lindegaard, S. Hagen, R. Nesbakken, I. Holme, K. Kristiansen, A. Torvik, G. Notter, M. Lipecki, S. Lindgren, O. Arnason, S. Littbrand, N. E. Säterborg, L. Johansson, G. Beneditsson, B. Spännare, A. Berthelsen, H. Busch, E. Grønbæk, J. Rygard, J. Haase, E. Lambretsen, S. Midholm. P. Sehested, M. Heikkinen, P. Taskinen, S. Nystrøm, M. Mäntylä, O. Mella, B. Rosengren, J. Ganz, R. Ringkjøb, K. Elgen, R. Hammer, Jensen, S. T. deGaris, I. Matheson, A. Brun

The first stage of the Scandinavian multicentre study, published in 1981, confirmed the value of postoperative irradiation. This second trial includes two methods of postoperative irradiation, with and without a radiosensitizer (Misonidazole), and a subsequent study of the additional effect of CCNU as adjuvant chemotherapy.

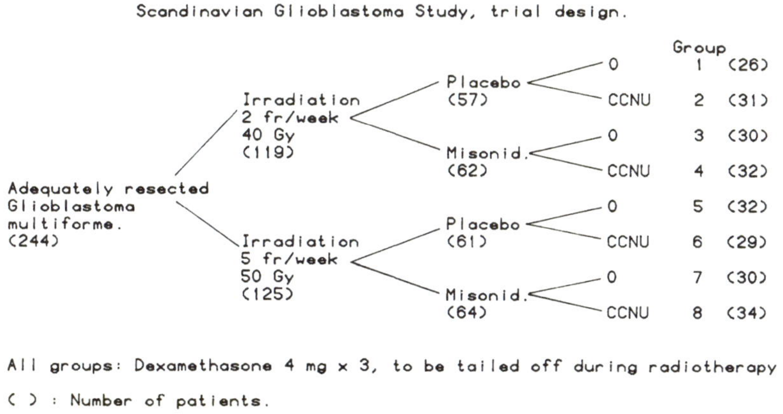

Fig. 1 The trial was arranged as a 2^3-factorial design. The whole material can be used to evaluate the effect of the two fractionation schedules, misonidazol vs. placebo, and the effect of CCNU vs. no adjuvant chemotherapy.

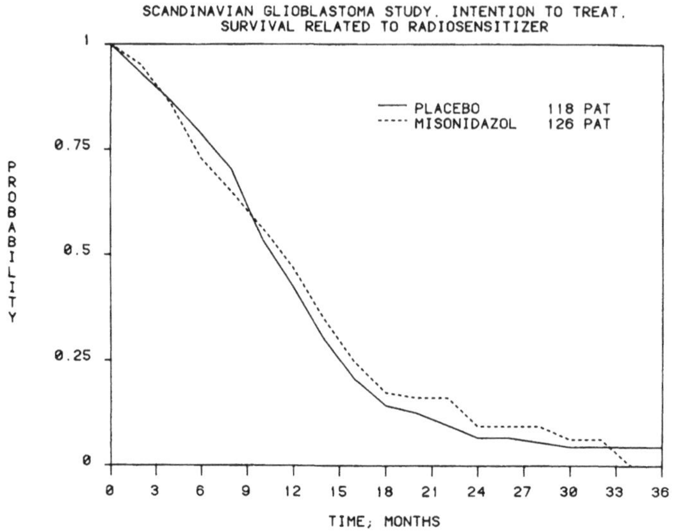

Fig. 2 All patients randomized to receive misonidazole are compared to the placebo group. No difference is seen.

The trial was performed as a 2^3-factorial design. A series of 244 patients were randomized and divided into 8 groups. One half of the patients received total brain irradiation, 40 Gy, 2 fractions per week, one half total brain irradiation, 50 Gy, 5 fractions per week. Total time was 5 weeks.

The effect of misonidazole was compared to placebo in both radiation groups.

Adjuvant chemotherapy with CCNU was given after three months to one half of the series. All patients received steroids during the radiation treatment.

No difference was found between the eight subgroups with regard to survival rates or functional capacity. Randomization procedures, statistical processing and side effects of the treatment are discussed.

Chemotherapy of gliomas in adults and of medulloblastoma in children

H. J. G. Bloom, J. P. Glees

Adults

By virtue of their lipid solubility and low molecular weight the nitrosoureas are able to penetrate the blood-brain barrier. Since they are active against both proliferating and non-proliferating tumour cells, they would be expected to be particularly effective against gliomas because of the low growth fraction of such tumours. Indeed, to date these agents have proved to be the most consistently active cytotoxic agents against cerebral gliomas in both experimental animals and in man. However in the treatment of recurrent high grade cerebral hemisphere astrocytomas, which constitute the most common primary brain tumour in adults, these drugs have proven largely ineffective.

Nitrosoureas for recurrent gliomas – Royal Marsden Hospital study

A consecutive series of 80 patients with recurrent gliomas, mainly of high grade malignancy, have been treated with CCNU (73 patients) or BCNU (7 patients). All patients had tumour recurrence after previous radical radiotherapy with or without surgery. Chemotherapy in standard dosage was the only specific treatment. The clinical response rate for all 80 patients, irrespective of type and grade, was 25% with a duration of 6–73 months (tab. 1). In 62 patients who survived long enough to receive 2 or more courses of chemotherapy the response rate reached 32%: in 9 patients the benefit lasted for 2 or more years. Only 7% of all 55 patients with

Table 1 Royal Marsden Hospital recurrent gliomas BCNU/CCNU treatment alone (80 adult patients) [11]

Benefit	Patients (%)		Mean survival (months)
None	55(69)		4.0
Doubtful	5(6)	} 31%	14.0
Definite	20*(25)		24.7

* For 6, 8+, 9, 9, 9, 11, 15, 17, 17, 19, 20, 24, 24+, 25, 28, 28+, 38, 57, 57, 73 months.

verified high grade astrocytomas responded to this treatment (tab. 2). On the other hand, results in 15 patients with verified gliomas of lesser malignancy (8 grade I–II astrocytomas, and 7 oligodendrogliomas) were more encouraging with 11 (73%) patients showing a definite objective response to treatment. These results for treatment of glioblastoma with nitrosoureas are far less encouraging than those from the United States [14, 15] where responses of up to 40% have been reported. This may be due, at least in part, to small numbers of patients in individual series and to different criteria used in case-selection and for defining objective response. To qualify for an objective response in our series of patients with verified gliomas it was necessary that steroids should be discontinued; examples of so-called stabilization without clinical improvement were not included. In the overall assessment, all patients were accounted for including those receiving only one course of chemotherapy before deterioration and death. All patients had recurrent tumours and received only chemotherapy with no other specific treatment. Apart from marrow depression following the use of BCNU, there may be serious additional risks such as fatal lung fibrosis [16] but this complication was not observed among our patients.

In various centers other established cytotoxic drugs are being tested alone or in combination programs against gliomas. These include VM 26, DTIC, procarbazine, dianhydrogalactitol, bleomycin, cis-platinum, and hydroxyurea, the last compound acting as both cytotoxic drug and possible radiosensitizer. In our experience, a combination of CCNU, procarbazine and vincristine for recurrent high grade astrocytomas has provided no more effective treatment than CCNU alone. From reported data, no single or combination of agents has emerged as being clearly more effective than members of the nitrosourea group. Recently, Levin et al. [17], using a revised schedule of CCNU, procarbazine and vincristine, have reported an objective response rate of 17% (2 of 12) for patients with recurrent glioblastoma, and 26% (12 of 46) for patients with other types of malignant glioma. Sklansky et al. [18] reported a response rate of 38% in patients with intracranial tumours following treatment with VM 26. Further studies with this agent alone [19] and in combination with CCNU

Table 2 Royal Marsden Hospital recurrent gliomas CCNU/BCNU treatment: Benefit by tumour type [11]

Gliomas	No.	%
Astrocytoma (grade III+IV)	4*/55	(7%)
Astrocytoma (grade I+II)	7†/	(87%)
Oligodendroglioma	4/7	(57%)
Unverified	4/9	(44%)
Microglioma	1/1	—
Total	20/80	(25%)

* 3 of 4 were grade III.
† 6 of 7 were grade II.

[20] or with CCNU and adriamycin [21] appeared promising: but results in a series of childhood cases were disappointing with no responses in 17 patients with residual or recurrent gliomas [22]. One of the latest cytotoxic agents undergoing investigation for brain tumour therapy at the present time is cis-platinum: in a preliminary communication, Khan et al. [23] report responses in 6 of 8 children with various types of intracranial glioma and a teratocarcinoma of the pineal region.

Chemotherapy as adjuvent primary treatment

While the nitrosourea agents undoubtedly cause tumour regression and promote clinical improvement in some patients with recurrent gliomas, from various studies, especially those of the Brain Tumour Study Group in the United States [24, 25] and the EORTC group in Europe [26], they appear to be of little value as adjuvants in the primary treatment of high grade astrocytomas. The drugs are clearly far less affective than radiotherapy, and no consistent and significant improvement has so far been demonstrated when they are combined with irradiation [25–29] (tab. 3). On the other hand, preliminary observations regarding dianhydrogalactitol (DAG) in a controlled study have been promising [30]: the median survival of 22 patients with grade III and IV astrocytomas treated by whole brain irradiation and DAG was 67 weeks,

Table 3 Malignant glioma B.T.S.G. adjuvant trials [24, 25]

Adjuvant Treatment	Total Patients	Mean survival (weeks)
1 Controls	96	26
Mithramycin		21
2 Controls	225	14
BCNU		18.5
Radioth.		36
BCNU + radioth.		34.5
3 Controls	167	17
BCNU		25
Radioth.		37.5
BCNU + radioth.		40.5
4 MeCCNU	263	23
Radioth.		37
MeCCNU + radioth.		43
BCNU + radioth.		52

Results from 4 controlled studies concerning post-operative adjuvant therapies carried out by the Brain Tumour Study Group (BTSG). Controls = surgery alone with or without steroids. Radiotherapy is the most effective single post-operative treatment. In the fourth study the combination of radiotherapy and BCNU appears better than radiotherapy alone, but this advantage was not found in the previous studies.

compared with only 35 weeks for 20 receiving irradiation alone. This observation requires confirmation since other contemporary experience concerning DAG for high grade gliomas has not been encouraging.

From scattered reports in the literature, involving small numbers of patients, it appears that CCNU, vincristine, methotrexate (intrathecally, or systematically in high dose with citrovorum rescue), procarbazine and VM-26 have each, and in different combinations, produced beneficial responses in up to 60%–70% of children with various types of recurrent brain glioma [31–36]. Controlled trials have now been established in Europe and in the United States to determine the value of adjuvant multiple agent chemotherapy in the primary treatment of medulloblastoma and some preliminary results are encouraging.

Children

Medulloblastoma is the most common type of brain cancer in children, consistuting some 25% of all intracranial tumours in patients under age 16. Post-operative irradiation has been and still remains the most effective adjuvant treatment available for this disease. To achieve the maximum therapeutic effect, radiotherapy must be carefully planned and executed ensuring complete coverage of the entire contents of the cerebrospinal axis with a maximum dose, compatible with reasonable safety, delivered to the posterior fossa where risk of tumour recurrence is greatest. With modern post-operative radiotherapy, survival rates up to 35–40% at five years, and 25–30% at ten years have been reported during the past decade in substantial numbers of childhood cases. Greater survival rates have been reported by some authors, but patient numbers in these series have generally been very small, ranging from 6–14.

Tumour recurrence in the posterior fossa, with or without spinal spread, is found in 80% of treatment failures. The risk to life and to cerebral function associated with radical surgery for medulloblastoma imposes serious limitations on attempts at total tumour excision. Furthermore, the maximum dose of irradiation which can be delivered without serious risk to normal brain tissue, especially in very young children, is also restricted. Thus, the efforts of both neurosurgeon and radiotherapist to eradicate medulloblastoma cannot be expected to advance much further using conventional methods of treatment. Since medulloblastoma is an embryonic tumour with a rapid growth rate and a high mitotic index, it may, like other primitive tumours in childhood, be expected to respond to chemotherapy. Gliomas rarely produce systemic spread, and chemotherapy in such cases is therefore directed towards assisting irradiation to eradicate residual primary tumour and any seedlings along the CSF pathways. Chemotherapy may also have a secondary role in destroying occult systemic metastases which occur in about 5% of all patients with medulloblastoma and in some 15% of those with CSF shunts.

Royal Marsden Hospital Pilot Study

In 1970 a pilot study was started to determine whether adjuvant chemotherapy was feasible and perhaps promising in a multimodality approach to the curative treatment of children with medulloblastoma. We have now treated 40 children with primary disease between 1970 and 1982 using principally CCNU and Vincristine. The survival of the children receiving adjuvant chemotherapy was considerably greater than that of an historical group of 87 patients who were treated prior to 1970 without chemotherapy at the same centre: at five years, 70% of the chemotherapy group were alive compared with 32% of the historical controls, a highly significant difference ($p < 0.0001$), (fig. 1). Historical controls are unsatisfactory, but our pilot study served to show that adjuvant chemotherapy in children treated by craniospinal irradiation was feasible and, with the usual precautions, reasonably safe, at least in the short term.

S.I.O.P. Study

In 1975 the Brain Tumour Committee of The International Society of Paediatric Oncology started a multicentre randomised trial to assess the value of adjuvant chemotherapy in children with medulloblastoma. Over the subsequent five years 44 centres from 15 countries entered 287 children under age 16 into the study. The treatment protocol and also the membership of the brain tumour committee and the list of participating centres and principal coordinators are given in the first report of the trial [12]. By September 1979 the difference between the disease-free survival rate for the chemotherapy and control groups of children with medulloblastoma reached a level of statistical significance ($p = 0.005$) and the study was closed to further case-entry on ethical grounds. 142 children were randomised to receive adjuvant

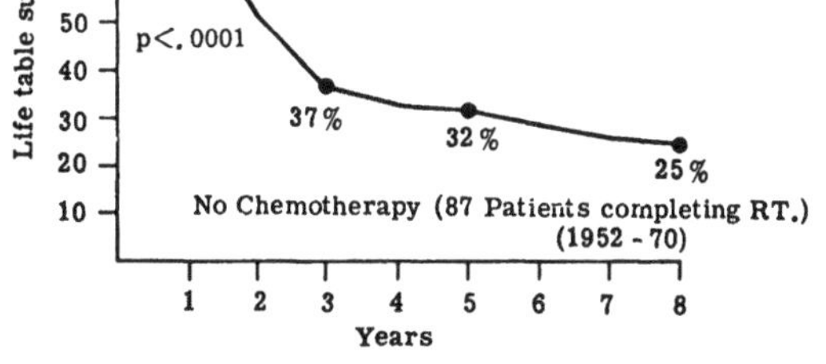

Fig. 1 (After Bloom [11]).

chemotherapy during irradiation and subsequently as maintenance treatment and 145 to no chemotherapy. Two patients were lost to follow-up leaving 285 children for analysis. There were 209 boys (73%) and 76 girls (27%). 26 children (9.1%) were under age 2 years, 190 (66.7%) between 2 and 9, and 69 (24.2%) between 10 and 15.

Protocol radiotherapy consisted of whole cerebrospinal axis megavoltage or cobalt 60 irradiation to be started within three weeks of operation. The maximum tumour dose to the posterior fossa was 5000–5500 rads and 3500–4500 rads to the remainder of the brain in 7–8 weeks. The spinal cord received 3000–3500 rads in 5–6 weeks. Treatment was daily, 5 days per week. In children under age 2 years the dose was reduced to 4000–4500 rads to the posterior fossa with 3000–3500 rads to the rest of the brain in 6–7 weeks and 3000 rads to the cord in 6 weeks. Protocol chemotherapy consisted of weekly injections of vincristine (1 mg/m^2) during radiotherapy, followed by eight courses of intermittent maintenance treatment with oral CCNU (100 mg/m^2 on day 1) and intravenous vincristine (1.5 mg/m^2 on day 1, 8 and 15), commencing one month after completing irradiation and cycled every six weeks over appromimately 1 year.

Analysis of survival data from time of operation was carried out strictly according to the original case randomisation. There have been no exclusions due to failure to carry out the randomised treatment nor to any protocol deviations. All results reported here refer to disease-free survival based on the log rank test (Mantel-Haenszel analysis).

The results, as reported to the Brain Tumour Committee and to the S.I.O.P. annual conference in Bern, September 1982 [13], revealed a difference in disease-free survival rate between the two principal arms of the trial in favour of patients receiving adjuvant chemotherapy. At three years 63% of the chemotherapy group were alive, compared to 51% of those in the non-chemotherapy group; at 5 years the corresponding figures were 51% and 40%, respectively. The difference reached only nominal significance at the 5% level ($p = 0.046$). In practically all major and subgroup comparisons the survival of patients receiving chemotherapy was superior to that of the control groups, although frequently the difference did not reach the generally accepted level of statistical significance. However, significant results, or at least important trends, in favour of chemotherapy were obtained in certain high risk sub-groups, namely in children age < 2 years ($p = 0.058$), in those having macroscopically incomplete tumour excision ($p = 0.002$), and in those with evidence of brain stem involvement at the time of operation ($p = 0.003$). Of the 176 patients (62% of the entire series) possessing one or more of these three high risk factors, the five-year survival rate for those receiving chemotherapy was 53%, compared to only 25% for control patients ($p = 0.001$). Chemotherapy was generally well tolerated, although on many occasions CCNU administration had to be delayed or reduced in dosage owing to a low blood count.

Conclusions

Survival rates in children with medulloblastoma have increased in major radiotherapy centres during the past two decades as a result of improved techniques in surgery and radiotherapy. However, the limits of modern surgery and megavoltage radiotherapy now appear to have been reached and more intensive use of these modalities may increase the risk to life and to cerebral function without improving the duration and quality of survival. From a pilot study at the Royal Marsden Hospital and the preliminary results of the S.I.O.P. trial, there is hope that adjuvant chemotherapy will lead to further advances in treatment. Whereas CCNU and vincristine may not improve the survival of low risk cases, this combination appears to be of value in children with one or more high risk factors. It is important to stress that the Royal Marsden study was not a controlled investigation and that in the S.I.O.P. trial the nominal significance of the overall difference in survival between the chemotherapy and control arms ($p = 0.043$) is not impressive and is based on the last of five annual analyses. In addition, two risk factors, brain stem involvement and extent of surgery were not stratified prior to analysis. Nevertheless, these observations should serve as an encouragement to pursue this line of investigation and to search for more active drugs and more effective schedules.

Late effects: there is concern regarding possible late neurological, psychosocial and endocrine disturbances in young children treated for brain tumours with irradiation or chemotherapy, especially when both agents are used together. In addition, there may be late sequelae from prolonged chemotherapy in other organs such as the marrow, lungs and kidneys. Consequently, the identification and selection of high risk cases of medulloblastoma for additional and perhaps more hazardous treatment would be of considerable value. A successful chemotherapy regime may ultimately permit a reduction in the dose of prophylactic irradiation to brain and spinal cord. This may lessen the risk of late neurogenic effects and help to preserve marrow function, which may give even greater scope for chemotherapy. At present, however, the dose of irradiation, especially to the primary tumour site, is of paramount importance and should not be reduced.

Since the number of children with medulloblastoma seen annually in any one medical centre is limited, it is essential for paediatric groups to join forces, share resources and establish cooperative, multicentre pilot studies and trials if meaningful results are to be obtained within a reasonable time.

References

[1] Bloom, H. J. G., E. N. K. Wallace, J. M. Henk: The treatment and prognosis of medulloblastoma in children: A study of 82 verified cases. Am. J. Roentgenol. **105** (1969) 43–62.

[2] Bloom, H. J. G.: Concepts in the natural history and treatment of medulloblastoma in children: increasing survival rates and possible risks with current therapy techniques. C.R.C. Crit. Rev. Radiol. Sci. **2** (1971) 89–143.

[3] Bloom, H. J. G.: Combined modality therapy for intracranial tumours. Cancer **35** (1975) 111–120.

[4] Bloom, H. J. G.: Medulloblastoma: Prognosis and prospects. Int. J. Radiat. Oncol. Biol. Phys. **2** (1977) 1031–1033.

[5] Bloom, H. J. G.: Medulloblastoma and ependymoma: Treatment principles and prognosis. Presentation at 9th Annual Conference of International Society of Paediatric Oncology (SIOP), Philadelphia, Sept. 1977.

[6] Bloom, H. J. G.: Management of some intracranial tumours in children and adults. In: Recent Advances in Clinical Oncology (T. A. Hazra, M. C. Beachley, eds.), pp. 55–84. Alan R. Liss Inc., New York 1978.

[7] Bloom, H. J. G.: Adjuvant therapy for residual disease in children with medulloblastoma. In: Recent Results in Cancer Research (G. Bonadonna, G. Mathe, S. E. Salomon, eds.), pp. 412–422. Springer, Berlin–Heidelberg–New York 1979.

[8] Bloom, H. J. G.: Intracranial secondary carcinomas and disseminating gliomas: Treatment and prognosis. In: CNS Complications of Malignant Disease (J. M. A. Whitehouse, H. E. M. Kay, eds.), pp. 329–355. McMillan Press Ltd., London 1979.

[9] Bloom, H. J. G.: Recent results and research in the treatment of intracranial gliomas. In: Tumours of the Central Nervous System: Modern Radiotherapy in Multidisciplinary Management (C. H. Chang, E. M. Housepian, eds.). Masson Publishing, New York–Paris 1981 (in press).

[10] Bloom, H. J. G., R. D. Bugden: Radiation and misonidazole in children with brain stem gliomas and supratentorial glioblastoma: A pilot study. In: Progress in Radio-Oncology, II EDF (K. H. Karcher, H. D. Kogelnik, G. Reinartz, eds.), pp. 203–211. Raven Press, New York 1981.

[11] Bloom, H. J. G.: Intracranial Tumours: Response and resistance to Therapeutic Endeavours, 1970–1980. Int. J. Rad. Oncol. Biol. Phys. **8** (1982) 1083–1113.

[12] Bloom, H. J. G., H. Thornton, O. Schweisugth: S.I.O.P. Medulloblastoma and high grade ependymoma therapeutic clinical trial: Preliminary results (1975–1981). In: Paediatric Oncology (C. Raybaud et al., eds.), pp. 309–322. Excerpta Medica, Amsterdam 1982.

[13] Bloom, H. J. G., H. Thornton: Proceedings 13th International Congress of Chemotherapy, Vienna, 28th August to 2nd September 1983.

[14] Rosenblum, M. L., A. F. Reynolds, K. A. Smith, et al.: CCNU in the treatment of malignant brain tumours. J. Neurosurg. **39** (1973) 306–314.

[15] Wilson, C. B., P. Gutin, E. B. Boldrey, et al.: Single agent chemotherapy of brain tumours: a five year review. Arch. Neurol. **33** (1976) 739–750.

[16] Sweet, D. L., F. J. Hindler, K. Hanlon, et al.: Treatment of grade 3 and 4 astrocytomas with BCNU alone and in combination with VM 26 following surgery and radiation therapy. Cancer Treat. Rep. **63** (1979) 1707–1711.

[17] Levin, V. A., M. S. Edwards, D. C. Wright, et al.: Modified procarbazine, CCNU and vincristine (PCV3) combination chemotherapy in the treatment of malignant brain tumours. Cancer Treat. Rep. **64** (1980) 237–241.

[18] Slansky, B. D., R. S. Mann-Kaplan, A. F. Reynolds, et al.: PTG (VM 26) in the treatment of malignant intracranial neoplasms. Cancer **33** (1974) 460–467.

[19] Kessinger, A., H. M. Lemon, J. F. Foley: VM 26 as a second drug in the treatment of brain gliomas. Cancer Treat. Rep. **63** (1979) 511–512.

[20] Seiler, R. W., F. Vassella, H. Markwalder: Combination chemotherapy with VM 26 and CCNU in primary malignant brain tumours. Surg. Neurol. **11** (1979) 237–242.

[21] Pouillart, P., G. Mathe, T. Hoang Thy, et al.: Treatment of malignant gliomas and brain metastases in adults with a combination of adriamycin, VM 26 and CCNU. Cancer **38** (1976) 1909–1916.

[22] Sullivan, M. P., J. van Eys, J. Herson, et al.: Nonresponsiveness of brain tumours to VM 26 therapy in children. Cancer Treat. Rep. **63** (1979) 155–156.
[23] Khan, A., D. McCullough, F. Borts, et al.: Update on use of cis-platinum in CNS malignancies. Abstracts Proc. AACR and ASCO, C283, 1980.
[24] Walker, M. D.: Brain Tumour Study Group: A survey of current activities. In: Modern Concepts in Brain Tumour Therapy: Laboratory and Clinical Investigations. Natl. Cancer Inst. Monogr. **46** (1977) 209–212.
[25] Walker, M. D., T. A. Strike: The treatment of malignant glioma in controlled trials. In: Multidisciplinary Aspects of Brain Tumour Therapy (P. Paoletti, M. D. Walker, G. Butti, R. Knerich, eds.), pp. 267–274. Elsevier/North Holland, Biomedical Press, Amsterdam–New York–Oxford 1979.
[26] Hildebrand, J.: The results of the EORTC Brain Tumour Group. In: Multidisciplinary Aspects of Brain Tumour Therapy (P. Paoletti, M. D. Walker, G. Butti, R. Knerich, eds.), pp. 235–243. Elsevier/North Holland, Biomedical Press, Amsterdam–New York–Oxford 1979.
[27] Brisman, R., E. M. Housepian, C. Chang, et al.: Adjuvant nitrosourea therapy for glioblastoma. Arch. Neurol. **33** (1976) 745–750.
[28] Gehan, E. A., M. D. Walker, Prognostic Factors for Patients with Brain Tumours. In: Modern Concepts in Brain Tumour Therapy: Laboratory and Clinical Investigations. National Cancer Inst. Monograph No. 46, pp. 189–195. US Govt. Printing Office, Washington 1977.
[29] Reagan, T. J., H. F. Bisel, D. S. Childs, et al.: Controlled study of CCNU and radiation therapy in malignant astrocytoma. J. Neurosurg. **44** (1976) 186–190.
[30] Eagan, R. T., D. S. Childs, D. D. Layton, et al.: Dianhydrogalactitol and radiation therapy. J. Am. Med. Assoc. **241** (1979) 2046–2050.
[31] Kumar, A. R. V., J. Renaudin, C. B. Wilson, et al.: Procarbazine hydrochloride in the treatment of brain tumours: Phase 2 study. J. Neurosurg. **40** (1974) 365–371.
[32] Lassman, L. P., G. W. Pearce, J. Gang: Effect of vincristine sulphate on the intracranial gliomata of childhood. Brit. J. Surg. **53** (1966) 774–777.
[33] Newton, W. A., M. P. Sayers, L. D. Samuels: Intrathecal methotrexate therapy for brain tumours in children. Cancer Chemoth. Rep. **52** (1968) 257–261.
[34] Rosenstock, J. G., A. E. Evans, L. Schut: Response to vincristine of recurrent brain tumours in children. J. Neurosurg. **45** (1976) 135–140.
[35] Shapiro, W. R.: Chemotherapy of primary malignant brain tumours in children. Cancer **35** (1975) 965–972.
[36] Sumer, T., A. I. Freeman, M. Cohen, et al.: Chemotherapy in recurrent non-cystic low grade astrocytomas of the cerebrum in children. J. Surg. Oncol. **10** (1978) 45–54.

Combined radiation and polychemotherapy (COMP) in the postoperative treatment of high-grade supratentorial gliomas

D. Volc, K. Jellinger, W. Grisold, R. Weiss, H. Flament, G. Wöber, G. Alth

Introduction

Malignant gliomas grade III and IV accounting for about one-third of all adult brain tumours have a uniformly fatal course with a historical mean life span of 4–6 months after operation and an additional mean of 4–6 months after postoperative radiotherapy or adjuvant single-agent chemotherapy, while combined radiation and single-agent chemotherapy prolong the median survival up to 14 months with a range between 32 and 69 weeks [2, 4, 10–13]. Encouraging results of multimodality treatment have been reported, but both toxic side-effects and chronic cerebral dysfunctions have to be considered [7, 8, 12]. In Vienna, since 1975, postoperative multiple-agent chemotherapy according to the COMP protocol [3] and since 1977, simultaneous megavoltage radiation and COMP chemotherapy has been performed [6]. The present paper reports the results of both postoperative protocols in comparison to radiotherapy and postoperative supportive care, based on a controlled, non-randomized, prospective study.

Material and methods

Between January 1975 and March 1983 290 non-randomized, consecutive patients entered into the study, 267 of them were evaluated. All fulfilled the same criteria: all except for two malignant lymphomas had histologically confirmed supratentorial grade III and IV gliomas, mainly anaplastic astrocytomas and glioblastomas (tab. 1), maximum feasible tumour resection except for a few patients with biopsy, minimum postoperative survival of two months, postoperative Karnofsky performance over 50, absence of severe secondary disease, normal blood and platelet counts, liver and kidney function tests. None had received previous antitumour treatment. Histology was evaluated according to the WHO Classification of Brain Tumours [14], and

Table 1 Histological classification of malignant supratentorial gliomas

Tumour Type	Grade	Support. Care	Radio-therapy	COMP-Chemo	Radioth. + COMP	Total
Astrocytoma anaplastic	III	29	31	20	38	118
Oligoastrocyt. anaplastic	III	–	6	1	3	10
Oligodendrogl. anaplastic	III	1	–	1	3	5
Ependymoma anaplastic	III IV	–	–	1	3	4
Glioblastoma	IV	35	32	20	39	126
Gliosarcoma	IV	–	–	–	2	2
Mal. lymphoma (high-grade)	IV	–	–	–	2	2
Total		65	69	43	90	267

confirmed by the Brain Tumour Reference Centre of the German Association of Neuropathology. The patients were divided into 4 groups (tab. 2):

I. *Supportive care:* 65 patients, most of them receiving steroids intermittently;
II. *Radiotherapy:* 69 patients received total doses of 40–66 Gy in fractions of 150–200 cGy, 5 days/week over 7–8 weeks, delivered to large opposing fields (no whole brain) using telecobalt or 25 and 43 MeV photon beam (betatron) without radiosensitzers.
III. *Polychemotherapy* – COMP protocol: 43 patients received oral CCNU (lomustine), 90–100 mg/sqm on day 1, procarbazine (Natulan) i.v. 100 mg/sqm on day 2–13; vincristine (Oncovin) 1.4 mg/sqm i.v. on day 1 and 8, MTX 20 mg/sqm i.v. on day 3, 7, 10, and 20 mg methyl-prednisone daily. The drugs were given in 15-day cycles beginning two weeks after operation, and were repeated after six weeks and then every three months.
IV. *Combined radiation and COMP therapy:* 90 patients received radiation using the same modalities as in group II with simultaneous COMP chemotherapy; 70 patients died, while 20 have survived for at least 6 months.

The patients were sequentially allocated to be above treatment procedures. There was no major difference in mean age, sex, tumour location, symptom duration, tumour resection, postoperative Karnofsky performance, and tumour grade; the mean age was highest in group I, group I and IV had comparatively large numbers of grade IV gliomas. Most patients of group IV, but less than half of those in group II received radiation of about 60 Gy. All patients were evaluated before and during the

Table 2 Characteristics of postoperative treatment groups

Protocol	Supportive care	Radio-therapy	COMP-Chemoth.	Radiation + COMP Ther. Total	Dead	Alive
N. of pat.	65	69	43	90	70	20
Male:Female	3:2	3:2	78:22	3:2	7:3	2:3
Age (years)	37–73	22–74	27–69	22–73	22–72	25–68
Age, mean	56.6	52.4	50.5	50.7	51.1	50.3
Age > 50 yr (%)	80	55	58	62	64	55
Grade 3:4 (%)	64:54	54:46	51:49	4:6	38:52	1:1
Preop. symp. ≷ 1 year (%)	8:92	9:91	8:92	1:9	1:9	1:9
Location (%)						
Rt:Lft:Bilat.	46:44:10	35:62:3	22:64:7	44:49:7	40:53:7	60:35:5
Frontal	35	27	53	28	29	25
Temporal	32	45	21	28	30	20
Parietal	26	17	23	19	18	20
Occipital	7	6	7	19	16	30
Corp. call	–	–	3	2	3	–
Bas. ganglia	–	5	3	4	4	5
Resect. Total: part:biopsy (%)	76:21:3	79:20:1	76:22:2	89:9:2	80:7:3	95:5:0
N. operat. (%)						
One	48	51	30	39	30	70
Two	48	45	39	37	39	30
Three	4	3	25	19	24	–
More	–	1	6	5	7	–
Radiat. Dose (%)						
> 40 Gy		33		11	14	–
> 50 Gy		22		2	3	–
> 60 Gy		45		87	83	100
N. COMP courses						
One (%)			26	9	10	5
Two			14	23	21	25
Three			18	46	47	50
More			40	22	22	–

course of treatment. Second or more tumour resections were performed in 49–70% of all patients, least frequent in groups I and II (tab. 2). In most patients steroids were given after operation, during radiation and chemotherapy or intermittently. Analysis included the *progression-free intervals,* i.e. the time between operation and the first clinical and/or CT evidence of a new or increased tumour mass, and *survival time,* both by September 1, 1983. Statistical evaluation was performed using variance analysis and Wilcoxon rank-sum test [3, 6, 7].

Results

The results are summarized in table 3 and figures 1–4.

Progression-free intervals in all treatment groups (mean 6.9–11.6 months) were significantly longer than in the supportive care group (mean 3.5 months), and showed a clear-cut correlation with the long-term prognosis. The longest delay in disease progress was seen in survivors of the multimodality group with a mean recurrence free interval of 18.5 months (range 3–36 months plus) (tab. 3).

Mean survival after both radiation and COMP chemotherapy was similar (12.3 and 13.2 months, respectively), with one-year survival rates of 63% and 77%, and 2-year survival rates of 19% and 22%, respectively. Although there was no survival over 24 months, these results were superior to the supportive care group I showing a mean survival of 7.2 months, with one-year survival in 15% and survival over 18 months in 5%. While no major differences were seen between groups II and III, the best results were observed in the multimodality group with a mean survival for the total sample of 19.1 months, 31% surviving over 2 years, 16% over 3 years, and 9% over four years. While the mean survival for the 70 deceased patients was 17.3 months, with a two-year survival of 23%, 3-year survival rate of 14% and a 4-year survival of 5%, 20 patients living over 6 months show a mean survival of 25.2 months with a one-year survival of 95%, and survival rates over 2 years of 53%, over 3 years of 47% and over 4 years of 12% (tab. 3). Comparison of the survival curves shows an improvement in all treatment groups compared to operation alone, with a 50% survival increasing from 5 months in group I to 10–11,3 months in groups II and III to 14 months in group IV, and a 10% survival increasing from 13 months in group I to 24 months in groups II and III and 48 months in the multi-modality group IV (fig. 1). The duration of progression-free intervals after operation

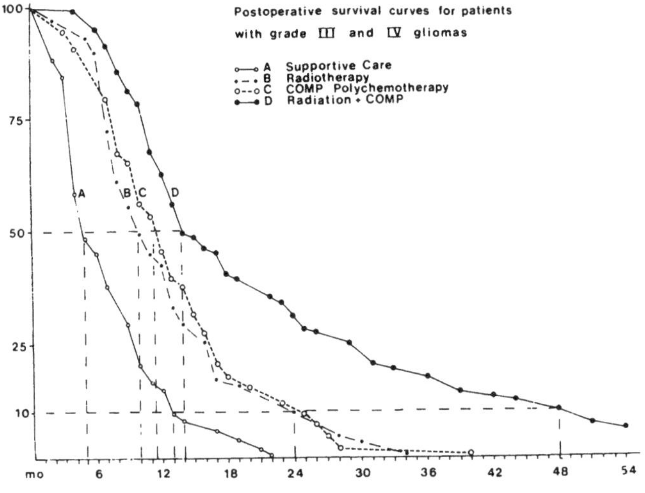

Fig. 1

Table 3 Recurrence-free intervals and survival (month) in patients with malignant gliomas

Protocol	Supportive Care			Radiotherapy (45–67 Gy)			COMP-Polychemo-therapy			Radiation + COMP-Polychemotherapy Dead			Alive (>6 mo)			Total Group		
Tumour Grade	3	4	3+4	3	4	3+4	3	4	3+4	3	4	3+4	3	4	3+4	3	4	3+4
N. of Pat.	30	35	65	37	31	68	22	21	43	27	43	70	10	10	20	37	53	90
Recurr. free	3–16	0–9		5–30	2–12		4–25	0–16		5–45	0–18		7–52+	3–36+		5–52+	0–36+	
Mean	6.9	2.3	*3.5*	9.3	5.8	*7.8*[a]	7.8	5.5	*6.9*[a]	12.6	6.2	*9.2*[a]	32.0	15.0	*18.5+*[b]	15.8	8.0	*11.6+*[b]
Survival	4–21	3–14		8–34	5–17		7–27	3–19		10–63	6–27		9–54+	6+–39+		9–56+	6–56	
Mean	10.7	4.2	*7.2*	15.4	8.6	*12.3*[a]	16.8	9.4	*13.2*[a]	25.0	12.4	*17.3*[b]	33.0+	17.3	*25.2+*[b]	27.1	13.7+	*19.1+*[b]
% Survival																		
> 6 mos	83	14	46	95	84	90	100	81	91	100	93	96	100	100	100	100	94	97
> 12 mos	30	3	15	63	19	43	77	28	53	85	42	59	100	90	95	89	52	67
> 18 mos	10	–	5	30	–	16	27	9	19	63	14	32	80	60	65	67	19	40
> 24 mos	–	–	–	19	–	13	22	–	12	44	12	23	80	50	53	54	15	31
> 36 mos	–	–	–	–	–	–	–	–	–	22	–	14	70	20	47	35	2	16
> 48 mos	–	–	–	–	–	–	–	–	–	15	–	5	40	–	12	22	–	9

[a]) Difference from group I $p<0.01$;
[b]) Difference from groups I–III $p<0.01$

shows a similar shift to the right in all treatment groups (fig. 2). Irrespective of treatment, much longer progression-free intervals and much longer survival was seen in patients with anaplastic grade III gliomas than for grade IV glioblastomas (figs. 3 and 4). The influence of age on survival in the multimodality group, demonstrated in figure 5, shows a better prognosis for patients under age 50 than for those over age 50 years, which is in agreement with other studies [2, 4, 11–13].

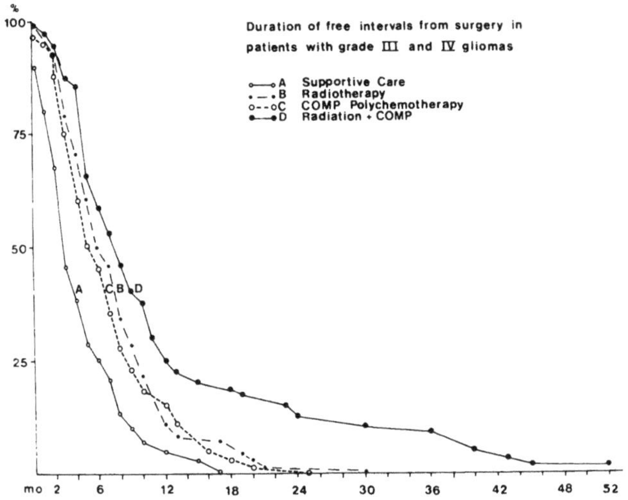

Fig. 2

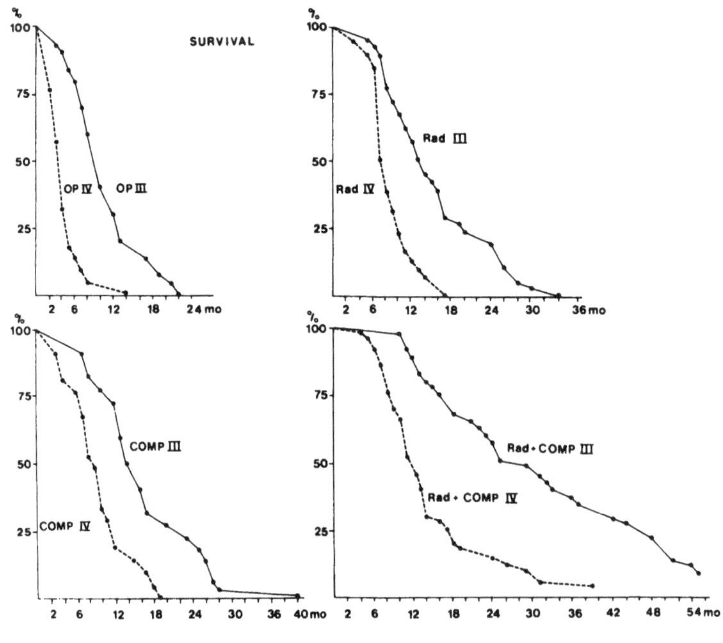

Fig. 3

Adverse effects: Evidence of toxicity only evaluated for groups III and IV (tab. 4) included the well known haematological and GI lesions, polyneuropathy, and a series of CNS complications, including rare cerebral haemorrhage, inflammatory lesions, radionecrosis of the brain, and the rather frequent occurrence of space-occupying cerebral cysts due to tumour and tissue necrosis often simulating tumour recurrence. Surgical treatment may produce transient clinical improvement, while patients harbouring cysts communicating with the ventricles show a rapid fatal outcome often with generalized seeding of the tumour throughout the CSF spaces (tab. 6).

It appears of interest that a 25 to 50% dose reduction of procarbazine considerably decreased both the haematologic and gastrointestinal toxicity, and the incidence of severe skin and mucosal lesions (tab. 4; figs. 6–7). On the other hand, the dose reduction of procarbazine in multimodality treatment had no essential negative influence on the progression-free intervals or survival time in grade III and IV glioma patients, the differences between patients receiving 100% PCZ and those receiving 50–75% PCZ not being statistically significant (tab. 5).

Long-term prognosis of patients with malignant gliomas is poor, and 10–30% of the long-term survivors may develop progressive dementia and brain atrophy [6–8, 12]. Among 27 patients of our group IV surviving over two years (i.e. 30% of the eva-

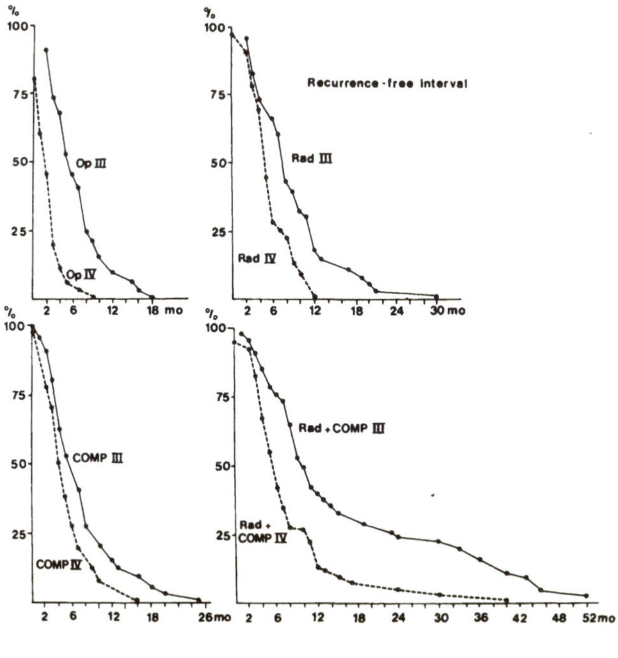

Fig. 4

Table 4 Side effects of COMP and combined radiation and COMP therapy of gliomas

Side Effects		C.O.M.P. n = 43 142 courses	C.O.M.P. + Radiotherapy n = 100; 261 courses Total	PCZ 100% (n = 54) 160 courses	50–75% (n = 46) 101
Gastrointestinal[a])	mild	20.0	30.0	42.6	15.2
	moderate	17.1	18.0	30.0	4.2
	severe	0	9.2	16.7	0
Skin + mucous membranes[a])	mild	17.1	10.0	9.3	10.9
	moderate	5.7	8.0	13.0	2.1
	severe	8.5	9.0	16.7	0
Haemorrhages extracranial[a])	mild	0	0	0	0
	moderate	2.9	3.0	3.7	2.1
	severe	0	1.0	1.9	0
Anaemia[b]) (Erythrocytes $\times 10^6$)	> 4	7.3	26.9	28.8	24.0
	> 3	2.5	1.2	1.9	0
	> 2	0	0	0	0
Leucopaenia[b]) (WBC $\times 10^3$)	> 3	25.0	40.0	40.6	38.0
	> 2	11.3	16.3	20.6	18.0
	> 1	5.6	7.2	20.8	2.0
Thrombocytopaenia[b]) (platelets $\times 10^3$)	> 100	4.0	10.3	15.0	3.0
	> 50	5.8	3.5	3.7	3.0
	> 25	1.6	1.9	2.5	1.0
Polyneuropathy[a]) (Clin./NCV)	mild	54.3	20.0		
	moderate	2.9	12.0		
	severe	4.6	5.0		
Cerebral cysts[a])		7.0	14.0		
Haemorrhage into tumour[a])		5.0	2.0		
Radionecrosis brain[a])		0	3.0		
Brain abscess/encephalitis[a])		0	3.0		
Internal hydrocephalus[a])		7.0	19.0		
Graft vs host reaction[a])		0	1.0		

[a]) percent age of cases
[b]) percent age of courses

luable cases), 18 (two-thirds) died of tumour recurrence or the sequelae of further operations with a median survival of 164 weeks (range 105–275 weeks), while 9 patients (one-third) are alive with a mean survival of 164.2 weeks (range 112–228 weeks) (tab. 6). One-third of the long-survivors had grade IV glioblastomas. While most of the deceased patients underwent further operation for tumour recurrence, only two of the surviving patients had a second operation. The performance status

Table 5 Recurrence-free intervals and survival in patients treated with radiation and COMP-polychemotherapy using different doses of procarbazine (PCZ)

	100% PCZ (n = 48)		50–75% PCZ (n = 42)		Total Group (n = 90)	
	Grade 3	Grade 4	Grade 3	Grade 4	Grade 3	Grade 4
Free interval (mean) mos	16.0	8.1 +	15.0	7.3	15.8	8.0
Survival (mean), mos	28.5 +	13.8 +	26.9 +	13.1 +	27.1 +	13.7 +
Difference	N. S.	N. S.	N. S.	N. S.		

Table 6 Patients with malignant gliomas surviving at least two years combined radiation and COMP-chemotherapy group N = 90

Total		N = 27 (30%)	Deceased N = 18	Alive N = 9
Tumour type	Astro III	13	8	5
	Oligo-Astro III	5	4	1
	Astro IV	9	6	3
Location	Right	17	10	7
	Left	10	8	2
	Frontal	11	7	4
	Temporal	7	6	1
	Parietal	5	3	2
	Occipital	4	2	2
N of operations	one	9	2	7
	two	8	6	2
	tree	8	8	–
	more	2	2	–
Survival (weeks)	Range	105–275	105–275	112+ – 228+
	Mean	164	164	164.2+
Karnofsky Rating (Mean)	3 mos after surg.		87	93.3
	after 2 years		61	90
	last (alive)		–	64.4
	4 weeks before death		23.9	
Complications	Tumour recurrence	17	16	1
	Recurrence + generalization		(5)	–
	Int. hydrocephalus[a)]	7	4	3
	Progressive dementia (a)	6	4	2
	Radionecrosis	2	2	–

[a)] same patients

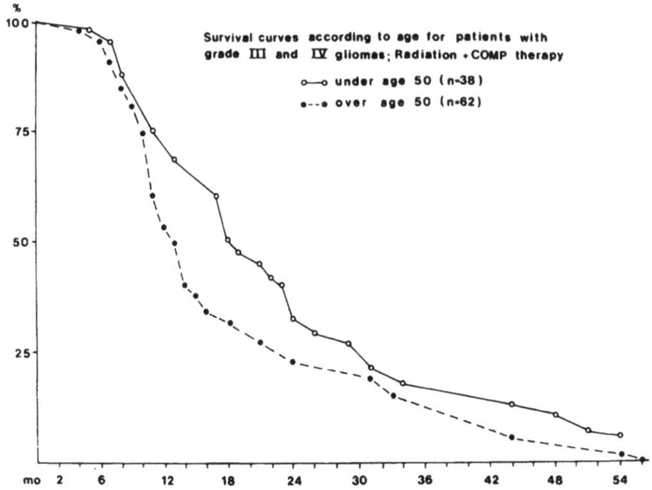

Fig. 5

remained fairly stable during the first two years, but afterwards showed a progressive decrease with rapid disease progression within a few weeks before death. Of the long-survivors 25–30% developed progressive cerebral dysfunction, dementia, and brain atrophy or internal hydrocephalus with or without tumour recurrence, while two patients died of delayed radionecrosis of the brain. Only five patients, i.e. 18% of the long-survivors or 5.6% of the total multimodality treatment group are doing well with a mean Karnofsky performance of 64 (tab. 6).

Conclusions

Radiation and chemotherapy cannot cure malignant gliomas, but they can produce considerable delay in progression of the disease and an increase in life span and quality of survival. From the presently available data the combination of operation, megavoltage irradiation, and multiple-agent chemotherapy seems to be the most suitable approach for malignant supratentorial gliomas, currently providing a 2–4 year survival with reasonable quality of life in 7–15% of these patients, while a 5-year survival, increasingly observed in medulloblastomas and malignant lymphomas of the CNS [5, 6, 9, 11], is almost never achieved in malignant gliomas [7, 12, 13]. However, it should be kept in mind that about 10% of the malignant gliomas, usually of anaplastic type III, without further treatment have been reported to show a two-year life-span after operation, while 1–3% are still alive five years after operation alone [1]. Further success with a better rate of tumour kill and improvement of both life span and quality of survival will only come after greater sophistication in combined treatment techniques with modification of system toxicity.

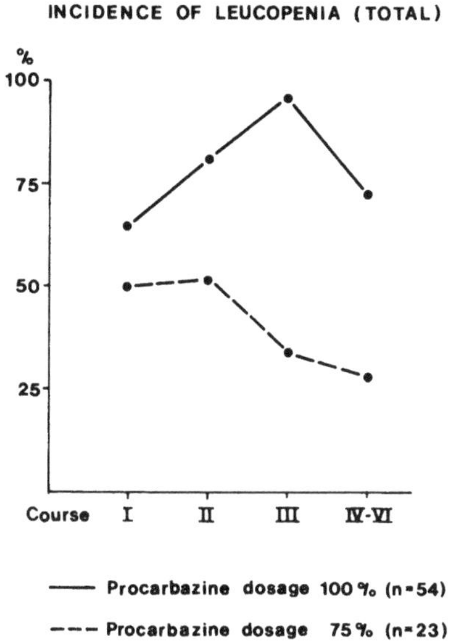

Fig. 6

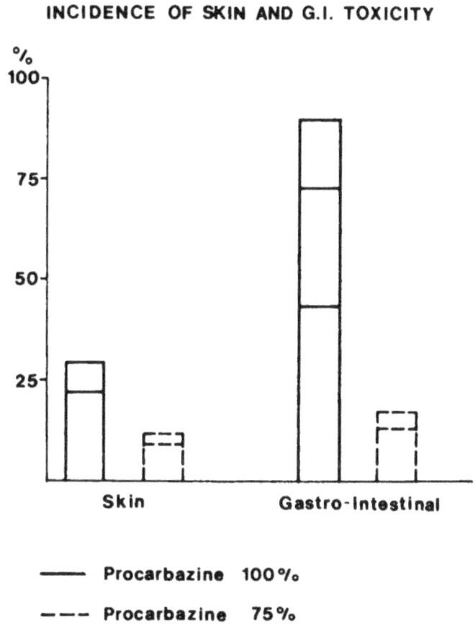

Fig. 7

Summary

A controlled, non-randomized study of 267 age-matched patients with histologically verified grade III and IV supratentorial gliomas, maximum feasible tumour resection, postoperative Karnofsky performance over 50, and minimum survival of eight weeks compares the results of supportive care with intermittent steroid administration (65 patients), megavoltage irradiation of 40 to 66 Gy (69 patients), polychemotherapy – COMP protocol (CCNU, procarbazine, vincristine, MTX, methylprednisone in 15-day cycles) – (43 patients), and simultaneous irradiation and COMP chemotherapy (90 cases including 20 survivors). Median recurrent-free intervals in the treatment groups (6.9 to 11.6 months) were significantly longer than after supportive care (3.5 months). Mean survival with supportive care (7.2 months) was significantly shorter than after radiation or COMP chemotherapy (12.3 and 13.2 months) and 17.3 to over 25.2 months with multimodality treatment, where the two-year survival rates were 23% and 55% (survivors), the 3-year survival rates 14% and 47%, and the 4-year survival rates 5% and 12% (survivors). Toxic side effects of multimodality treatment were more frequent and more severe than after chemotherapy alone, but haematologic, gastrointestinal, and mucosal toxicity was considerably decreased by 25% to 50% dose reduction of procarbazine without impairment of tumour prognosis. In addition to space-occupying cerebral cysts often simulating tumour recurrence (7–14%), rare radiation necrosis, CNS haemorrhage and infections, about 25% of long-term survivors developed progressive intellectual dysfunction with brain atrophy in the absence of tumour regrowth. Despite promising results of multimodality treatment of malignant gliomas, currently providing a 2–4 year survival with reasonable quality of life in 7–15% of tumour hosts, the results generally are unsatisfactory and need further improvement.

References

[1] Elvidge, A. R., J. G. Roth: Glioblastoma multiforme, Review of 219 cases with regard to natural history, pathology, diagnosis, methods and treatment. J. Neurosurg. **15** (1960) 489–503.

[2] Green, S. B., D. P. Byar, M. D. Walker, et al.: Comparison of carmustine, procarbazine, and high-dose methylprednisolone as addition to surgery and radiotherapy for the treatment of malignant glioma. Cancer Treatm. Rep. **67** (1983) 121–132.

[3] Heiss, W. D., M. Turnheim, B. Mamoli: Combination therapy of malignant gliomas. Europ. J. Cancer **14** (1978) 1191–1202.

[4] Hildebrand, J.: Chemotherapy of malignant supratentorial gliomas in adults. A ten-year experience of the E.O.R.T.C. Brain Tumour Group. Proc. 13th Int. Congr. Chemother. S. E. 12. 1/17, Part 249, 1–4, Vienna 1983.

[5] Jellinger, K.: Primäre und sekundäre Lymphome des Zentralnervensystems. In: Verhandl. Dtsch. Ges. Neurol. (D. Seitz, P. Vogel, eds.), Bd. 2, pp. 14–48. Springer, Berlin–Heidelberg–New York 1983.

[6] Jellinger, K., D. Volc, W. Grisold, et al.: Ergebnisse der Kombinationsbehandlung maligner Hirngeschwülste. Neuropsychiat. Clin. **2** (1983) 21–41.

[7] Jellinger, K., D. Volc, W. Grishold, et al.: Kombinationsbehandlung maligner Gliome. Wien. Klin. Wschr. **95** (1983) 407–416.

[8] Lieberman, A. N., S. H. Foo, J. Ransohoff, et al.: Long term survival among patients with malignant brain tumours. Neurosurg. **10** (1982) 450–453.

[9] Mertens, H. G., U. Bogdahn, D. Dommasch, et al.: Diagnostik und Therapie cerebrospinaler Manifestationen von Leukosen und malignen Lymphomen. In: Verhandl. Dtsch. Ges. Neurol. (D. Seitz, P. Vogel, eds.), Bd. 2, pp. 49–69. Springer, Berlin–Heidelberg–New York 1983.

[10] Neumann, J.: Zur Prognose des Glioblastoma multiforme heute. Nervenarzt **54** (1983) 191–196.

[11] Paoletti, P., M. D. Walker, G. Butti, et al. (eds.): Multidisciplinary aspects of brain tumour therapy. Elsevier, Amsterdam 1979.

[12] Seiler, W.: Die undifferenzierten Astrozytome des Großhirns. Springer, Berlin–Heidelberg–New York 1982.

[13] Walker, M. D. (ed.): Oncology of the nervous system. Martinus Nijhoff Publ., Boston–The Hague–Dordrecht–Lancaster 1983.

[14] Zülch, K. J.: Histological types of the tumours of the CNS (International Histological Classification of Tumours, Nr. 21). WHO, Geneva 1979.

Combined chemotherapy of inoperable and operable malignant gliomas

P. Krauseneck, H. G. Mertens, E. Richter, M. Schmidt, E. Halves, U. Bogdahn, L. Kappos, D. Seybold

Introduction

Since 1977 we have been treating inoperable malignant gliomas with a combination of Bleomycin and BCNU. Bleomycin possesses only minimal bone-marrow toxicity, as a G-2 phase specific agent it is a radio-sensitizer and it is reported to be effective in malignant gliomas [1, 10]. Therefore it seemed to be an ideal agent to combine with BCNU, an alkylating substance effective in all phases of the cell cycle, likewise radio-sensitizing and with cumulating dose-limiting bone-marrow toxicity [3].

Although in series of autopsies of Bleomycin-treated patients drug-related histological changes were described in up to 60% [2], the likelihood of symptomatic interstitial pneumonitis was estimated to be as how as 3.4%–10% [1, 7] and of definite pulmonary fibrosis as 2% [1]. Pulmonary toxicity of BCNU was been reported in only a few cases [6].

However, because of the unexpectedly high incidence of pulmonary toxicity in our series, we even had to consider the possibility, that the combination would produce a shorter survival time than BCNU alone. Furthermore we wanted to investigate the pulmonary toxicity of BCNU alone and of the combination of BCNU with VM 26 as a possible more effective chemotherapy in malignant gliomas.

Methods

Four groups of patients (pts.) with malignant brain tumours were treated. All groups were irradiated with 60 Gy tumour dose within 7–11 weeks. Group 1 (N = 16) and 2 (N = 17) were operated on and received as chemotherapy BCNU + VM 26 or BCNU alone. Group 3 (N = 23)* and 4 (N = 50)** could not be operated on, and

---

* In cooperation with the Neurological Department of the Medical School Hannover.

** In cooperation with the Neurological Department of the University of Homburg/Saar.

BCNU alone or in combination with Bleomycin, was administered. Clinical (Karnofsky rating), haematological (WBC, RBC, platelets, SMA 12 + 6, GOT, GPT, γ-GT) and pulmonary (chest X-ray, pulmonary function test) conditions were closely monitored. Fifteen non-operated, only irradiated patients collected from previous years were compared to the inoperable groups as historical controls.

Patient selection

The groups were treated consecutively and patients were not randomized. In the operated groups all had a histologically verified malignant glioma at least partially resected (56% and 76% glioblastoma), a Karnofsky-score of 50% or more and no major reduction of pulmonary function. In the inoperable groups selection criteria were: history, clinical findings, CT and angiography indicative of a malignant glioma, no sign of systemic malignant disease and operation not considered by the neurosurgeon. The autopsy findings, which were available for 50% of the patients revealed only one case without a verified malignant brain tumour (no cerebral lesion detected). Sixty-three percent of the tumours in group 3 and 77% of group 4 were glioblastomas. Inoperable patients with minor preexisting pulmonary disease were excluded from Bleomycin treatment. No chemotherapy was given to patients with severe pulmonary disease. Starting from July 1980 we selected only patients with a Karnofsky score of at least 50%. Until then patients with lower ratings had also been treated. Selection criteria were the same for the historical control group as for the inoperable groups.

Chemotherapy

BCNU (80 mg/m^2) was given on three consecutive days every six weeks, starting with day of radiotherapy. This dose was reduced to 70%, only when severe thrombocytopaenia (< 30 000/μl) or leucopaenia (< 1000/μl) occurred. However, in case of toxicity the next cycle was delayed until the WBC returned to 3500/μl and platelet count to 10 000/μl. BCNU was continued as long as the CT showed a tumour mass and bone marrow and pulmonary function were adequate. Bleomycin was given initially 4 × 15 mg weekly during the irradiation only. After having treated 12 patients the dose was reduced to 15 mg twice weekly because of severe pulmonary toxicity. Pulmonary function tests were performed before every chemotherapy pulmonary restriction occurred or the diffusion capacity for CO dropped below 50%. VM 26 in a dose of 50 mg/m^2 was given simultaneously with BCNU on days 1 and 2 of the cycle. Limitations were the same as for BCNU. Dexamethasone was used to treat brain oedema as required and usually during the radiation therapy. It was given in doses as low as possible and discontinued as soon as possible.

For evaluation of pulmonary toxicity the patients were divided into three groups: BCNU + Bleomycin (N = 19), BCNU alone (N = 23) or BCNU + VM 26 (N = 14).

Whole body plethysmography was used to monitor pulmonary function with supplementary equipment to measure diffusion capacity of CO in steady state. Patients were evaluated, when at least three examinations had been recorded.

Results

No statistical differences were found for the 5 groups in sex distribution and Karnofsky scores (fig. 1) but the patients in group 3 were significantly older and had a smaller radiation dose, namely 50.7 Gy as against at least 57.0 Gy in the other groups. This is partially due to selection for pre-existing lung disease. Follow-up period (tab. 1) in group 1 at 42 weeks is considerably shorter.

As in group 1 only four patients died the follow-up will show if the combination with VM 26 is more favourable than BCNU alone. In this preliminary evaluation of the operated patients the life-table analysis [4] shows slightly longer survival times than the randomized studies of the American BTSG [5, 11, 12] (fig. 2).

In spite of the additional toxicity of Bleomycin the survival of group 4 is similar to that of group 3, which however is negatively selected by age and lower radiation dose. Both groups lived longer than the 4–5 months reported in the literature for operated patients without radio- or chemotherapy [8, 11]. The differences in survival time are significant only between the operated and non-operated groups.

Considering only those patients who have received the complete irradiation series and two or more cycles of chemotherapy as a 'valid study group', the mean and

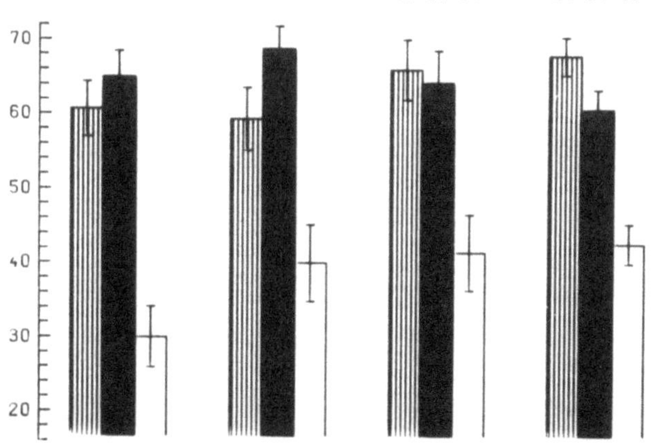

Fig. 1 Pre-treatment Karnofsky-scores (striate column), mean scores (Black) and scores four weeks before death (white column) in the four chemotherapy groups.

Table 1 Actual Survival of the four chemotherapy groups

group	N	Age mean	Survival (wks) mean	median	alive	more than ... months 12	18	24
1 OP + VM 26	16	50.2	42	36.5 +	12	4 + (25%)	1 + (6%)	?
2 Op	17	53.8	62	60	7	12 (71%)	6 (35%)	1 (6%)
3 no Op	23	58.6	37	31	7	5 (22%)	2 (9%)	1 (4%)
4 no Op + Bleo	50	53.2	31	20	5	9 (18%)	6 (12%)	3 (6%)

All groups had 60 Gray radiation and BCNU every 6 weeks

median survival is as long as the 9–10 months reported for operated patients with additional irradiation of 60 Gray [8, 11] (tab. 2).

The comparison with the control group of inoperable patients – irradiated only – shows that somewhat younger patients with higher Karnofsky scores live considerably longer with completed chemo-/radiotherapy. Older patients with lower Karnofsky scores seem to have a higher risk of complications and of not completing the initial phase of combined treatment, so eventually doing better with radiotherapy alone. However, this needs further examination.

Toxicity was not different in the four groups as regards bonemarrow depression, infections and impairment of liver and renal functions. Renal toxicity was not seen at all, nor in autopsy evaluations. Liver toxicity was mild and did not require any dose reduction. Some problems were caused by chronic relapsing or septic infections, in four cases they were responsible for an untimely death. There were several thromboembolic complications (two strokes, two myocardial infarctions, seven pulmonary embolisms) not accumulating in any group.

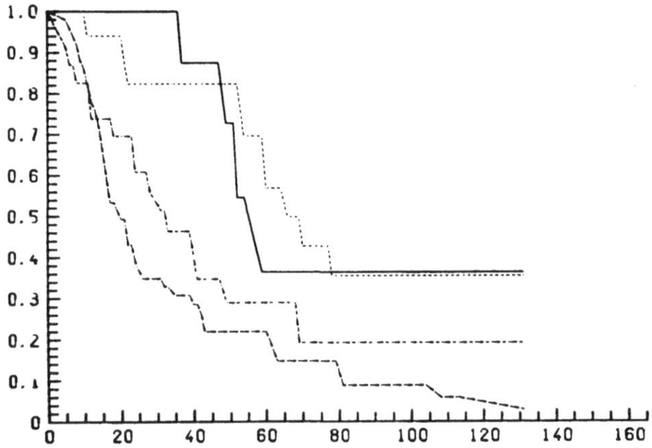

Fig. 2 Life-table analysis of the four chemotherapy groups (survival times in weeks).
——— = BCNU + VM 26
..... = BCNU (op.)
–·–·– = BCNU (not op.)
– – – = BCNU + Bleomycin

Table 2 Survival of non-operated patients: historical only irradiated control group, incompletely treated group and 'valid study group'

group	N	Age	Survival (wks)		Karn. pre.	≥ 18 months
		mean	mean	median		
only radiation 60 Gy	15	49.7	28	25		0
< 60 Gray < 2 × chemotherapy	27	58.9	18	13	57%	1 (4%)
≥ 60 Gray ≥ 2 × chemotherapy	46	52.5	41	34	72%	7 (15%)

Significantly different in the chemotherapy groups was the pulmonary toxicity (table 3). Indeed, in all three groups pulmonary function decreased and showed a partial reversibility. However, in the Bleomycin group the decrease of the diffusion capacity as the most specific indicator of drug-related toxicity was significantly greater and toxicity occurred considerably earlier (table 4). Cytostatic therapy had to be interrupted more often in the Bleomycin group and one patient who was in a good state of remission died of acute pulmonary fibrosis. In four other cases the pulmonary problems contributed to the fatal outcome, in contrast to one case in both other groups. Other significant differences between the pulmologically monitored groups were not detected.

Conclusions

Inoperable patients with malignant glioma should be treated with a combined radiotherapy/chemotherapy as the median survival time may reach that of patients irradiated after operations. Although a carefully established clinical diagnosis is fairly safe, a stereotactic biopsy is preferable in these cases.

Table 3 Course of pulmonary function during chemotherapy

test	group	before ther.	minimum	last exam.
Vital Capacity	I	3896 ml	−30.6%	−24.9%
	II	4557 ↑	−26.9%	−21.4%
	III	3843	−19.2%	− 9.9%
Total Lung Capacity	I	6316 ml	−29.3%	−24.1%
	II	7213 ↑	−22.1%	−15.9%
	III	6582	−11.4%	−11.7% ↑
Diffusion Capacity	I	108%	−46.3%	−37.9% ↑
	II	100	−32.0%	−19.0%
	III	97	−36.1%	−25.8%

group I = BCNU + Bleo, II = BCNU, III = BCNU + VM 26
(↑ = significantly different from the other groups)

Table 4 Time interval (in days) between pre-treatment pulmonary function test and lowest value during chemotherapy

group	mean	median interval (days)
BCNU + Bleo	142.3	79.0
BCNU	276.1	281.5 ↑
BCNU + VM 26	186.5	160.5

(↑ the difference BCNU, and BCNU + Bleomycin is significant)

In spite of a good theoretical basis the combination of BCNU with Bleomycin in patients with malignant glioma does not produce a longer or better survival than BCNU alone. The combination is also accompanied by a high rate of toxicity.

In malignant glioma the effectiveness of polychemotherapy remains unproven. As the cytostatic drugs available have high toxicity but low effectiveness any combination bears the risk merely of being more toxic. Therefore in this field pilot studies with regard to toxicity are especially necessary.

Until now in 16 patients the combination of BCNU and VM 26 was in no respect more toxic than BCNU alone. The follow-up is too short to determine a possible higher effectiveness.

As shown here pulmonary function regularly decreases under BCNU therapy with only partial reversibility. Therefore treatment with BCNU requires monitoring of pulmonary function to prevent a potentially lethal pulmonary fibrosis.

References

[1] Blum, R. H., S. K. Carter, K. Agre: A Clinical Review of Bleomycin – A New Antineoplastic Agent. Cancer **31** (1973) 903–14.

[2] Burkhardt, A., J. O. Gebbers, W.-J. Höltje: Die Bleomycin-Lunge. DMW **102** (1977) 281–289.

[3] Carter, S. K., J. W. Newmann: Nitrosoureas: 1,3 – bis (chloroethyl) -1- nitrosourea (BCNU) and 1-(2-chloroethyl) -3- cyclohexyl -1- nitrosourea (CCNU) – Clinical Brochure. Cancer Chemother. Rep. **1** (1968) 115–151.

[4] Cutler, S. J., F. Ederer: Maximum Utilization of the life-table method in analyzing survival. J. Chron. Dis. **8** (1958) 699–712.

[5] Green, S. B., D. P. Byar, M. D. Walker, et al.: Comparisons of Carmustine, Procarbazine, and High-Dose Methylprednisolone as additions to surgery and radiotherapy for the treatment of malignant glioma. Cancer Treat. Rep. **67** (1983) 121–132.

[6] Holoye, P. Y., D. E. Jenkins, S. D. Greenberg: Pulmonary toxicity in long-term administration of BCNU. Cancer Treat. Rep. **60** (1973) 1691–1694.

[7] Ichikawa, T., S. Tsubak, I. Hirokawa: Statistical observations of the side effects of Bleomycin. The First National Hospital of Tokyo Monograph, pp. 1–16 (1968).

[8[Jellinger, K., D. Volc, I. Podreka, et al.: Ergebnisse der Kombinationsbehandlung maligner Gliome. Nervenarzt **52** (1981) 41–50.

[9] Luna, M. A., C. W. M. Bedrossian, B. Lightiger, et al.: Interstitial pneumonitis associated with Bleomycin therapy. Am. J. Clin. Path. **58** (1972) 501–510.

[10] Takeuchi, K.: A clinical trial of intravenous Bleomycin in the treatment of brain tumours. Int. J. Clin. Pharm. **12** (1975) 419–426.
[11] Walker, M. D., E. Alexander Jr., W. E. Hunt, et al.: Evaluation of BCNU and/or radiotherapy in the treatment of anaplastic gliomas: a Cooperative Clinical Trial. J. Neurosurg. **49** (1978) 333–343.
[12] Walker, M. D., S. B. Green, D. P. Byar, et al.: Randomized comparisons of radiotherapy and nitrosoureas for the treatment of malignant glioma after Surgery. N. Engl. J. Med. **303** (1980) 1323–1329.

Mono-treatment of malignant glioma with a derivate of nitrosourea, ACNU (first results)

D. Voth, N. Hüwel, S. Al-Hami, A. Kuhnert

Introduction

Derivates of nitrosourea on their own, or in combination with other chemicals are widely used in the treatment for malignant glioma [15, 20, 21, 22]. However in the course of recent years the optimistic note in judging the efficiency of this treatment has decreased considerably. Some authors report no beneficial effect at all [5, 14] while others stating an improvement in survival rate [1, 3, 4, 7, 8, 9, 12, 18, 19].

With the development of a water soluble and stable derivate, the substance *ACNU* (Nimustin) a more effective [37] and also a more favourable substance concerning side effects seemed possible. The chemical composition of the compound is 1-(4 amino-2-methyl-5-pyrimidinyl)methyl-3-(2-chloraethyl)3-nitrosourea-HCL.

A phase I study started in October 1974, a phase II study was carried out in Japan between 1975–1978 [11, 23]. At the beginning of 1980 the substance became available in Europe and we used it persistently in chemotherapy of malignant glioma. On account of its marked lipophilia, ionisation tendency and minimal protein binding capacity we used the substance as the sole therapy, which we could interrupt at will, in case no therapeutic effect was noted.

Selection of patients and methodology

Chemotherapy with ACNU followed operation and radiotherapy. The operation [32] aimed at total (macroscopically) tumour resection or at least a considerable reduction of tumour mass. In the early post-operative phase dexamethasone was administered but was terminated during radiotherapy.

The *radiotherapy* was a convential one, reaching 50–60 Gy for a focal tumour dose. During radiation each patient was examined in regular intervals (oncology outpatients) and the course of the disease process recorded. Computer-Tomography was carried out three or four times in the first year with greater intervals later on.

ACNU-chemotherapy was supervised in outpatients, the mode of treatment will be reported separately (N. Hüwel, D. Voth). After finishing the course of radiotherapy, the ACNU treatment started (fig. 1) and 2–3 mg/kg i.v. were administered in intervals of 4–6 weeks. The general practioner measured twice weekly the following parameters; haemoglobin, red and white cell counts, differential blood cell counts, thrombocytes, SGPT and γ-GT. Before this therapy started a pulmonary test was performed, to screen vulnerable patients for the possible complication of interstitial pulmonary fibrosis.

To be admitted to the mono-therapy study the following conditions had to be fullfilled:

1. The tumour has to be verified histologically and its malignancy grading ascertained.
2. The patient must be older than 16 years.
3. Administration of steroids (dexamethasone) had to be stopped at least 12 days postoperative and used only occasionally during irradiation.
4. The condition of the patient at the start of chemotherapy has to correspond at least to a Karnofsky-index of 60%. The success of the treatment is judged, a) by the survival time, b) the interval between operation and the re-appearance of tumour tissue (free interval), c) the clinical condition of the patient in comparison to Karnofsky-index.

After a series of 6–8 cycles the medication was interrupted for 3 months and than continued for the same number of cycles. After two of such periods chemotherapy was stopped altogether in patients free from tumour regrowth.

The *classification of patients* into treatment groups: A) operation, B) operation and radiotherapy, C) operation + radio- and chemotherapy. The number of patients in the glioblastoma groups were 121; 21 in A, 66 in B, 34 in C. The astrocytoma III and

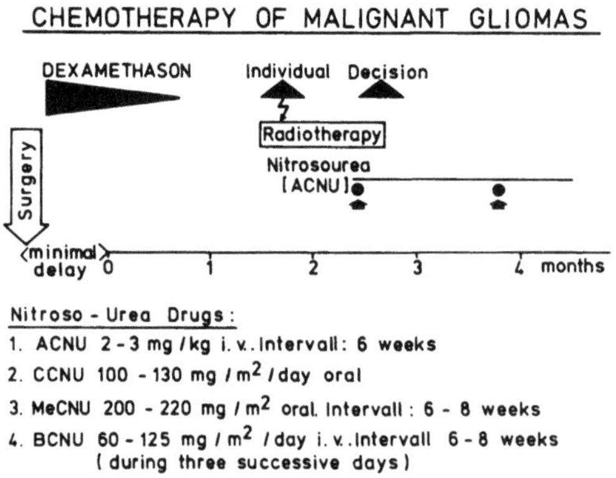

Fig. 1 Diagramatic presentation of therapeutic planning. Dosage and plan of therapy of other nitrosourea derivates are illustrated in lower half of illustration.

IV cases, intentionally separated from the glioblastomas numbered 12 in A; 33 in B; 13 in C. The oligodendrogliomas, which will not be considered in this context numbered 27 in A; 21 in B; 7 in C. Other tumours such as ependymomas and rare forms of gliomas have not been considered.

A comparison of groups showed no disturbing variation regarding age and sex within the types of tumour classification. The control groups A (operation) and B (operation and radiotherapy) were patients treated before we introduced ACNU monomedication. For this reason no comparable controls in time course or clinical history were available. To avoid this inherent disadvantage, all calculations were made against a small group of patients closely related in time to each therapeutic groups. This procedure has been necessary, as the classification of astrocytomas III and IV has been altered by the WHO classification. The consequences of this new definition for judging the different therapeutic effects has been characterised by Gullotta (p. 21); when the new classification was published in 1979 we had to reclassify our previous groupings.

We report in the present paper the results of the ACNU treatment as these are shown in the *post-operative survival times. The statistical evalution* was carried out by Mrs. S. Kuhnert of the Dept. of Medical Statistics and Documentation of the University of Mainz, a co-author of the paper, using 1. the generalized Wilcoxon (Breslow) and 2. the generalized Savage (Mantel-Cox) procedures. A $P < 0.001$ was considered to be the significance level.

Results

Glioblastomas

Using a life-table analysis after Cutler and Ederer the ACNU treatment for the total number of patients with glioblastoma and astrocytoma III and IV showed a positive effect, although not a dramatic one (fig. 2). A further analysis of the data resulted in a much clearer picture. Considering the glioblastoma group on its own, no age factor on the prognosis of the operated patients (A) is detectable (fig. 3a). Patients in group C however survive significantly longer if their age at the disease onset is under 50 years (fig. 3b).

A similar behaviour can be detected concerning the *sex of the patient.* This factor is of no significance for survival if the patient has only been operated on (A) (fig. 4a). However female patients survive distinctly longer if the operation is followed by irradiation and chemotherapy (group C). This influence on prognosis by a sex and age factor becomes apparent when additional chemotherapy is applied (fig. 4b), while operation and irradiation (group B) has no influence on survival by belonging to one of the sexes.

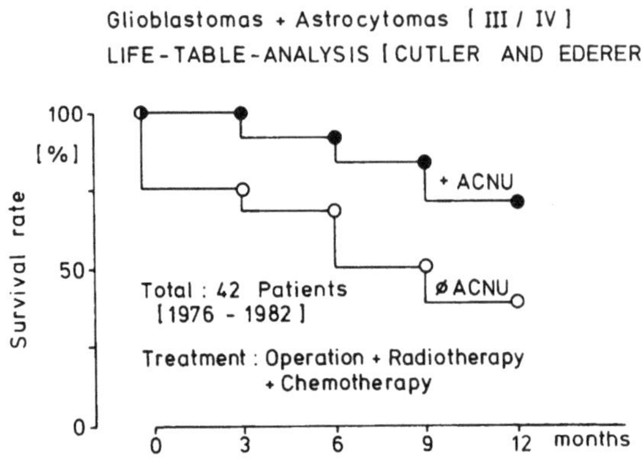

Fig. 2 Life-table-analysis for the total number of patients suffering from glioblastomas and astrocytomas grad III and IV shows a global improvement of life expectancy for ACNU.

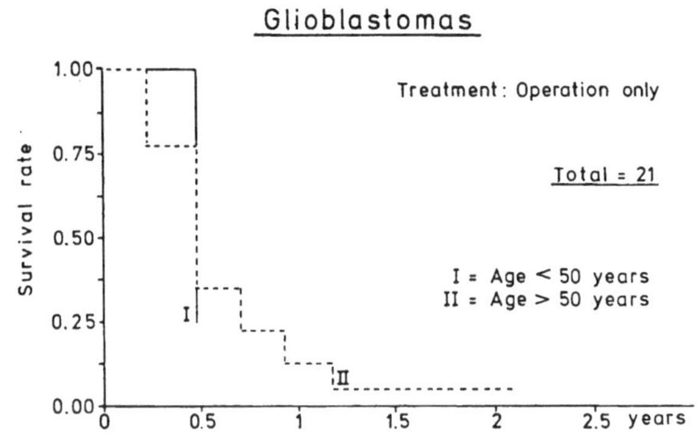

Fig. 3a Age of operated patients has no influence on survival. However additional radio- and chemotherapy reveal a prognostic significance of this parameter.

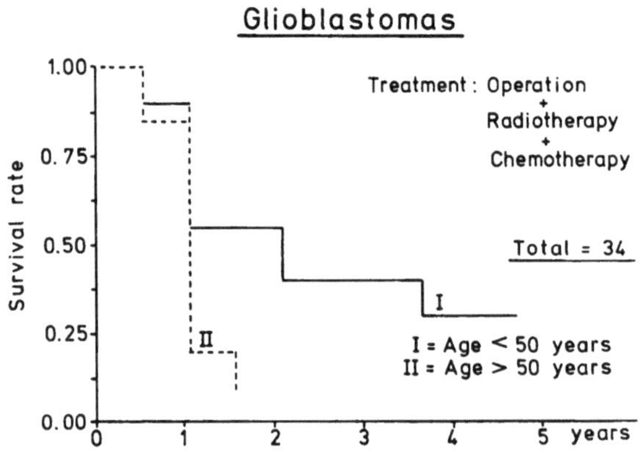

Fig. 3b A favourable prognostic factor is not evident – although reported previously – for lower age groups in our therapeutic approach A, however present in approach C.

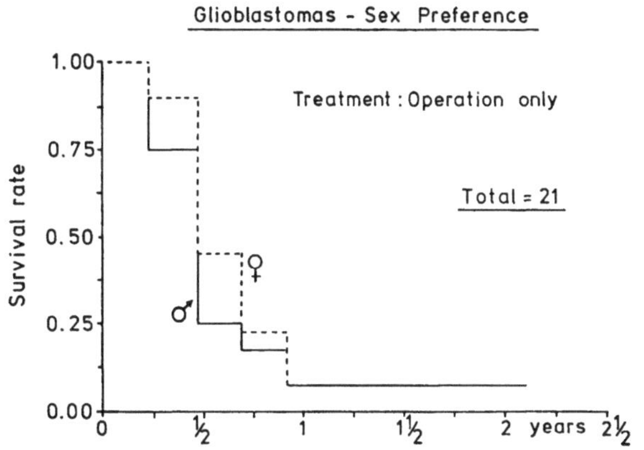

Fig. 4a A previously reported favourable prognostic "female" factor is not evident for patients operated on only.

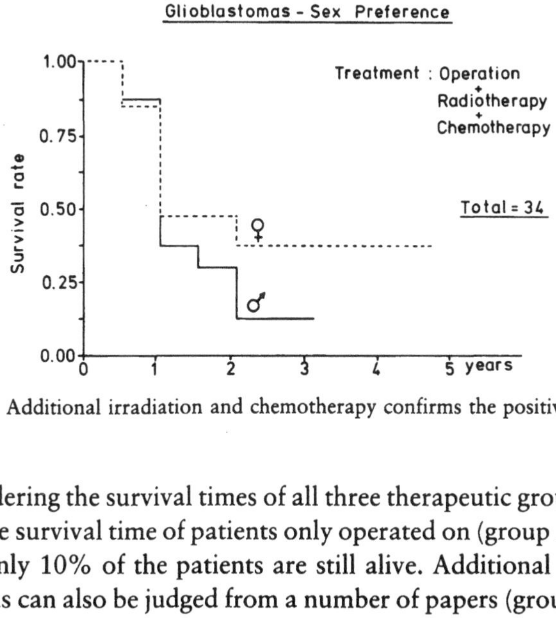

Fig. 4b Additional irradiation and chemotherapy confirms the positive "female" factor.

Considering the survival times of all three therapeutic groups (fig. 5) it becomes clear that the survival time of patients only operated on (group A) is minimal, for after one year only 10% of the patients are still alive. Additional radiotherapy improves results, as can also be judged from a number of papers (group B). In this group 50% of patients are still alive after one year, but after 2 years the survival rate is below 10%. An additional therapy with ACNU (group C) has no significant effect on survival. Only a small number of patients survive longer than two years and no difference exists between B and C. These relationships mirror the middle and mean values obvious between group A on the one hand and groups B and C on the other, but not between group B and C.

The findings permit the statement, that additional chemotherapy for the treatment of glioblastoma shows no effect on survival time. This is clear, if the results of group B

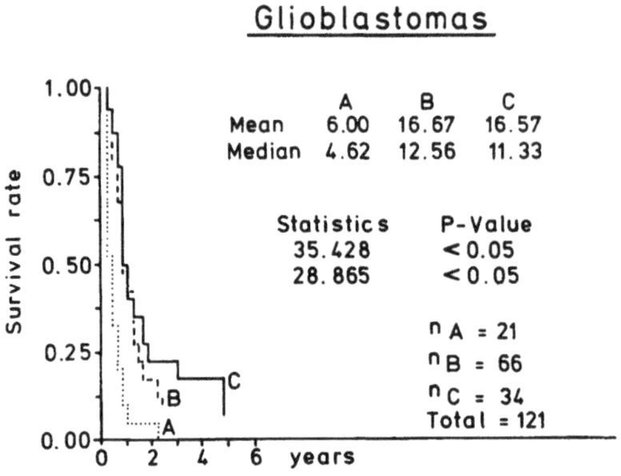

Fig. 5 Survival rates of glioblastoma-patients subjected to all three forms of therapy. Median and middle values show that chemotherapy (approach C) does not improve results in group B.

and C are contrasted using a different scale (fig. 6). It means at the same time that the glioblastomas as such are not responsible for the favourable effect of ACNU treatment, as it seems to be the case from the life-table-analysis.

Astrocytomas

The group of astrocytomas I and II (old nomenclatur) will be discussed only briefly, as they are not of malignant nature. From the 800 patients suffering from glioma we have isolated those patients with benign astrocytomas. A first survey shows their survival time to be much higher and that those patients only operated on, half of them survived longer than five years (fig. 7). Additional irradiation, usually carried out if the tumour could only partially removed or was located in an unaccessible region did not alter the outcome. A comparison of both therapeutic groups A and B showed no significant differences (fig. 7a)).

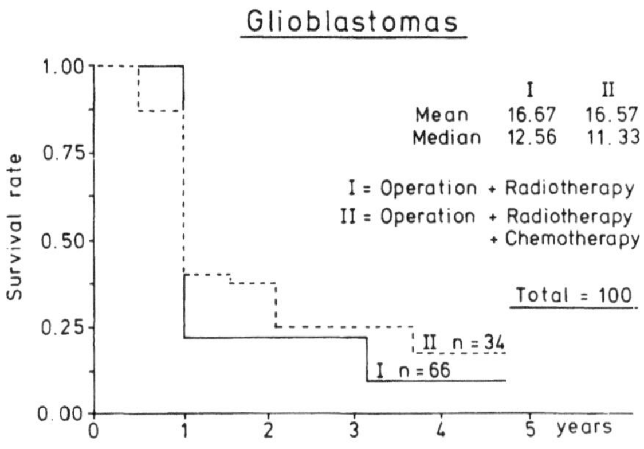

Fig. 6 ACNU therapy in glioblastoma is ineffectual and even more evident when extending the time axis.

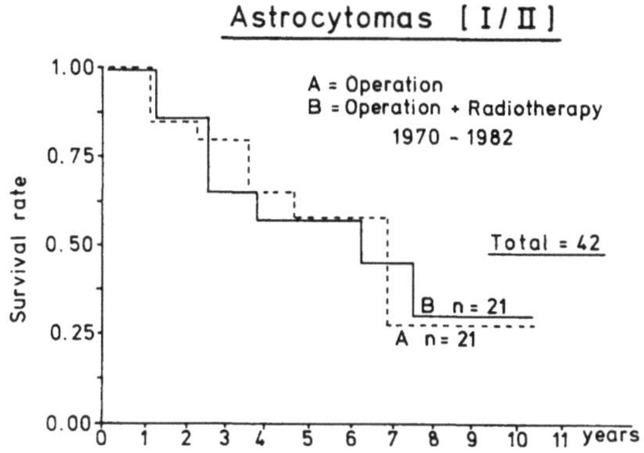

Fig. 7 Survival time of operated patients for "benign" astrocytoma (A) is not improved by radiotherapy (B).

The results in the patients group (astrocytoma III or IV) (s. fig. 8) were surprising. Survival time after operation only (A) is as bad as in cases of glioblastoma. After one year only 10% of the patients survived, but additional irradiation improved survival for the first year by 75%. The end of the second year showed no survivor in group A, but group B had 30% survivors. Group C had the best results. End of the first year 90% were still alive, at the end of the second year 70% and 50% lived longer than 3 years. The therapeutic group C has so far been followed up for 3½ year only. Statistical examination of the numbers confirms these findings with a significance level P below 0.0001. In this connexion it may be mentioned that as far as oligodendrogliomas are concerned, no differences between the 3 therapy types have been found. (A = 27, B = 21, C = 7 patients). For all 3 groups the 50% survival rate is at six years.

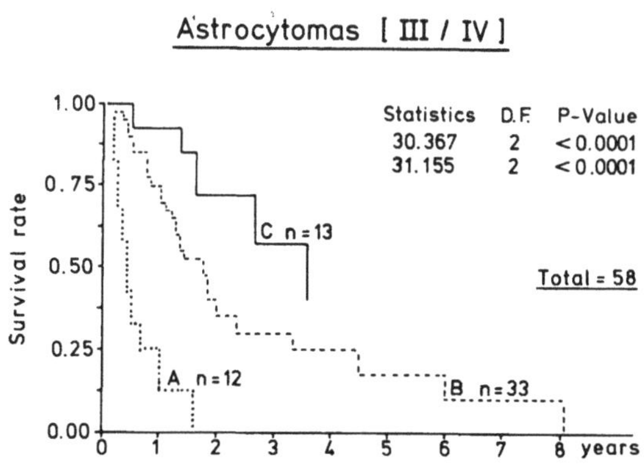

Fig. 8 Cases of astrocytoma III and IV of group A are not better placed than glioblastoma patients. Radiotherapy (B) has a significantly favourable effect still improving if chemotherapy (C) is added.

Therapeutic side effects

The degree of side effects was controlable enabling outpatient treatment. Acute side effects were vomiting, nausea and fatigue but after 3 days they subsided. During the following week a third of the patients complained of a reduction in well being, similar to a mild virus infection. A number of patients were able to follow their profession. In case a patient felt very unwell we reduced the drug to half the dose and sometimes shortened the interval between two injections, provided the blood values permitted.

Besides these acute and on the whole harmless side effects the action on the bone marrow is more serious. Bone marrow depression however is at the same time an indicator of the efficiency of the therapy and present in a high proportion. In 70% of the patients undergoing ACNU treatment the number of thrombocytes decreased below 100 000/mm^3; in 70% of the patients the white cell counts dropped below 4000/mm^3. An impairment of renal or liver function was not noticed, although transaminases were slightly increased in 50% of our patients.

In 7% of patients severe bone marrow damage was noted after several treatment cycles, forcing cessation of treatment and blood transfusion due to severe anaemia. In two patients this condition lasted several months. Several transfusions were needed and hospitalisation for a short period. No fatalities however were recorded.

Pulmonary tests before and after ACNU treatment showed no evidence of fibrosis, although the number of treated patients might have been too small.

The time course for side effects regarding bone marrow depression was characterised by the low values for white cell count and thrombocytes in the 3rd week but showed a tendency to normalisation in the 4th week. The intervals of six weeks between the single injections proved to be adequate.

Discussion

The results of the ACNU treatment for the *glioblastomas* [28] are clearly disappointing. It has not been possible to prolong survival time beyond the time, which can be gained by operation and irradiation alone. This fact forced us to terminate this type of treatment for glioblastoma and search for better ways [16, 17, 26, 30, 36].

A questionable, but perhaps not an unimportant aspect is the small percentage of a group of long survivors. The number of long surviving glioblastoma patients undergoing chemotherapy is bigger than the number of the two other groups treated. This aspect will be dealt with in a separate publication (N. Hüwel, D. Voth). It was to be expected that chemotherapy might not be rewarding in cases of benign astrocytomas (I type of the old, II of the WHO classification) [10, 13] as older observations reporting therapeutic effects could not be confirmed. In our therapeutic approaches irradiation proved also ineffectual and we see for astrocytomas of malignancy grading of II (WHO) no indication for irradiation or chemotherapy.

Concerning *astrocytomas grade III and IV* the results from our studies proved to be surprising [33]. These tumours responded to monotherapy with ACNU in a highly significant way regarding survival, well beyond the good effect of radiotherapy. The findings of the phase I and phase II studies had already revealed a favourable effect on neurogenic tumours. Although the treatment results of glioblastomas forces one to a considerable scepticism, it must be emphasize that the chemotherapy in this approach shows without any doubt a better survival time with ACNU.

We are aware that in this study some inherent difficulties are hidden. There is the problem of terminology changes and grading of 1979, which in particular for astrocytomas caused a devaluation of historically established controls for the valuation of therapeutic effects. This change will necessitate new or very cautious grading, as has been emphazized by Gullotta (p. 21) and Stochdorph (p. 19).

The neurosurgeon has to consider that the change in malignancy grading makes a comparison of different gliomas having the same malignancy grading most difficult. Furthermore that within a group of tumours, such as astrocytomas, the diagnosis of a grad III glioma has been made more frequently since 1979, in contrast to the earlier application of the malignancy grading after Kernohan or Ringertz. Some of these grade III tumours were in earlier times classified as grade II tumours.

It is therefore possible that recent studies show a higher survival rate only on account of the old terminology and a four step grading simulating a therapeutic effect. This trap can be avoided by either employing a strictly time-equal control group, as this is the case in a double blind or randomised study, or the controls have to be started from the onset of the new malignancy grading. The most labour consuming and final way would be the renewed evaluation of the tumour slides and regrading after the WHO recommendation.

We have tried solving these problems by revaluation of the slides, when this was possible and to take account of the present control groups as a whole, or to divide them into two parts one before 1979 and one after and scrutinise these groups against each other. In case there was no difference, the total group could be used for further evaluation. We are of course aware that only a study with time-equal controls can solve the problems raised above. This means furthermore the need for a multicenter study to re-examine our findings on the therapeutic effect of ACNU.

In spite of this cautious view we believe our results to be encouraging as far as astrocytomas are concerned [17, 29, 34], while the results for glioblastomas are not encouraging, confirming that a glioblastoma is biologically speaking different from an anaplastic astrocytoma.

The extent of side effects appears to be more favourable than those occuring when the treatment was carried out with BCNU, CCNU or MeCNU [1, 2, 4, 13, 24, 25, 29]. The impression is gained that among the nitrosourea derivates ACNU can be adapted more easily and with controlable side effects, but having to some extent all the undesirable side effects of this group of substances. The controlable side effects make it possible to treat patients under outpatient conditions at a period of life when their time spend at home is most appreciated and valued. For these reasons ACNU should be seriously considered as one of the therapeutic measures in spite of all the disappointments in chemotherapy.

Summary

The present paper reports the results of chemotherapy for glioma with the nitrosourea derivate ACNU. ACNU has been administered in a single dose of 2–3 mg/kg i.v. in six weeks intervals.

This mono-therapy with ACNU is ineffectual in patients suffering from glioblastoma. In patients with malignant astrocytoma (III and IV grading, WHO) a highly significant improvement in survival has been seen. These findings however have to be critically viewed against the background of the change in tumour terminology and malignancy grading. Our results regarding astrocytoma treatment, hopeful as they are, ought to be reviewed in a multi-center-study. Concerning side effects, ACNU is the most favourable among derivates of nitrosourea.

References

[1] Avellanosa, A. M., Ch. R. West, Y. Tsukuda, et al.: Chemotherapy of non-irradiated malignant gliomas. Phase II Study of the combination of methyl-CCNU, vincristine, and procarbacine. Cancer **44** (1979) 839–844.

[2] Band, W. R., B. Weir, R. C. Urtasun, et al.: Radiotherapy and CCNU in grade III and IV astrocytoma. ASCO abstract **15** (1974) 161.

[3] Cooper, J. S., T. L. Borok, J. Ranshoff, et al.: Malignant glioma. Results of combined modality therapy. JAMA **248** (1982) 62–65.

[4] Edwards, M. S., V. A. Levin, C. B. Wilson: Brain tumour chemotherapy: an evaluation of agents in current use for phase II and III trials. Cancer Treat. Rep. **64** (1980) 1179–1205.

[5] EORTC Brain tumour group: Effect of CCNU on survival rate of objective remission and duration of free interval in patients with malignant brain glioma: final evaluation. Eur. J. Cancer **14** (1978) 851–856.

[6] Fewer, D., C. B. Wilson, E. B. Boldrey, et al.: The chemotherapy of brain tumours. Clinical experience with carmustine (BCNU) and vincristine. JAMA **222** (1972) 549–552.

[7] Fulton, D. S., V. A. Levin, W. M. Wara, et al.: Chemotherapy of pediatric brainstem tumors. J. Neurosurg. **54** (1981) 721–725.

[8] Green, S. B., D. P. Byar, M. D. Walker, et al.: Comparisons of carmustine, procarbazine, and high-dose methylprednisolone as additions to surgery and radiotherapy for the treatment of malignant glioma. Cancer Treat Rep. **67** (1983) 121–132.

[9] Gutjahr, P., D. Voth, M. Neidhardt: Ergebnisse der kombinierten Behandlung (Operation, Radio-

und Chemotherapie) bei 132 Kindern mit primären ZNS-Tumoren. Therapiewoche **28** (1978) 4346–4352.

[10] Gutjahr, P., D. Voth: Treatment and prognosis of childhood brain tumours: experience with 140 cases. Verhdlg. Deutsch. Krebsges. **2** (1979) 434–435.

[11] Hasegawa, H., T. Hayakawa, M. Hori, et al.: Antineoplastic effects of nitrosoureas on experimental gliomas. Comparison of ACNU, a water-soluble agent, and Methyl-CCNU, a lipid-soluble agent. No-to-Shinkei **29** (1977) 891–898.

[12] Heiss, W. D.: Chemotherapy of the effect of polychemo- and CCNU-therapy. Acta neurochirurg. **42** (1978) 109–115.

[13] Hildebrand, J., J. Brihaye, L. Wagenknecht, et al.: Combination chemotherapy with CCNU, vincristine and methotrexate in primary and metastatic brain tumors. Eur. J. Cancer **11** (1973) 585–589.

[14] Hildebrand, J. (ed.): Evaluation of CCNU, VM-26 plus CCNU, and procarbazine in supratentorial brain gliomas. Final evaluation of a randomized study. J. Neurosurg. **55** (1981) 27–31.

[15] Hildebrand, J., D. Zegers de Beyl: Rationale of combined chemotherapy of brain tumours. In: Tumours of the central nervous system in infancy and childhood (D. Voth, P. Gutjahr, C. Langmaid, eds.), pp. 374–377. Springer-Verlag, Berlin–Heidelberg–New York 1982.

[16] Hill, S. A., E. A. Neuwelt: Intra-arterial chemotherapy following blood-brain barrier disruption in a patient with malignant glioma. J. Neurosurg. Nurs. **14** (1982) 94–97.

[17] Hochberg, F. H., L. M. Parker, T. Takvorian, et al.: High-dose BCNU with autologous bone marrow rescue for recurrent glioblastoma multiforme. J. Neurosurg. **54** (1981) 455–460.

[18] Jellinger, K., D. Volc, I. Podreka, et al.: Ergebnisse der Kombinationsbehandlung maligner Gliome. Vergleiche postoperative Strahlen-, Polychemo- sowie kombinierte Strahlen- und Polychemotherapie. Nervenarzt **52** (1981) 41–50.

[19] Jellinger, K., D. Volc, W. Grisold, et al.: Kombinationsbehandlung maligner Gliome. Wien. Klin. Wschr. **95** (1983) 407–416.

[20] Kornhuber, B.: Cytostatic monotherapy of tumours of the central nervous system in children. In: Tumours of the central nervous system in infancy and childhood (D. Voth, P. Gutjahr, C. Langmaid, eds.), pp. 367–373. Springer-Verlag, Berlin–Heidelberg–New York 1982.

[21] Levin, V. A., C. B. Wilson: Chemotherapy: The agents in current use. Semin. Oncol. **2** (1975) 63–67.

[22] Levine, M. A., M. D. Walker, H. D. Weiss: Intravenous methyl-CCNU in the treatment of malignant glioma (Phase II). ASCO abstract **15** (1974) 167–172.

[23] Nagourney, R. A., P. Fox, P. S. Schein: A comparison of the biological and biochemical properties of 1-(4-Amino-2-methylpyrimidin-5-yl)methyl-3-(2-chlorethyl)-3-nitrosourea and 2-(3-[2-Chlorethyl]-3-nitroso-ureido)-D-glucophyranose. Cancer Research **38** (1978) 65–68.

[24] Reagan, T. J., H. F. Bisel, D. S. Childs, et al.: Controlled study of CCNU and radiation therapy in malignant astrocytoma. J. Neurosurg. **44** (1976) 186–190.

[25] Rosenblum, M. L., A. F. Reynolds, K. A. Smith: Chloroethyl-cyclohexyl-nitrosourea (CCNU) in the treatment of malignant brain tumors. J. Neurosurg. **39** (1973) 306–314.

[26] Salcman, M., R. S. Kaplan, G. M. Samaras, et al.: Aggressive multimodality therapy based on a multicompartmental model of glioblastoma. Surgery **92** (1982) 250–259.

[27] Scherer, E., U. Schulz: Möglichkeiten und Grenzen der Strahlentherapie bei Geschwülsten der vorderen Schädelgrube. Onkologie **4** (1981) 322–327.

[28] Shehata, W. M., R. L. Meyer, F. K. Jazy, et al.: Management of glioblastoma multiforme by irradiation and chemotherapy. IMJ **163** (1983) 30–34.

[29] Taylor, S. G., L. Nelson, D. Baxter, et al.: Treatment of grade III and IV astrocytoma with dimethyl triazeno imidazole carboxamide (DTIC, NSC-45388) alone and in combination with CCNU (NSC-79037) or methyl CCNU (MeCCNU, NSC-95441). Cancer **36** (1975) 1269–1276.

[30] Urtasun, R. C., P. Bond, J. D. Chapman, et al.: Radiation and high dose metronidazole (Flagyl) in supratentorial glioblastomas. New Eng. J. Med. **294** (1976) 1364–1367.

[31] Voth, D., P. Gutjahr, C. Landmaid: Tumours of the central nervous system in infancy and childhood. Springer-Verlag, Berlin–Heidelberg–New York 1982.

[32] Voth, D.: Standard methods and microneurosurgery: the operative treatment of supra- and infratentorial tumours. In: Tumours of the centralnervous system in infancy and childhood (D. Voth, P. Gutjahr, C. Langmaid, eds.). Springer-Verlag, Berlin–Heidelberg–New York 1982.

[33] Voth, D., N. Hüwel, S. Al-Hami, et al.: Brain tumour chemotherapy with ACNU – prevention and treatment in cases of recurrence. Proc. 13th Internat. Congr. Chemother. Vienna (1983).
[34] Walker, M. D., E. Alexander, W. E. Hunt: Evaluation of BCNU and/or radiotherapy in the treatment of anaplastic gliomas. A cooperative clinical trial. J. Neurosurg. 49 (1978) 333–343.
[35] Wilson, C. B., P. Gutin, E. B. Boldrey, et al.: Single-agent chemotherapy of brain tumors. Arch. Neurol. 33 (1976) 739–744.
[36] Witman, G., E. Cadman, D. Kapp, et al.: The use of cisplatinum for treatment of malignant glioma. Med. Hypotheses 8 (1982) 335–341.
[37] Yoshida, J., N. Shibuya, T. Kobayashi, et al.: Sensitivity to 1-(4-amino-2methyl-5-pyrimidinyl)methyl-3(2-chloroethyl)-3-nitrosourea hydrochloride (ACNU) of glioma cells in vivo and in vitro. Cancer 50 (1982) 410–418.

Retrospective study on the effect of CCNU and radiotherapy in 44 patients with malignant glioma

H. W. Ilsen, W.-D. Heiss

Introduction

Several therapeutic schedules for the treatment of malignant gliomas have been used in the Neurological Clinic in Köln-Merheim since 1975. From 1975 to 1977, the patients received a combination chemotherapy with CCNU, VM 26 and adriamycin, as introduced by Pouillart et al. [5]. This treatment resulted in a median survival time of 6.5 months [2, 4]. 1978 and 1979 we continued by giving CCNU alone instead of a combination therapy, for it had become obvious by recent publications [6, 7] that CCNU alone (also BCNU alone) was at least as effective as our previous combination therapy.

In 1979, the therapeutic procedure for our malignant glioma patients was changed again, since new encouraging results (median survival time 10.7 months) were obtained by the COMP (CCNU, vincristine, amethopterine, procarbazine) protocol [1, 3]. However, after the first experience with the COMP schedule in Köln-Merheim, the impression was gained that this therapy was frequently accompanied by severe side effects, especially polyneuropathy, bone marrow disturbances and allergic resp. toxic skin manifestations. This was the reason why several of our patients who had started to receive the COMP schedule continued with CCNU alone. Some of these patients also received modified COMP therapy (without amethopterine or without vincristine).

In 1981, we decided to stop the COMP therapy on account of its severe side effects and to give CCNU only in combination with high dose (50 Gy) radiotherapy.

For the present meeting we studied the patient files from 1979–1982 and summarize our experience with the CCNU- and the COMP-protocol.

Material and methods

44 patients (34 men, 10 women), aged between 24 and 68 years (mean age 47.4 years), were evaluated for this study. All patients suffered from malignant gliomas. At the beginning of the chemotherapy, they were in a good general clinical condition

and free from severe neurological symptoms and had an estimated life expectancy of more than 6 weeks.

Tumour diagnosis

In 28 cases the tumour was treated (removed) neurosurgically before the beginning of the chemotherapy. The time interval between operation and chemotherapy was between 2 and 6 weeks. The histological diagnosis of the 28 pre-operated patients is listed in table 1 (12 glioblastomas, 16 grade III gliomas). 2 of these patients had been operated twice, and one patient had been operated 3 times before included into this study. In these three cases, the primarily operated tumours had been gliomas of low malignancy degree, and no chemotherapy or radiotherapy had been given before the second resp. third operation.

In the remaining 16 cases, the tumour was considered to be inoperable due to its unfavourable localization or size. In these cases, the diagnosis (malignant glioma) was established by clinical and radiological findings (X-ray CT, cerebral angiography, positron emission tomography, exclusion of an extracerebral malignant tumour). 3 of these patients were operated during or after the time course of this study. In all of them the histological finding confirmed a glioblastoma. In 3 further patients, the diagnosis could be confirmed by post-mortem-autopsy. Thus, 10 cases remained with unknown histology.

Therapy schedules

28 patients were treated with CCNU (120 mg/m^2 orally in a two-day-cycle). The first 3–4 cycles were given at 6–8 weeks intervals, the later cycles in 8–12 weeks intervals. Between the first and the second cycle radiotherapy of 50 Gy was administered.

10 patients were treated according to the COMP protocol in 15-days-cycles as shown in table 2. The therapy cycles were repeated in the same rhythm as in the CCNU-protocol.

The remaining 6 patients received a "mixed" therapy, i.e. after 1–3 cycles of the COMP protocol their treatment was continued with CCNU alone as explained in the

Table 1 Diagnoses in 44 patients with malignant gliomas

44 patients	
28 after surgery (tumour removed)	16 without surgery (tumour inoperable)
12 glioblastomas	3 glioblastomas (verified by later neurosurgery)
9 astrocytomas III	3 tumours verified by autopsy (1 glioblastoma, 2 astrocytomas III)
6 oligodendrogliomas III	10 tumours without histology
1 mixed glioma III	

Table 2 The COMP protocol

CCNU	100 mg/m² p. o.	1 day
Vincristine	1.4 mg/m² i. v.	1. + 8. day
Amethopterine	10 mg/m² i. m.	3., 7., 10., 14. day
Procarbazine	100 mg/m² i. v.	2.–15. day

introduction. Both the COMP therapy and the "mixed" therapy patients had 30 Gy radiotherapy between the first and the second cycle.

In all cases the chemotherapy was continued either until the patient's death or until a survival of more than 2 years was reached. However, if severe bone marrow depression (white blood cells below $2000/mm^3$) or other complications (see below) occurred the inter-cycle interval was prolonged to allow sufficient recovery.

Results

Number of applied therapy cycles

The 28 patients who received CCNU and radiotherapy had a total number of 157 therapy cycles. For a single patient, the number of applied cycles ranged between 1 and 13 with an average of 5.7 cycles per patient. The 10 COMP patients received 42 cycles (1–8 cycles per patient; average 4.2). The 6 "mixed" therapy patients had 10 COMP cycles and 15 CCNU cycles (1–7 cycles per patient; average 4.1).

Survival times

The survival curve of the 28 patients with CCNU therapy is shown in figure 1. As seen, the curve median (indicating 50% survival) is 10.5 months. After 30 months 6 patients (= 21.4%) were still alive. – The survival curve of the 16 patients who received either the COMP protocol or the "mixed" therapy looks very similar (fig. 2). However, near the 50% level this curve exhibits a slight shifting to the right resulting in a curve median of 11.4 months. After 30 months 3 patients (18.75%) were still alive.

When comparing tumour types with different malignancy degrees, the median survival time of the glioblastoma patients was found to be distinctly shorter (8.5–9.5 months with CCNU, n = 10; 7.5–8.2 months with COMP, n = 6) than that of the grade III glioma patients (18 months with CCNU, n = 13; 24 months with COMP, n = 5, see tab. 3).

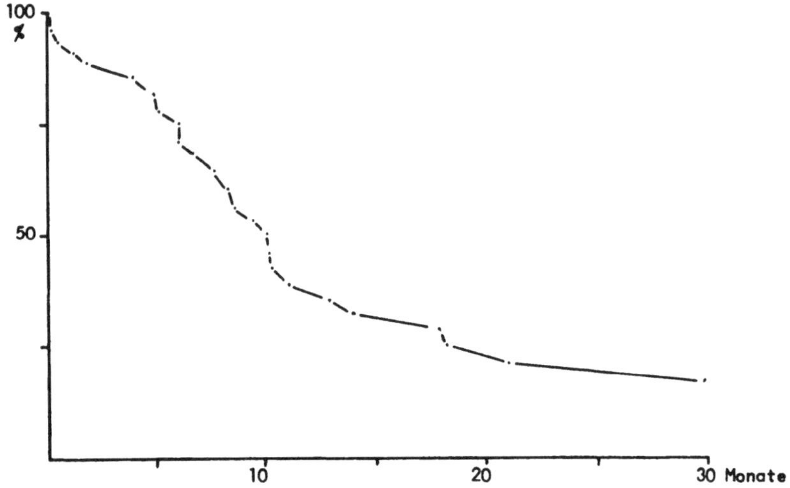

Fig. 1 Survival curve of 28 malignant glioma patients treated with CCNU. (Median survival time 10.5 months).

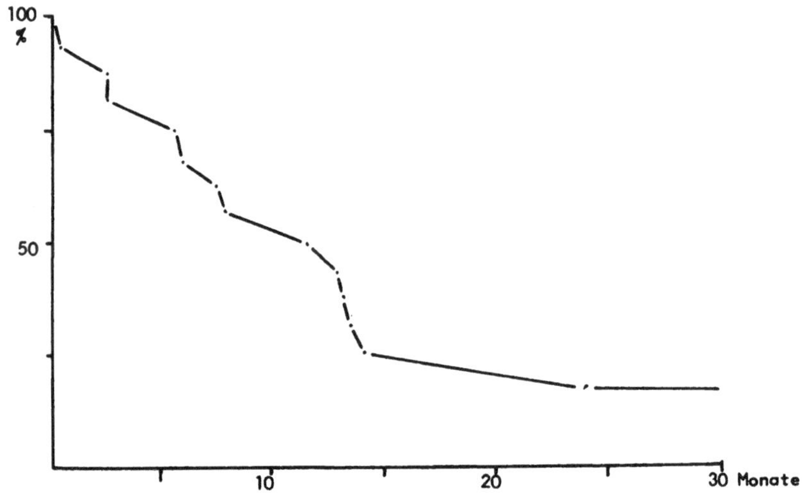

Fig. 2 Survival curve of 16 malignant glioma patients treated with the COMP protocol (including the "mixed" therapy patients). Curve median is 11.4 months.

Side effects

A list of the complications observed resp. unwanted effects is given in table 4. Only those disturbances were registered which were severe enough to cause specific measures (e.g. intercurrent hospitalization or delay of the next therapeutic cycle). As seen, bone marrow depression (leucopenia and/or thrombopenia) was the most frequent side effect. It occurred to a higher or lesser degree in all patients whose survival was

Table 3 Results (median survival time) after chemotherapy of malignant gliomas

	CCNU		COMP (incl. "mixed" therapy)	
	N	median (months)	N	median (months)
Glioblastomas	10	8.5–9.5	6	7.5–8.2
Grade III gliomas	13	18	5	24
without histology	5	10.5	5	12.8

long enough to administer 8–9 cycles and was reversible in all cases. Polyneuropathy and toxic skin manifestations (exanthema, purpura) were observed only after COMP therapy and not with CCNU alone. Both therapy protocols exhibited a relatively high frequency of infectious complications (herpes zoster, soor stomatitis, pleuritis).

Discussion

With CCNU and radiotherapy, we achieved for our malignant glioma patients a median survival time of 10.5 months. About 20% of the patients had more than 30 months of survival. This result is in the same order of magnitude as those of controlled studies on CCNU and radiotherapy [6] or BCNU and radiotherapy [8].

In comparison with our previously given polychemotherapy [2], a clear superority of the current therapeutic schedule is obvious (6.5 months median survival time with CCNU/VM 26/adriamycine versus 10.5 months with CCNU and radiation). However, since in both protocols CCNU is given in similar dosages, the significant differences seems to consist in the combination with radiotherapy which adds a further 4 months prolongation of survival time.

Table 4 Side effects of chemotherapy in malignant glioma patients

	CCNU alone (N = 28)	COMP incl. "mixed" therapy (N = 16)
Bone marrow depression	6 (21.4%)	2 (12.5%)
Polyneuropathy	0	5 (31.3%)
Herpes zoster	4 (14.3%)	2 (12.5%)
Increase of liver enzymes	3 (10.7%)	1 (6.25%)
Gastrointestinal disorders	1 (3.6%)	3 (18.75%)
Venous thrombosis	2 (7.2%)	1 (6.25%)
Exanthema, purpura	0	2 (12.5%)
Pleuritis	1 (3.6%)	3 (18.75%)
Candida-stomatitis (soor)	1 (3.6%)	3 (18.75%)
Nephrotic syndrome	1 (3.6%)	0

As for the COMP protocol a clear valuation of our data is difficult since our patients were treated rather inhomogenously (in some of them the COMP combination therapy was not completed because of severe side effects and was replaced by CCNU alone). However, we believe that the observed clinical treatment courses indicate that the COMP therapy may lead to further 1–2 months extension of median survival time in the grade III glioma but does not increase the rate of "long-time-survivors" (who survive more than 2 and ½ years). Furthermore, it is accompanied by severe side effects which reduce the benefit of longer survival.

Summary

44 patients with malignant gliomas received a cyclic chemotherapy with CCNU (120 mg/m^2 in a two-day-cycle; repeated every 6–12 weeks) and 50 Gy radiotherapy between the first and the second CCNU cycle. 16 of the patients additionally received vincristine, procarbazine and amethopterine (COMP protocol). The median survival time of the 28 CCNU patients was 10.5 months; that of the 16 COMP patients was 11.4 months. In both groups, about 20% of the patients survived more than 30 months. Toxic effects consisted in bone marrow depression, gastrointestinal disorders and infectious complications in both groups, whereas polyneuropathy and skin manifestations (exanthema, purpura) occurred in the COMP group only. A brief comparison with other publications is presented. It is concluded that the COMP protocol seems to be superior to CCNU alone in achieving a short prolongation of median survival time, but this effect is compensated by a number of severe side effects.

References

[1] Heiss, W.-D., M. Turnheim, W. Mamoli: Combination chemotherapy of malignant gliomas: effect of postoperative treatment with CCNU, vincristine, amethopterine, and procarbazine. Eur. J. Cancer **14** (1978) 1191–1202.

[2] Ilsen, H. W., J. N. Petrovici, H. D. Mennel, et al.: Die Wirkung kombinierter Chemotherapie (Adriamycin/VM 26/CCNU) bei hirneigenen Tumoren des Erwachsenenalters und im Tierexperiment. Fortschr. Neurol. Psychiat. 50 (1982) 73–90.

[3] Mennel, H. D., W.-D. Heiss, J. Petrovici: Vergleichsuntersuchungen mit verschiedenen chemotherapeutischen Behandlungsschemata bei malignen Gliomen. In: Therapie maligner Neoplasien des Gehirns (P. Krauseneck, H. G. Mertens (eds.). Perimed Fachbuch-Verlag, Erlangen 1983.

[4] Petrovici, J., H. W. Ilsen: Chemotherapy of brain tumors. In: Head Injuries. Tumors of the Cerebellar Region. Proceedings of the 28th Annual Meeting of the Deutsche Gesellschaft für Neurochirurgie (R. A. Frowein, O. Wilcke, A. Karimi-Nejad, M. Brock, M. Klinger, eds.). Springer-Verlag, Berlin – Heidelberg – New York 1978.

[5] Pouillart, P., G. Mathe, M. Poisson, et al.: Essai de traitement des glioblastomes de l'adulte et des metastases cerebrales par l'association d'adriamycine, de VM 26 et de CCNU. Noev. presse méd. 5 (1976) 1571–1576.

[6] Reagan, R. J., H. Bisel, D. S. Childs, et al.: Controlled study of CCNU and radiation therapy in malignant astrocytoma. J. Neurosurg. **44** (1976) 186–190.
[7] Rosenblum, M. L., A. F. Reynolds, K. A. Smith, et al.: CCNU (2-[2-Chloroethyl]-3-cyclohexyl-1-nitrosourea; NSC-79037) in the treatment of malignant brain tumors. J. Neurosurg. **39** (1973) 306–314.
[8] Walker, M. D., E. Alexander Jr., W. E. Hunt, et al.: An evaluation of BCNU and/or radiotherapy in the treatment of anaplastic gliomas. (A cooperative clinical trial) for the Brain Tumor Study Group. J. Neurosurg. **49** (1978) 333–343.

The treatment of brain tumours and brain metastases with a combination of Ifosfamid, BCNU and radiotherapy – preliminary results
(Brief communication)

W. Scheef, J. Schlechtingen

204 patients suffering from brain tumours or metastases were treated between September 1979 and May 1983. 124 patients had primary brain tumours, the remainders suffered from brain metastases (80 patients). The metastases originated from bronchial carcinomas of varying histo-pathology, breast-tumours, colon-rectal tumours and testicular tumours. The radiotherapy started with 300 rad, further 300 rad were applied during chemotherapy. 2 g/m^2 of Ifosfamid were given during five consecutive days and 20 mg/m^2 BCNU during days 1, 3, 5. On the average four treatment cycles were carried out, in cases where the initial treatment caused tumour regression. The therapy free intervals were arranged according to bone marrow reactions and lasted between 4–8 weeks. In 147 patients computertomography permitted the following assessment in cases of 101 primary brain tumours and 46 cases of secondaries: Among the cases of primary brain tumours 9 cases appeared to be fully recovered (9%) and 34 partially (33.4%). In further 14 patients (13.8%) a subjective improvement was reported but only little or no regression of tumour tissue was observable in CT. In 46 patients suffering from metastatic tumour, eight patients fully recovered (17.3%) and 20 patients (43.4%) partially.

Subjective compatibility was satisfactory if pre-medication and additional medication was well chosen. Late toxicity of BCNU demanded prolonged supervision after cessation of therapy. The great diversity of the disease process in the patients observed makes definite conclusions impossible and demands further systematic investigations.

Intra-arterial therapy of malignant gliomas with ACNU and BCNU in combination with phenobarbital protection (preliminary results)

H. Jaksche

Introduction

Intra-arterial therapy of malignant gliomas has been practiced since the discovery of cytotoxic drugs in the 1950s. The results during those first years were not very convincing, particularly in view of the toxic side-effects of the drugs. The cytotoxic treatment of gliomas is rarely used today. An unpublished report by Yamashita [7] however has renewed our interest in this possibility of treating gliomas. Since it is known that therapy with nitrosourea is accompanied by a depression of bone-marrow function after two to five weeks, an intravenous therapy with this powerful cytotoxic agent has to be used with considerable caution, and only few clinics treat malignant brain tumours with cytotoxic drugs. According to Levin et al. [5] and Müller et al. [6], it is possible to reduce bone-marrow depression by administering phenobarbital concomittant to the treatment with the cytostatic drug.

Cases

Nine patients with malignant gliomas were treated with intra-arterially administered ACNU and BCNU: 4 patients with computertomographically and angiographically diagnosed glioblastomas who had neither been operated on nor received radiotherapy, 2 patients with histologically verified glioblastomas without radiotherapy, 2 patients with histologically verified glioblastomas without radiotherapy, 2 patients with histologically established third degree astrocytomas without radiotherapy, and finally 1 patient with a polymorphous oligodendroglioma which had become malignant, and who had been operated on twice and received radiotherapy.

Methods

The patients were given alternating doses of either 100 mg ACNU or BCNU twice weekly. The cytostatic drugs were dissolved in 50 ml of distilled water and injected into the carotid artery or perfused through an angiographic catheter. 25 mg were administered during the first minute, the remaining 75 mg during the following 5 minutes. The patients received 4 × 100 mg phenobarbital daily beginning two days before treatment with the cytostatic drugs and continuing for the entire period of hospitalization. In addition, the patients were given 600 ml of 20% Mannitol 2 hours before the onset of treatment. The infusion of Mannitol should be concluded 1 hour before perfusion so that its therapeutic effect is maximal during application of the cytotoxic drugs. This preparatory treatment was designed to reduce tumour oedema and keep the penetration of the nitrosourea into the surrounding tissue at a minimum. The patients also received steroid in initially high, then progressively lower dosages.

Therapy with the cytostatic drugs was planned to last for two weeks and be repeated at monthly intervals. Following initial angiographic examination, the patients were monitored on a weekly basis by computertomography.

Case histories

Case 1: A 54 year old woman in poor condition was admitted for hospitalization. The patient had a slight hemiparesis of the left side and a beginning papilloedema. Tomography revealed a richly vascularized tumour on the right side with distinct collateral oedema and affinity for contrasting substances (fig. 2a). The angiogram showed such a highly vascularized tumour, which also had a media aneurysm, that the presence of an angioma was at first taken into consideration (fig. 1a). 100 mg of BCNU was administered twice.

According to subsequent computer scans, the tumour did not react, nor was the oedema reduced. Having procured ACNU, which was commercially available only in Japan at the time, the patient received 2 × 100 mg of this drug. Subsequent angiograms revealed a distinct reduction in the vascularization of the tumour (fig. 1b) and computer scans showed that the tumour itself (fig. 2b) as well as the extent of the collateral oedema had become smaller.

Case 2: A 35 year old man was initially admitted for hospitalization in 1979 at which time he was operated on for the removal of an oligodendroglioma in the right temporal area. A second operation was necessary in 1982 for a residual tumour. At that time the patient was also treated with 6000 rad radiotherapy. The patient was admitted to our clinic for hospitalization in 1983 with a second residual tumour on the right side and a further tumour in the left frontal region (fig. 3a). 100 mg of

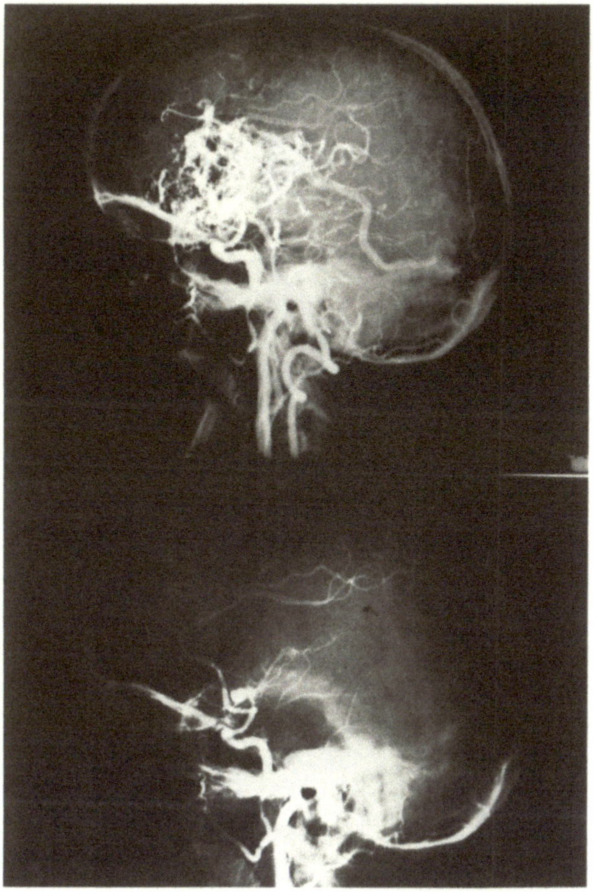

Fig. 1 The angiogram (case 1) showed a highly vascularized tumour.

ACNU was administered through both carotids twice weekly for two weeks. The neurological symptoms, e. g. hemiparesis, worsened. The man became comatose. In the hope that his condition could be favourably influenced by BCNU, as had been the case refered to above, the patient was given a single dose of BCNU. Subsequent computer scans (fig. 3e) revealed a reduction in the size of the tumour and the patient was sent home in markeldy improved condition after three additional doses of BCNU.

Results

Based on the encouraging experience gained with these two cases, we have begun treating additional tumour patients with regularly alternating doses of ACNU and BCNU. After only 5 months of this therapy, only preliminary results can be given.

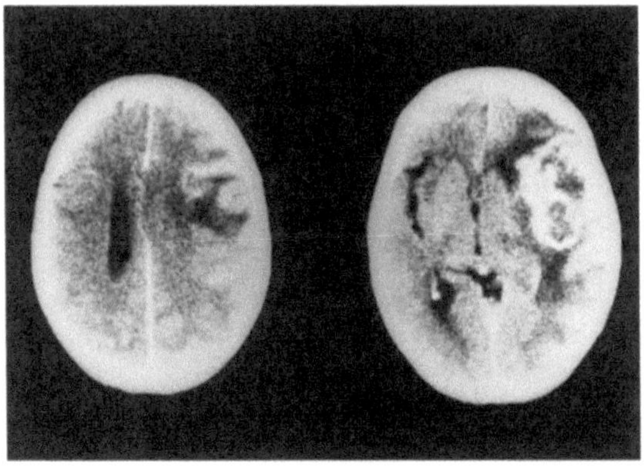

a)

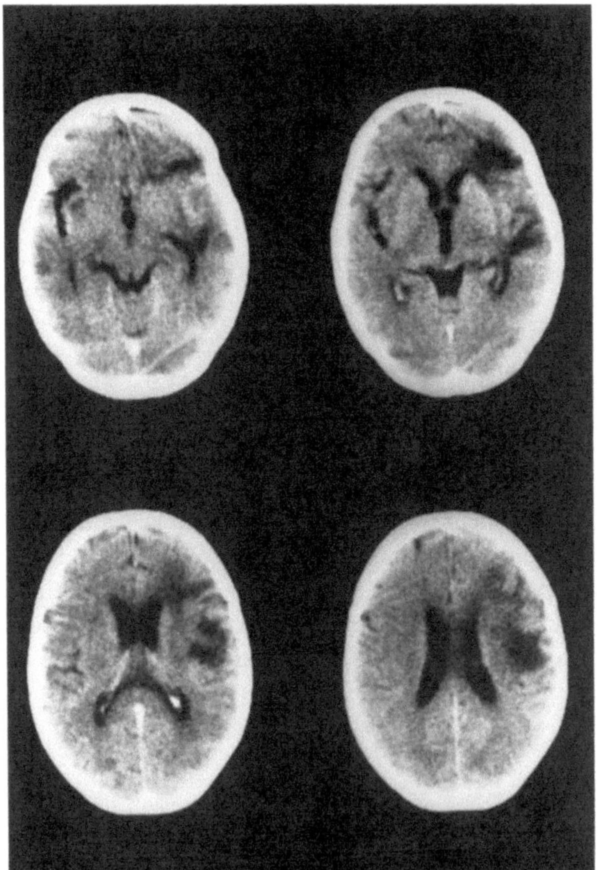

b)

Fig. 2 CT-findings (case 1): (a) a vascularized tumour with a collateral oedema and a strong enhancement. (b) After treatment with ACNU the tumour had become smaller.

One of our nine patients, after initial improvement, has died. There is a certain degree of bone marrow depression despite the treatment with phenobarbital. Thrombocyte counts (fig. 4) were reduced during therapy; granulocytes counts however, remained unchanged (fig. 5). Administration of ACNU has advantages over that of BCNU because in the former no pain occurs while intra-arterial perfusion of BCNU causes excrutiating pain in the eye on the side of the perfusion.

Discussion

The intra-arterial administration of cytostatic drugs was the method of choice in the hope that the systemic toxic effect could be reduced while simultaneously increasing the concentration of the cytotoxic agent in the tumour itself. In contrast to earlier

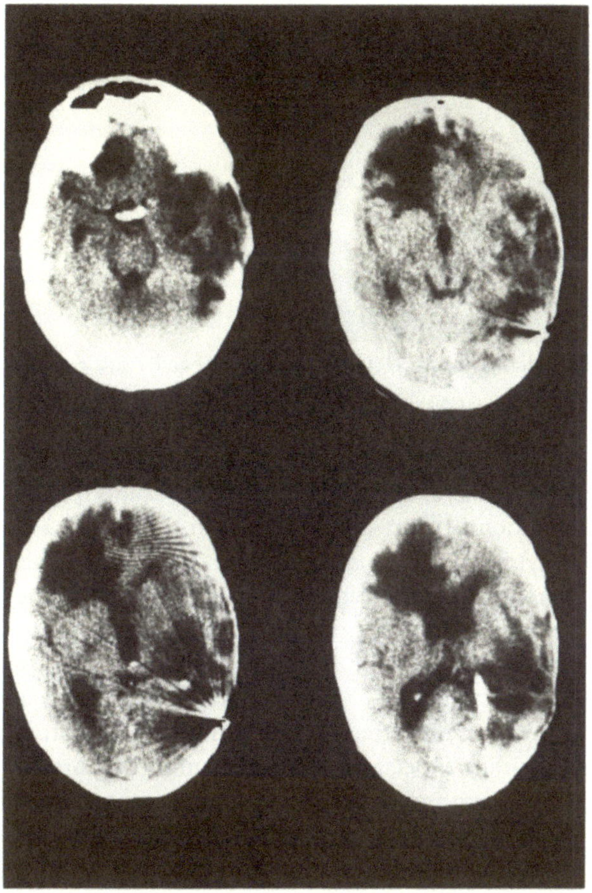

Fig. 3a

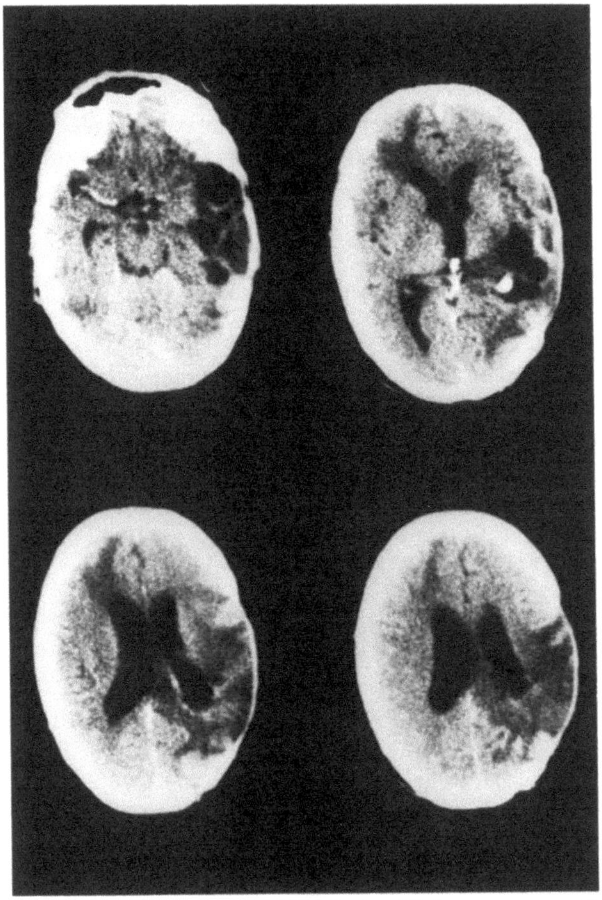

Fig. 3b CT (case 2) at the beginning (a) and after (b) the treatment with ACNU and a single dose of BCNU.

investigations, more recent pharmacokinetic research on monkey brains [4] has shown that intra-arterial administration of nitrosourea results in a three-fold increase in the concentration of the cytotoxic drugs in the tumour. On the one hand these compounds comply with the requirements set up by Blasberg [2] because they are selectively incorporated by the tumour. On the other hand, they are also particularly suited for intra-arterial perfusion because they have only a short half-life, another requirement set up by the same author [2]. BCNU has a half-life of only 15 minutes and ACNU one of 25 minutes. Intra-arterial administration of cytotoxic drugs to glioma patients lengthens their life expectancy [8]. These authors report that intravenously treated patients (i.e. systemic application) survived only an average of 9 months, whereas those who had been treated intra-arterially survived on the average 12½ months.

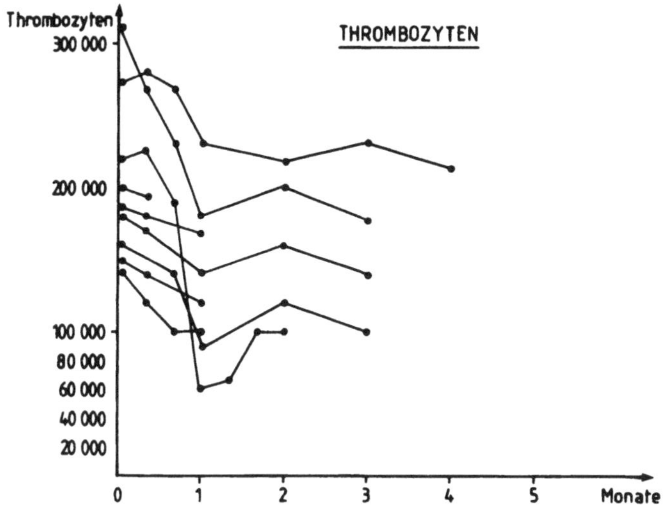

Fig. 4 Thrombocyte counts during the treatment (nine patients).

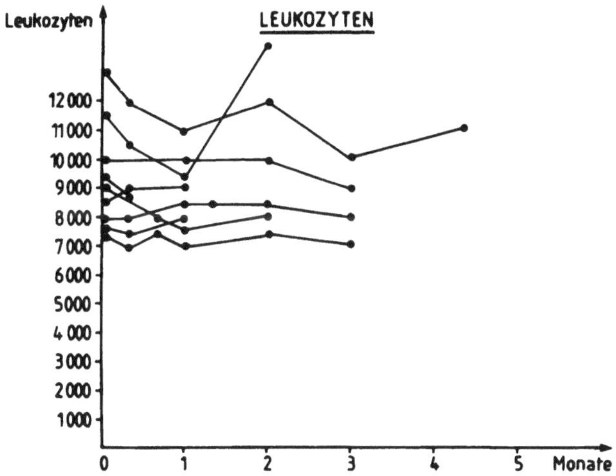

Fig. 5 Leukocyte counts of the same nine patients.

Summary

Nine glioma patients were treated with ACNU and BCNU. On the basis of our clinical experience, we believe that the combined use of these two nitrosourea compounds leads to better results than the use of either of them alone. Since the patients also received phenobarbital, bone marrow depression could be kept at a minimum. Although our results have so far been very encouraging, they should be regarded as preliminary until we have had additional clinical experience.

References

[1] Avellanosa, A. M., C. R. West, N. R. Barua, et al.: Treatment of malignant CNS gliomas by intra-arterial BCNU infusion. Proc. Am. Assoc. Cancer. Res. and ASCO. **20** (1979) 384.
[2] Blasberg, R. G.: Pharmacodynamics and the blood-brain barrier. Natl. Cancer. Inst. Monogr. **46** (1977) 19–27.
[3] French, J. D., P. M. West, F. K. von Amerongen, et al.: Effects of intracarotid administration of nitrogen mustard on normal brain and brain tumors. J. Neurosurg. **9** (1952) 378–389.
[4] Levin, V. A., P. M. Kabra, D. M. A. Freemann: Pharmacokinetics of intracarotid artery C-BCNU in the sqirrel monkey. J. Neurosurg. **48** (1978) 587–593.
[5] Levin, V. A., J. Stearns, A. Byrd, et al.: The effect of phenobarbital pretreatment on the antitumor activity of 1,3- bis (2-chloroethyl) 1-nitrosourea (BCNU), 1-(2-chloroethyl)-3-cyclohexyl- 1-nitrosourea (CCNU) and 1-(2-chloroethyl)-3-(2,6-dioxo-3-piperidyl)-1-nitrosourea (PCNU) and on the plasma pharmacokinetics and biotransformation of BCNU. J. Pharmacol. Exp. Ther. **208** (1979) 1–6.
[6] Muller, P. J., C. H. Tator, M. Bloom: The effect of phenobarbital on the toxicity and tumorcidal activity of CCNU in a murine tumor model. J. Neurosurg. **52** (1980) 359–366.
[7] Yamashita, J., K. Yumitori, H. Handa, et al.: Treatment of malignant brain tumors with ACNU and Phenobarbital (not yet published).
[8] Yamashita, J., H. Handa, Y. Tokuriki, et al.: Intra-arterial ACNU therapy for malignant brain tumors. J. Neurosurg. **59** (1983) 424–430.

Critical analysis of therapy in long-term surviving patients with glioblastoma multiforme

N. Hüwel, D. Voth, H. H. Göbel

Introduction

The aim of this scientific investigation was to examine critically the therapeutic results in glioblastoma-patients.

First of all we would like to explain the workings of the Oncological Outpatient Department at the University Clinic in Mainz, starting in 1976. It was our intention to utilise the new chemotherapeutic methods and conduct them with own tests.

Since 1976 we have treated a total of 131 patients in our Oncological Outpatient Department, 73 patients of these with glioblastoma multiforme. During the first 3 years we performed to some extent a polychemotherapy by administrating several drugs. Beside the nitrosourea derivatives obtainable at that time, like CiNU and BCNU [1–6, 19, 21–28, 30] we also used Methotrexat, VM 26, Vincristin, Adriblastin and DTIC. In some patients we have tried a combination therapy. It was one of our therapeutic principles to inject intrathecally at lumbar level Methotrexat to reach metastases at spinal level or in the liquor. In a number of glioblastoma-patients we also employed Ommaya-Reservoires and through these we applied cytostatica. Since 1980 we have given up this combined therapy using different chemicals and continued to administer the nitrosourea derivative ACNU [6–9, 16, 20]. In addition to this substance we gave only Methotrexat in such cases where spinal metastases were present or a dissemination into the spinal fluid.

Since 1976 the complete oncological therapy has been carried out in an outpatient department, arranging consulting hours once a week for clinical-neurological as well as neuro-radiological follow-up examinations.

Methods and patients

A significant aid in carrying out an oncological outpatient department is the cooperation of resident physicians. In each single case of these 131 patients we had weekly information about the actual blood picture and every four weeks, we were told of the total blood picture and the liver status. We are pleased to state that the cooperation between neuro-surgeon and physician for the follow-up treatment was excellent. It is in our outpatient department that the patients with malignant gliomas (oligodendrogliomas, astrocytomas grade III, and glioblastoma multiforme) receive their injection of 100 mg ACNU/qm body surface i.v. at intervals of 4 weeks. After the injection the patients are requested to stay in the clinica area for one hour in order to be observed and if necessary treated for allergic reactions. However, not a single case in the 131 patients developed an allergic reaction. The patients, who received chemotherapeutica intrathecally either by Ommaya-Reservoir or through lumbar puncture have also been seen in our outpatient-department.

In the course of these years our oncological outpatient-department got well established and relieved our general outpatient-department by observing treatment and control of tumour patients with malignant gliomas. Considerable time is needed for tumour patients regarding various advisory services, mainly those concerned with psycho-social problems. Here too we have to stress that tumour patients and their families have more need of social advisory service by clinical social workers, pastors and psychologists than is expected by the responsible authorities. We believe that social advisory work is an indispensable supplement to medial therapy and care. In many cases the contact between physician or surgeon and the patient is impaired by stress. It is unfortunate that we have first to inform the consulting patient and correct his expectations before we are able to approach slowly the problems concerning the patient himself. We also attach great importance to the discussion with his family in a very frank and responsible way about risks, therapy and results of treatment.

In the course of caring work we experienced that we take over quickly the tasks of a family doctor and become responsible for all the problems involved. This extends from providing expert's opinion in the social areas to the treatment of trivial disorders of family members.

Results

After these general remarks on the organisation and problems of the tumour outpatient-department, we shall now discuss the medical analysis in patients with glioblastoma or malignant gliomas grade III/IV. We emphasize that we changed from the initial polypraxy in the chemotherapeutical treatment to a more or less mono-therapy with nitrosourea derivatives, especially with ACNU.

The table 1 shows the case material, 73 patients with the neuropathological definite diagnosis of a malignant glioma grade III/IV or a glioblastoma multiforme (42 male and 31 female cases). The lowest line illustrates the age distribution curve with concentration on the 4th and 6th decade. All 73 patients have had a neuropatho-

Table 1 Number, age group and sex of the glioblastoma patients (Outpatient Department for Oncology, Neurochirurgische Universitätsklinik Mainz)

Glioblastoma multiforme 1. 1. 1976–15. 8. 1983	n = 73	42 ♂	31 ♀
Age distribution			
20–30 years	2		
30–40 years	9		
40–50 years	25		
50–60 years	26		
> 60 years	11		

logic-histologically diagnosis. In a few cases full surgery or tumour reduction was not possible, and we disposed of a biopsy specimen. There is not a single case included where tumour diagnosis was only made for neuro-radiogical reasons. In most cases chemotherapy was applied pre-operatively followed by radiation. Each one of these 73 patients had radiation, some with a dose under 6000 rad. Four to six weeks after radiation – in many cases with an intervention of neurological rehabilitation – we started the treatment and application of chemotherapeutics. Table 2 and 3 show what kind of cytostatics and chemotherapeutics were employed in the total

Table 2 Previous chemotherapy – Survey of therapeutically applicable cytotoxic drugs

Drugs used	Brain tumours Induction therapy	Relapse-prevention	Brain metastases	Total number
Nitrosourea				
– BCNU	4	1	3	8 (8.3%)
– CCNU	1	–	7	8 (8.3%)
Oxazaphosphorines				
– Endoxan	–	–	12	12 (12.5%)
– Ixoten	–	–	1	1 (1.0%)
– Holoxan	4	–	6	10 (10.4%)
Antimetabolites				
– S-Flourouracil/Ftorafur	–	–	2	2 (2.1%)
– Methotrexat	3	–	3	6 (6.3%)
– Alexan	–	–	3	3 (3.1%)
Vinca-Alkaloids				
– Vincristin	1	–	12	13 (13.5%)
– Vindesin	–	–	6	6 (6.3%)
– VP 16	–	–	6	6 (6.3%)
Antibiotics				
– Adriamycin	–	–	5	5 (5.2%)
– Bleomycin	–	–	1	1 (1.0%)

Table 3 Previous drugs taken – Continuation of summary of table 2

Drugs used	Brain tumours Induction therapy	Relapse-prevention
Other cytostatic drugs		
– TP 1	–	–
– Cis-Platin	–	–
– DTIC	–	–
– Litalir	–	–
– Iscador	–	–
Cortisone		
– Fortecortin	7	2
– Prednison	–	–
Hormones		
– Clinovir	–	–
Enzymes		
– Wobenzyme	–	–

number of our cases. Mainly those patients are listed who have been referred to us from other neurosurgical clinics for chemotherapy. Frequently chemotherapy had been applied which, according to our experience and judging from literature, could not be considered as first choice treatment of cerebral gliomas. The two relevant show at first no homogenous line in our case material. Usually we completed the multiple chemotherapy and continued with one or two drugs but since 1980 only with ACNU.

The following more selected considerations in some long-term surviving patients show that treatment of our patients can be described differently. Table 4 demonstrates which drugs could be disposed of considering their toxicity. The selected group of tumour patients is presented receiving a repeated prophylaxis with ACNU. The left side illustrates the number of applied drug courses (an injection stands for a course). Within a relatively short time you can see that a great number of patients has received a course and that with increasing periods of application the number of courses becomes more limited. The third line shows the minimum, maximum and the average value of the ACNU-dosage. One should not be deceived that the wanted dosage of 200 mg ACNU in intervals of four weeks is obtainable as a rule or can be given in general clinical practice.

Table 5 demonstrates that in the non-operated group of patients the same phenomenon was observed under chemotherapy as an induction therapy after radiation. Generally speaking it is not possible to reach the 4-weeks-Thythm of 200 mg ACNU-injections. Here too the average values are markedly lower whereas the number of patients is higher. The total number of cases is presented, and not only tumour patients with glioblastoma multiforme or malignant gliomas. The next picture

Table 4 Summary of ACNU-dosage in our number of patients after surgery and radiotherapy

No.	n	Minimum dose	Maximal dose	Mean value	< 80	80–99	100	101–120	> 120
1	19	91	143	117	–	1	1	10	7
2	14	50	143	107	2	1	1	5	5
3	12	50	125	88	5	2	–	3	2
4	11	53	125	90	3	3	1	3	1
5	11	45	125	70	8	1	–	1	1
6	9	45	105	80	4	1	2	2	–
7	6	45	105	78	3	–	1	2	–
8	5	45	105	72	3	–	1	1	–
9	5	45	105	72	3	–	1	1	–
10	4	45	105	76	2	–	1	1	–
11	1	–	–	100	–	–	1	–	–
12	1	–	–	100	–	–	1	–	–
13	1	–	–	100	–	–	1	–	–
Total	99	45	143	91	33	9	12	29	16

(tab. 6) shows our results concerning tolerance of drugs. In the induction therapy group as well as in the group of repeated prophylactic therapy the following criteria for tolerance tests were observed, namely by the patient and objectively by the examining physician. We find that in patients with inoperable gliomas the tolerance is declared to be good or moderate, compared to those patients subjected to repeated prophylactic treatment. When trying to substantiate the statements of the examining physician, the same result is found in the group of induction therapy patients. To our great surprise the group which had repeated therapy showed a good or moderate tolerance more frequently than the patient himself was able to state.

Table 5 Statements on ACNU-therapy in our oncologic outpatient department

No.	n	Minimum dose	Maximal dose	Mean value	< 80	80–99	100	101–120	> 120
1	54	66	133	107	1	3	17	30	3
2	37	56	120	98	5	4	12	16	–
3	24	50	118	91	5	5	6	8	–
4	18	50	118	98	3	–	6	9	–
5	13	56	118	94	3	2	3	5	–
6	10	50	118	95	2	1	2	5	–
7	5	50	111	84	2	1	–	2	–
8	4	44	59	52	4	–	–	–	–
9	3	29	56	45	3	–	–	–	–
10	1	–	–	29	1	–	–	–	–
11	1	–	–	29	1	–	–	–	–
12	1	–	–	29	1	–	–	–	–
Total	171	29	133	96	31	16	46	75	3

Table 6 Judgement on tolerance of ACNU-therapy in the view of the patient and attending physcian

Judgement	Degree	Brain tumours Induction therapy	Relapse-prevention
subjective/patient	good	34	4
	average	3	5
	bad	5	6
	not able to judge/missing	12	4
objective/physician	good	24	7
	average	14	7
	bad	5	1
	not able to judge/missing	11	4

Table 7 represents a sketch showing how many treatment courses per patient could be attained. The first line shows that in a great number of induction therapy patients one course could be given that however the desired 14 courses which we tried to achieve at intervals of 7 injections per 28 weeks were not attainable. Especially in glioblastoma patients with the monotherapy with ACNU we were not successful in a single case obtaining a frequency of 14 injections. In this connection the time span between diagnosis and operation and radiation as well as the beginning of ACNU-therapy illustrated in table 8 during many months, are very important for judging the success of the therapy. It clearly shows that significantly later the average value in induction therapy are reached than in the therapy of repeated preventive treatment. This is due to the fact that patients with inoperable gliomas have been referred to our department from other clinics in a great number of cases and were available for

Table 7 Summary of the number of courses per patient

Number of courses	Brain tumours Induction therapy	Relapse-prevention
1	17	5
2	11	2
3	8	1
4	5	–
5	3	2
6	5	3
7	1	1
8	1	–
9	2	1
10	–	3
11	–	–
12	1	–
13	–	1

Table 8 Summary of time span (weeks) between first diagnosis of glioblastoma and the beginning of chemotherapy with ACNU

Degree/	Brain tumours	
Designated number	Induction therapy	Relapse-prevention
Minimum	0	2
Maximum	121	9
Median	4.0	5.3
Average	9.6	5.1
< 3	24	3
4 – 6	12	11
7 – 12	9	3
13 – 24	3	–
> 24	6	–
Missing data	–	2

therapy only much later. It would be desirable to start the therapy of both groups earlier.

An important factor in the analysis of prognosis and success in therapy of long-term surviving patients with glioblastomas is the *quality of life*. For this reason it became a routine to refer to in our oncological outpatient-department the Karnofsky-Index. Table 9 is a survey of our patients who had the initial ACNU-therapy and it is apparent that the majority of patients can be found within an activity index according to Karnofsky from 100 to 60%.

It has to be emphasised that most of the patients with glioblastomas have been treated since 1980 with ACNU only.

Table 9 Condition of patient at the beginning of treatment with ACNU, specified by the Karnofsky-Index. Most patients show a value above 60%

Karnofsky-Index	Brain tumours	
	Introduction therapy	Relapse-prevention
100%	5	2
90%	5	4
80%	7	3
70%	8	8
60%	12	2
50%	7	–
40%	7	–
30%	1	–
20%	–	–
Missing data	2	–

Why did we prefer the drug ACNU, still not freely available in contrast to other nitrosourea derivatives. The reason is that we have been convinced by Japanese results that the attainable concentration of these hydrosoluble nitrosourea compound reaches the highest possible level of concentration in malignant glioma tissue. This is illustrated in figure 1. Thirty patients were examined, their weight was between 60 and 80 kg and received a push-injection of 200 mg ACNU. At the surgical exstirpation of tissue the desirable level of the drug of about 4 μg/g brain tissue was attainable. These values are clearly higher than those obtainable from BCNU, CiNU and CCNU. We also want to draw attention to our experiences of side-effects occurring in the treatment with these nitrosourea derivatives, resulting in cases of Herpes-Zoster. In a single case therapy had to be stopped since a level of myelotoxidity was reached forbidding further use of nitrosourea derivatives but in a total number of 131 patients we consider this to be a favourable sign for controlling of the side affects of nitrosourea derivatives.

Before discussing the satisfactory results of the therapy we would like to mention that we were not only motivated to a critical attitude by the nature of our work but we were forced to a radical criticism by the statistical analysis. Chemotherapy, whether applied as poly-, oligo- or monotherapy in glioma patients has been appalling regarding its success. All our efforts to attain essential improvements have so far not been effective. Therapeutic results in cases of astrocytomas grade III and IV are statistically significant and satisfactory. Therapeutic results in glioblastomas multiforme are, however still appalling. Table 10 represents our satisfactory results and failures in chemo-therapeutic treatment of glioblastoma-patients. The survival times in 73 patients with a histologically sound diagnosis of glioblastomas multiforme or of brain gliomas (grade IV) can be seen in the last line of table 10. 45 patients have a

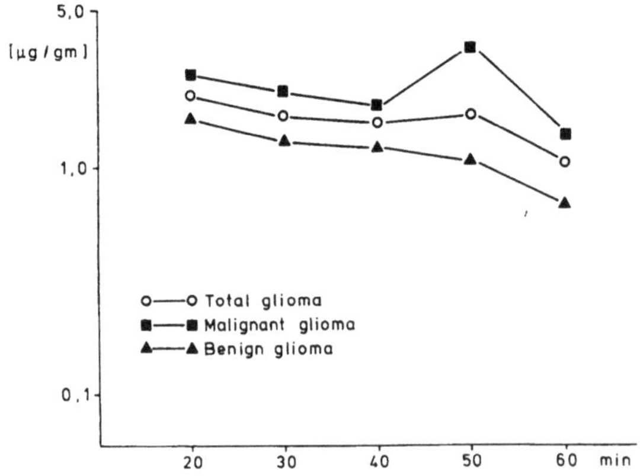

Fig. 1 Presentation of ACNU-concentration in tumour tissue after one injection of 200 mg ACNU. Values are considerably above the concentration which can be reached with other nitrosourea derivates. (The picture has been taken from K. Harada et al. [7].).

Table 10 Tabular summary of attained survival times (Outpatient Department for Oncology, Neurochirurgische Universitätsklinik Mainz)

Glioblastoma multiforme 1. 1. 1976–15. 8. 1983	n = 73
< 1 year	45
> 1 year	19
2 years	3
3 years	2
4 years	2
5 years	1
6 years	1

Further details can bee seen in the publication of our working group in this book on pages 361 – 372 (Voth, Hüwel, Al-Hami, Kuhnert).

survival time of less than 1 year, 19 patients survived more than 1 year and only 3 patients reached a survival time of 2 years. However 2 patients have been surviving 3 years, 2 patients with a survival time of 4 years, one patient surviving 5 years and one patient has still survived after the diagnosis of a glioblastoma multiforme, the operation, radiation and chemotherapy for the last 6 years. When we add those patients from the total of 73 who survived 2 years or more, it amounts to 9 which is more than 10%. At first glance this seems surprising but unfortunately it cannot be expressed in statistically significant numbers.

Case reports

We submit in the following the case histories of patients with the longest survival time. Of special interest is a female patient surviving with her tumour for more than 6 years. Age of this patient is 45 years who was operated on in our clinic 7 years ago for a right frontal tumour which could be removed without any neurological deficit. Following operation the patient received radiation of 6000 rad. and subsequently a 4-weeks neurological course of rehabilitation. Afterwards a cytostatic therapy was started with the available CCNU and then with CiNU. Already then we tried to reach a 2 × 7 application rhythm, giving 220 to 200 mg CCNU or CiNU at 6-weeks intervals. The patient received a total of 1600 mg CCNU and 1400 mg CiNU, spread over a period of 3 years after operation. The operation was in 1977 and the last application of cytostatica in October 1980. The patient, who is still being treated in our outpatient-department, has an activity index of 90% and is fully occupied by her household duties. These include the care for her husband, a wheel-chair patient due to multiple sclerosis. Our radiological control examination as well as our clinical neurological findings and the electrophysiological findings have not revealed up to now a recurrent tumour.

Our next detailed case report is a 50 year old patient whose initial operation in 1976 was under the diagnosis of cerebral haemorrhage revealing a spontaneous intracerebral haemorrhage right frontally. During the emergency operation for a haemorrhage some cerebral tissue was histologically examined which showed an astrocytoma. Further diagnostic investigation revealed a glioma apoplecticum and a second operation was performed the same year. Through a right frontal lobectomy a large tumour was removed which was histologically a glioblastoma multiforme. Preoperatively the patient received a total radiation of 6000 rad. Medication with CCNU, total of 1400 g orally in 6 individual doses, followed. We observed a leuco- and thrombocytopenia, present for years forcing us to end the CCNU administration. The patient is still without recurrence of tumour, in good health and working in an academic position.

The third patient we wish to record is a 30 year old women who has been operated on for a glioblastoma multiforme, (left parieto-occipital) in 1978. Pre- and postoperatively the patient showed a reduced visual field and a mixed aphasia. This patient too was radiated with 6000 rad. and medicated with following chemotherapeutics: Intrathekal 70 mg Methotrexat in 7 times of 10 mg each through lumbar puncture, in addition a total of 2000 mg DTIC parenterally and then 2 series of 7 applications of 200 mg CINU per os each. Chemotherapy was ended 3 years after operation. Since that time the patient has been seen in our department for regular controls without showing signs of tumour recurrence. The patient has to look after 2 small children and a husband and is able to manage this without difficulties. The Karnofsky-Index is 100%. Various problems had to be solved by her regarding orientation in a room caused by a reduced visual field with homonymous hemianopsia to the right. However, this patient is able to drive her own car and to walk in a room without difficulty. She has learned to compensate completely her reduced vision. Her small children are going to school and she is able to help them with their homework. She has a mixed aphasia, her writing, reading and counting were faulty. For this reason she is unhappy when shopping and had problems in explaining to the teacher that she was unable to help fully her children with their homework. We arranged for her an intensive logopedic treatment which she has followed over the years until now. The patient speaks now without hesitation and is able to instruct and correct her children with their homework, at least at elementary school level. No psychologic problems so far have arisen.

Table 10 shows that 2 glioblastoma patients surviving for 4 years, 2 patients with survival time of 3 years and 3 patients with a survival time of 2 years. These patients are still in our care. Only one patient with a survival time of 4 years has now a recurrence of the tumour. All patients have been treated with ACNU only but in none of the patients the complete total dosage i.e. 14 injections could not be achieved. Life quality of these patients differs between 60 and 100% according to Karnofsky. The patient with the recurrence of tumour has a Karnofsky-Index of 60%.

Discussion

We have been observing a number of patients for several years who have survived the fatal diagnosis of a glioblastoma multiforme. Out of 73 patients nine had a survival time of 2 years and longer amounting to more than 10% who reached a survival time of 2 years. The question arises whether the general stress caused by chemotherapy is worthwhile the result – i.e. to visit the clinic every 4 weeks, to see the family doctor every week for blood tests. The patient suffers from the loss of appetite after the injections and nausea and vomiting can occur. From the 73 patients under our care 9 had for more than 2 years a reasonable existence under the circumstances.

The last reflection should be of course which way we intend to follow now. Many therapeutic methods are available, many working groups have been established and have a claim on multicentric support. Nevertheless, we believe on the basis of our experiences that perhaps the way of chemotherapy in astrocytomas III may be successful, although it is still not satisfactory. It is also obvious that polychemotherapy in glioblastomas does not convince with successful results, even though we may be very proud to have kept alive 9 patients over 2 to 7 years. We should anticipate with interest future developments on this field. We want to emphasize that especially the unification of neuropathologic judgement and valence should take absolut precedence of all efforts. Not until each pathologist can determine the same tumour qualification and we dispose of a neuropathologic standard, the basis for real comparative tests at all centres would be given. Here surely the Neuropathologic Society is called upon to make every possible effort for a standardization in cooperation with the World Health Organization (WHO). Additional biologic examinations, like measurements of cerebral blood flow or metabolic investigations in glioma tissue, should also be called upon.

Summary

The organisation and management of an oncological outpatient-department has been described and its inherent problems and some successful results are analysed. Special attention has been given to long-term surviving glioblastoma patients, whose number so far is about 10%, with survival times of more than 5 years.

Provided the diagnosis of a glioblastoma was justified, these unusual long survival times encourage the search for further therapeutic exploration into the treatment of the highly malignant glioblastoma multiforme.

References

[1] Arakawa, M., F. Shimizu, N. Okada: Effect of 1-(4-amino-2-methyl-pyrimidine-5-yl)methyl-3-(2-chloroethyl)-3-nitrosourea hydrochloride on leukemia L-1210. Gan **65** (1974) 191.

[2] Calogero, J., C. D. Crafts, C. B. Wilson, et al.: Long-term survival of patients treated with BCNU for brain tumours. J. Neurosurg. **43** (1975) 191–196.

[3] Fewer, D., C. B. Wilson, E. B. Boldrey, et al.: Phase II study of CCNU (NSC 79037) in the treatment of brain tumors. Cancer Chemother. Rep. **56** (1972) 421–427.

[4] Garrett, M. J., H. J. Hughes, R. D. H. Ryall: CCNU in brain tumors. Clin. Radiol. **25** (1974) 183–184.

[5] Hansch, C., N. Smith, R. Engle, et al.: Quantitative structure activity relationships of antineoplastic drugs. Nitrosoureas and triazeno-imidazoles. Cancer Chemother. Rep. **56** (1972) 443–456.

[6] Hara, M., K. Takeuchi: Pharmacokinetics analysis of ACNU in brain tumors. No To Shinkei **31** (1979) 1289–1293.

[7] Harada, K., K. Kiya, T. Uozumi: Pharmacokinetics of a new watersoluble nitrosourea derivate (ACNU) in human gliomas. Surg. Neurol. **15** (1981) 410–415.

[8] Hasegawa, H., T. Hayakawa, M. Hori, et al.: Chemotherapy of experimental glioma with nitrosourea-comparison of water soluble ACNU and lipid soluble Me-CCNU. No To Shinkei **29** (1977) 891–898.

[9] Kato, T., T. Fujikawa, K. Ota: Effects of various anticancer agents, especially ACNU on intracerebral L_{1210} leukemia. Gan To Kagakuryoho **3** (1976) 945–951.

[10] Levin, V. A., W. R. Shapiro, T. P. Clancy, et al.: The uptake distribution and antitumor activity of 1-(2-chloroethyl)-3-cyclohexyl-1-nitrosourea in the murine glioma. Cancer Res. **30** (1970) 2451–2455.

[11] Levin, V. A.: The permeability characteristics of capillaries in the edematous brain adjacent to intracerebral tumors. Neurology **24** (1974) 390.

[12] Levin, V. A., M. Freeman-Dove, H. D. Landahl: Permeability characteristics of brain adjacent to tumors in rats. Arch. Neurol. **32** (1975) 785–791.

[13] Levin, V. A., P. Kabara: Effectiveness of the nitrosoureas as a function of their lipid solubility. The chemotherapy of experimental rat brain tumours. Cancer Chemother. Rep. **58** (1974) 787–792.

[14] Levin, V. A., C. B. Wilson: Pharmacological considerations in brain tumor chemotherapy. In: Brain Tumor Chemotherapy (D. Fewer, C. B. Wilson, V. A. Levin, eds.), pp. 42–74. Thomas, Springfield, Ill., 1976.

[15] Mellett, L. B.: Physicochemical considerations and pharmacokinetics behavior in delivery of drugs to the central nervous system. Cancer Chemother. Rep. **61** (1977) 527–531.

[16] Mori, T., K. Mineura, R. Katakura: A consideration on pharmacokinetics of a new water-soluble antitumor nitrosourea, ACNU. No To Shinkei **31** (1979) 601–606.

[17] Nakamura, T., M. Sasada, M. Tashima, et al.: Mechanism of action of 1-(4-amino-2-methylpyrimidin-5-yl)methyl-3-(2-chloroethyl)-3-nitrosourea (ACNU) in leukemia cells. Gan To Kagakuryoho **5** (1978) 991–1000.

[18] Oliverio, V. T.: Pharmacology of the nitrosoureas: an overview. Cancer Treat. Rep. **60** (1976) 703–707.

[19] Rosenblum, M. L., A. F. Reynolds, K. A. Smith, et al.: Chloroethyl-cyclohexyl nitrosourea (CCNU) in the treatment of malignant brain tumors. J. Neurosurg. **39** (1973) 306–314.

[20] Saito, Y., Y. Nakaya, K. Muraoka, et al.: Chemotherapy of brain tumors with nitrosourea derivative (ACNU). Gan To Kagakuryoho **5** (1978) 779–794.

[21] Shimizu, F., M. Arakawa: Effects of 3[(4-amino-2-methyl-5-pyrimidinyl) methyl]-1-(2-chloroethyl)-1-nitrosourea hydrochloride on lymphoid leukemia L-1210. Gan **66** (1975) 149–154.

[22] Spozo, R. W., V. H. Bono, V. T. Oliverio: The physiologic distribution of radioactive 1-(2-chloroethyl)-3-(4-methyl-cyclohexyl)-1-nitrosourea (Me-CCNU) in man. Proc. Am. Assoc. Cancer Res. **13** (1973) 1154–1159.

[23] Tanaka, M., E. Nakajima, T. Nishigaka, et al.: Studies on metabolism of 3-[(4-amino-2-methyl-5-pyrimidinyl)methyl]-1-(2-chloroethyl)-1-nitrosourea). A new water-soluble nitrosourea in rats and mice. Proceedings of the 10th International Congress of Chemotherapy, Zurich, Switzerland,

Sept. 18–23, 1977. In: Current Chemotherapy, pp. 1230–1232. International Society of Chemotherapy, 1978.

[24] Tator, C. H.: Chemotherapy of an experimental glioma with nitrosoureas. Cancer Res. **37** (1977) 467–481.

[25] Walker, M. D.: Nitrosoureas in central nervous system tumors. Cancer Chemother. Rep. **4** (1973) 21–26.

[26] Walker, M. D., E. Alexander Jr., W. E. Hunt, et al.: Evaluation of BCNU and/or radiotherapy in the treatment of anaplastic gliomas. A cooperative clinical trial. J. Neurosurg. **49** (1978) 333–343.

[27] Walker, M. D., J. Hilton: Nitrosourea pharmacodynamics in relation to the central nervous system. Cancer Treat. Rep. **60** (1976) 725–728.

[28] Wilson, C. B., E. B. Boldrey, K. J. Enot: 1,3-bis(2-chloroethyl)-1-nitrosoureas (NSC) in the treatment of brain tumours. Cancer Chemother. Rep. **54** (1970) 273–281.

[29] Wilson, C. B., P. Gutin, E. B. Boldrey: Single-agent chemotherapy of brain tumors. A five-year vew. Arch. neurol. **33** (1976) 739–744.

[30] Young, R. C., M. D. Walker, G. P. Canellos, et al.: Initial clinical trials with methyl-CCNU 1-(2-chloroethyl)-3-(4-methylcyclohexyl)-1-nitrosourea (me-CCNU). Cancer **31** (1973) 1164-1169.

Preoperative chemo- and/or radiotherapy: its possible role in the treatment of malignant brain gliomas
(Brief communication)

H. Müller, W. Roggendorf, M. Brock, H. Ernst

Surgical management of malignant supra-tentorial gliomas remains a problem. One of the difficulties is the ill defined demarcation zone between tumour and brain. An extended resection "in sano" is often either impossible or can lead to deleterious results, except when the tumour is polar.

Material and methods

In the early course of our studies on the biological behaviour of malignant gliomas, we were impressed at post mortem inspection of one of our patients treated by irradiation and chemotherapy (CCNU) without surgery that radiation therapy had apparently caused a sharp demarcation between the tumour and brain tissue. These changes, probably caused by radiotherapy and chemotherapy focused our attention on autopsy and biopsy findings in further cases treated similarly. Patients with inoperable or recurrent tumours were excluded from a randomized trial to study the value of CCNU in addition to surgery (S) and radiotherapy (RT) [1, 2]. Three brain autopsies and two brain biopsies were examined. Following fixation in 10% formalin solution, 5 μ paraffin sections or 25 μ celloidin sections were cut and stained with haematoxyline-eosin, Elastica staining van Gieson, Nissl, Kanzler stains or Weigert myelin-stain.

Results

The cytological picture corresponded in general to that of the glioblastoma multiforme, showing numerous polymorphic glial cell elements, giant or multiple nuclei, and cellular arrangements in palisadal fashion. Moreover, special staining techniques reveal an increase in the number of glial filaments in the borderzones of gliomas treated in this way. Markedly firmer consistency of the tissue occured but also necrotic areas with multiple small cysts were visible. Increased amounts of collagenous fibers are also encountered. These fibrillary changes could explain the firmer consistency of tumourous and necrotic areas. The central parts of the tumour contain large necrotic areas in which an increased number of blood vessels with hyalinosis, fibrosis, and fibrinoid necrosis are detectable. These vascular changes might be responsible for the extremely large necrotic areas seen in gliomas treated by radio- and chemotherapy alone.

These findings encouraged us to try a pre-operative lowdose radio- and chemotherapy in a patient with glioblastoma of the right temporal lobe. Pre-operative radiotherapy is often used for tumours of organs other than the brain (e.g., pulmonary sarcoma, hypernephroid carcinoma, head and neck tumours, carcinomas of the gastro-intestinal and the urinary tract, collum carcinoma, etc.). A comparable information is scarce for gliomas [3–5]. In the present case, the disease began with headaches and epilepsy, followed by leftsided hemiparesis two weeks later. Diagnosis was made by computerized tomography and confirmed by angiography. Initial medication consisted in 4 × 4 mg dexamethasone (DXM) and 2 × 100 mg CCNU complemented by 22 Gy.

Summary

The surgical treatment of malignant glioma remains problematic. Post-mortem findings in non-operated patients treated by irradiation and chemotherapy (CCNu) disclosed a well defined demarcation zone between the tumour and the surrounding brain tissue, as well as an increased tumour consistency. This is most likely the consequence of radiation- and/or chemotherapy. Such macroscopic changes were also noted in a patient with a glioblastoma of the right temporal lobe, deliberately pretreated with 22 Gy radiotherapy and a cytostatic drug (2 × 100 mg CCNU). We conclude that pre-operative (low-dose) radio- and/or chemotherapy may simplify and improve the surgical management of a malignant supra-tentorial glioma.

References

[1] Müller, H., F. Oppel, M. Brock: Kombinierte Behandlung operierter und nicht operierter maligner Astrocytome mit CCNU und Bestrahlung (Abstract). In: Bestandsaufnahme Krebsforschung in der BRD, Bd. III, p. 1541. Deutsche Forschungsgemeinschaft. Boldt, Boppard 1979.

[2] Müller, H., M. Brock: Long-term survival and recurrence-free interval in combined surgical, radio- and chemotherapy of malignant brain gliomas. 7th E.A.N.S. Congress, Book of Conference Abstracts (J. Brihaye, R. Vigouroux, J. Achslogh, et al., eds.), p. 193. Bruxelles 1983.

[3] Seiler, R. W., A. Zimmermann, H. Markwalder: Preoperative radiotherapy and chemotherapy in hypervascular, high-grade supratentorial astrocytomas. Surg. Neurol. 12 (1979) 131–133.

[4] Seiler, R. W.: Die undifferenzierten Astrocytome des Großhirns. Neurology Series 22. Springer-Verlag, Berlin – Heidelberg – New York 1982.

[5] Walker, M. D.: The next generation of brain tumor research – can we learn from the past? Abstracts of the 7th International Congress of Neurological Surgery (H. Dietz, E. Metzel, C. Langmaid, eds.), p. 274. G. Thieme Verlag, Stuttgart – New York 1981.

The present state of development of multistage treatment of cancer*

Fundamental principles of the two-stage regional hyperthermia technique, using the "Selectotherm" procedure, as well as the heat sensitisation of cancer tissue by means of hyperglycaemia (Brief communication)

M. von Ardenne

In the fight against cancer the therapeutic use of hyperthermia has been dedicated principally to this theme since its first appearance and in a series of papers (1964–1971) has aroused constantly increasing interest in international cancer research [1–8]. Since 1975 more than ten special symposia on cancer treatment with hyperthermia have taken place at national and international levels [9–11] and for 1984 three further international symposia about hyperthermic oncology have already been announced. In spite of this it is considered on several grounds that the *therapeutic use of hyperthermia against cancer* is still *in its infancy*. The significance of the combined use of synergistic or supporting adjuvant measures (hyperglycaemia, circulatory support with O_2, immunostimulation etc.) is not yet realised and hence is not used at all, or still not with appropriate timing. With regard to the aims and the solutions at the present time, the hyperthermia technique is still not completely standardised. Even with the most highly developed hyperthermia procedures the interplay between clinical research and the adaptations of the technique is still in such a dynamic stage that, in a short time, promising improvements seem to overlap. Even in phases with higher dynamic which are characteristic in the early years of a growing scientific area, it is important every so often to keep oneself informed about the present state of affairs.

In the case of hyperthermia, which generally acts on the host tissue at a temperature between 41.8 and 43.0 °C for a duration of several hours, there are several techniques which must be quite strictly distinguished from each other.

---

* Although hitherto no practical experiences of this group have been available, as regards the treatment of human gliomas, it seemed to us that this contribution is useful as a basis for discussion, including also the methods which have been used.

The Editors

The distinguishing feature of the multistage cancer treatment (CMT) which even at present is in its developmental stages, is the simultaneous use of the two-stage regional hyperthermia according to the "Selectotherm" method and the synergistic measure of producing selective hyperacidification of the cancer tissue through prolonged raising of the blood glucose level to about eight times its normal value. For destruction of remnants of cancer cells resistant to treatment and for prophylaxis against metastases, the existing main stages are supplemented by the process of O_2-immunostimulation also described. With this two-stage hyperthermia the 'core' temperature of the body is raised to 41 °C and a temperature of 42.5 °C is produced in that part of the body being treated. A homogenisation of the energy supply is brought about by movement of the scanner of the applicator in a circular track or by other measures. By combinations of the "stages" described, a selective irreversible occlusion of the capillaries of the carcinomatous tissue is attempted. Radiographs of the results of the treatment show that this target is clinically attainable (fig. 1).

With the usual treatment nowadays, as a result of O_2-deficiency and leucopaenia, encouragement of the formation of metastases occurs, to the point of wide-spread dissemination. Therefore, the technique of O_2-immunostimulation, in which measures against leucopaenia and O_2-deficiency are combined, is for that reason alone of general interest.

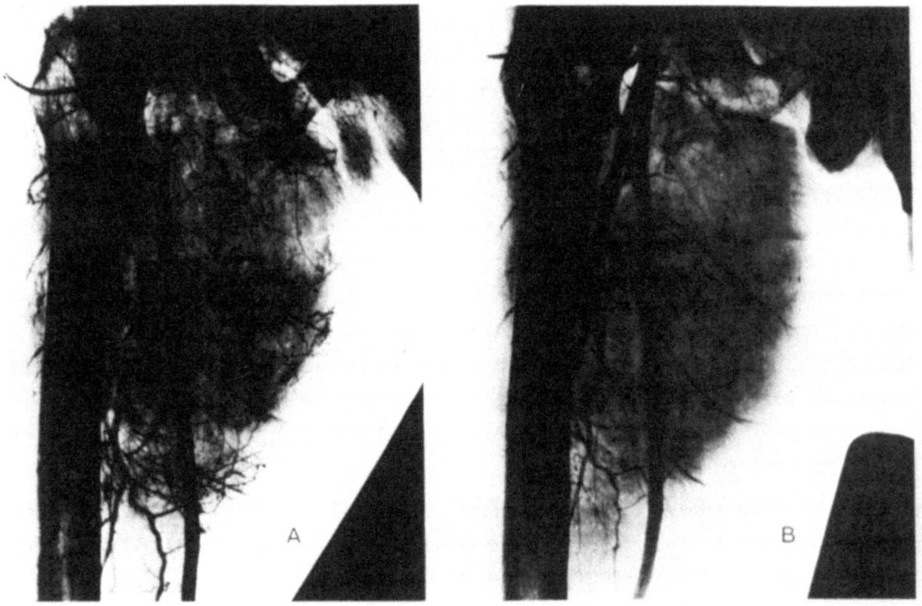

Fig. 1 Alfred P., age 61. Malignant histiocytoma, right femoral region. Follow-up after two fractions of CMT.
A = angiogram before treatment, B = four weeks later.
Result: Selective destruction of the finer blood vessels of the tumour through the induction of irreversible haemostasis.

References

[1] Ardenne, M. von: Theoretische und experimentelle Grundlagen der Krebs-Mehrschritt-Therapie, 2. Auflage. VEB Verlag Volk und Gesundheit, Berlin 1970/1971.
[2] Ardenne, M. von: Sauerstoff-Mehrschritt-Therapie, 3. Auflage. Georg Thieme Verlag, Stuttgart 1983.
[3] Ardenne, M. von: Grundlagen für die Bekämpfung der Krebs-Metastasierung durch Prozesse der O_2-Mehrschritt-Immunstimulation. M. Cancer Res. Clin. Oncol. **106** ^{2}(1984), in press.
[4] Ardenne, M. von, G. Böhme, E. Kell, et al.: Die Bedeutung der Wärmeleitung für die therapeutischen Grenzen der selektiven Lokalhyperthermie von Krebsgeweben. Radiobiol. Radiother. **20** (1979) 529–551.
[5] Ardenne, M. von, H. G. Lippmann, P. G. Reitnauer, et al.: Histological Proof for Selective Stop of Microcirculation in Tumour tissue at pH 6.1 and 41 °C. Naturwiss. **66** (1979) 59.
[6] Ardenne, M. von, P. G. Reitnauer: Verstärkung der mit Glykoseinfusion erzielbaren Tumorübersäuerung in vivo durch lokale Hyperthermie. Res. exp. med. **175** (1979) 7–18.
[7] Ardenne, M. von, P. G. Reitnauer: Selective Inhibition of Microcirculation in Tumour tissue. Naturwiss. **67** (1980) 154.
[8] Ardenne, M. von, P. G. Reitnauer: Vergleichende photoelektronische Registrierung des Einstromes von Evansblau in das Blutgefäßsystem von Normalgewebe und von Tumoren mit selektiv ausgelöster Hämostase. Arch. Geschwulstforsch. **50** (1980) 443–462.
[9] Gautherie, M., E. Albert (eds.): Biomedical Thermology. Alan Liss Inc., New York 1982.
[10] Pettigrew, R. T., J. M. Galt, C. M. Ludgate, et al.: Circulatory and biochemical effects of whole body hyperthermia. Br. J. Surg. **61** (1974) 727–730.
[11] Streffer, C. (ed.): Cancer Therapy by Hyperthermia and Radiation. Urban & Schwarzenberg, München – Baltimore 1978.

Hyperthermia-radiotherapy of the gliomas – a critical report

M. Herbst

Introduction

Independent of its localization, a glioblastoma is the most malignant and fastest growing tumour of the brain. The therapeutic results achieved with surgery, radiotherapy, chemotherapy and their combinations are very limited. The average survival time after extirpation of the lesion alone, is 4 to 6 months, in comparison with untreated patients, who have a life expectancy of 6 to 8 weeks only [5]. Postoperative radiotherapy and/or corticosteroids prolong the average life expectancy to between 9 and 12 months [4, 6]. Using a combination of surgery, radiotherapy and chemotherapy, it is possible to extend the average life expectancy, but side effects can be severe [5].

In view of these depressing results, all possibilities of improving the treatment of glioblastoma multiforme should be tried and we present here our approach to the problem.

Methods

At the Radiotherapy Department of the University of Erlangen-Nuremberg, 34 patients with advanced, inoperable tumours, some with confirmed histological diagnosis, were subjected to a combined treatment of hyperthermia and radiotherapy. The tumours comprised 5 glioblastomas, 3 astrocytomas, not further differentiated, 2 ependymomas, 1 oligodendroglioma, 1 medulloblastoma, 1 meningioma, a metastatic hypernephroma and 20 tumours of unknown histology. Of these latter 20 tumours, the computerized tomographic findings prompted an experienced neuroradiologist to make a presumptive diagnosis of glioblastoma in 13 patients.

The combination therapy was designed in such a way that hyperthermic treatment was given prior to radiotherapy and immediately thereafter. For hyperthermia, we employed a generator manufactured by the firm of Thermotime AG in Zug, Switzerland, which, employing a frequency of 13.56 MHz, operates in accordance with the condenserfield principle (fig. 1). The electrodes were applied to either side of the head, "straddling" the region of the tumour. In each case, the high frequency was applied gradually, increasing up to the threshold of tolerance, then being maintained for at least 30 minutes at a power level of more than 100 watts. This procedure was designed on the basis of temperature measurements performed on cadavers, which revealed a homogeneous temperature distribution within the brain with this technique [2], and on calculations dealing with the supply of energy necessary to achieve hyperthermia despite the haemodynamics operative within the brain [1].

Results

Fractioning of the hyperthermia varied considerably in this group. Nine patients were treated with 2, ten patients with 3, and twelve patients with 4, fractions per week. Radiotherapy was applied irrespective of the hyperthermia fractioning scheme, being given 5 times a week up to a total dose of 50 to 70 Gy, usually as whole-brain irradiation, with a 2 to 4 week pause after 40 Gy. The high dosage of radiotherapy was not reduced, hoping that the additional hyperthermia would improve the therapeutic effect by enhancing the total dose. With this combination treatment, no attempt was made to employ the additional heat therapy to achieve an identical effect at a reduced radiation dose.

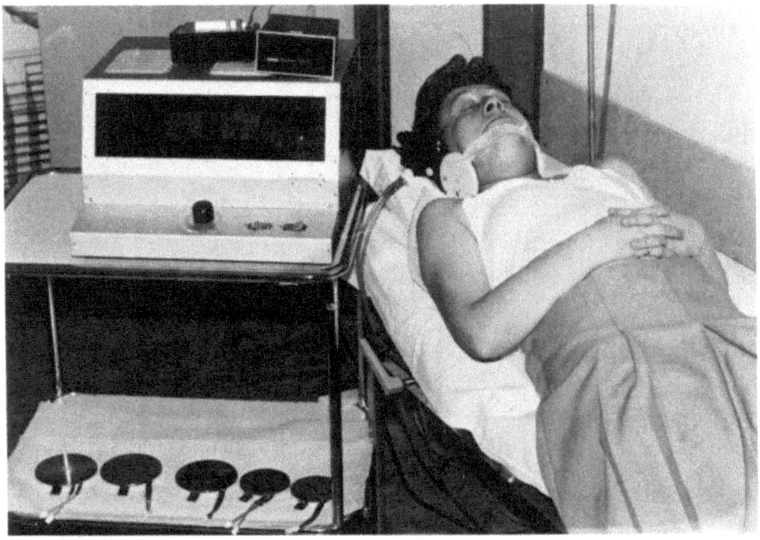

Fig. 1 Hyperthermia generator with electrodes applied to the patient. Here, the patient is being freated for a metastasis from a breast carcinoma.

In view of the advanced tumour stages present, hopes of achieving good therapeutic results were not very high. In nine patients the tumour was too advanced to permit any therapeutic effect, and treatment was abandoned. In four patients, complete remission was obtained, while in twelve patients partial remission was achieved, in seven patients no change in the size of the tumour was observed. In a further six patients, the tumour continued to progress. In some cases, the response of the glioblastoma at the start of combination therapy was much more marked, computer-tomographically (fig. 2), than has otherwise been observed under radiotherapy alone. With this form of therapy, 16 remissions were obtained, although no significant prolongation of survival rates was observed; two patients survived for more than 2 years.

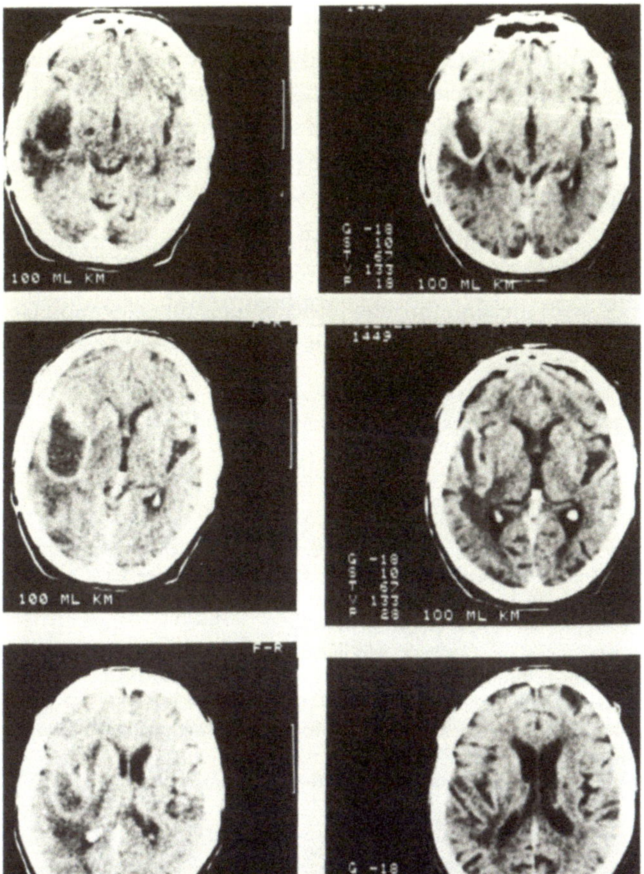

Fig. 2 Computer tomographic documentation of the therapeutic results achieved with a combination of hyperthermia and radiotherapy – pre-treatment situation and following the application of 30 Gy.

With respect to subjective side effects, 80% of the patients reported a marked, but still tolerable, local sensation of heat during hyperthermia. In addition, eight patients experienced a feeling of lassitude, and nausea, while orthostatic circulatory disturbances were objectified in two patients immediately following hyperthermia. It was, however, not possible to establish unequivocally whether these complaints were due to hyperthermia or to radiotherapy. Local changes in the skin and/or cranium brought about by hyperthermia were not observed. Thus, the combination therapy was well tolerated, and, employing cooled electrodes, never led to any critical increases in temperature of the skin or the underlying tissues.

Combination therapy employing hyperthermia and radiotherapy was partially abandoned for the following reasons:

1. The overall results obtained with this method were not very encouraging. With the split-course technique (40 Gy in 4 weeks, with a pause of 2 to 4 weeks and a subsequent "booster" to 60–70 Gy) we employed, it seemed to us that in five patients, tumour growth was accelerated during the pause in treatment.
2. In vitro results have since been published, which show that in human glioblastoma cells, hyperthermia leads to a lowering of tissue pH and thus to a reduction in the sensitivity of these cells to radiation [3].

Nevertheless, there may still be justification for this combination therapy if, in the initial phase of treatment, in the presence of large tumours, hyperthermia is employed only a few times, with the aim, through toxic temperature elevation (> 43 °C) of producing necroses within the tumour, and thus achieving a rapid reduction in the volume of the lesion.

References

[1] Allis, J. W., C. F. Blackman, M. L. Fromme, et al.: Measurement of microwave radiation absorbed by biological systems. Analysis of heating and cooling data. Radio Science **12** (1977) 1–8.

[2] Herbst, M., J. Bernhardt: Temperature distributions produced by 13.56 MHz EM radiation in various phantoms. Br. J. Cancer **45** Suppl. V (1982) 14–45.

[3] Röttinger, E. M., M. Medonca, L. E. Gerweck: Modification of pH-induced cellular inactivation by irradiation – glial cells. Int. J. Radiol. Oncol. Biol. Phys. **6** (1980) 1659–1662.

[4] Salcman, M.: Glioblastoma multiforme. Amer. J. med. Sci. **279** (1980) 84–89.

[5] Sellinger, K., D. Volc, W. Gisold, et al.: Kombinationsbehandlung maligner Gliome. Wiener klinische Wochenschrift **95** (1983) 407–416.

[6] Shapiro, W. R.: Treatment of neuroectodermal brain tumours. Am Neurol. **12** (1982) 115–119.

Planning, realization and evaluation of clinical trials: some statistical aspects

A. Neiss

Introduction

Clinical trials are generally aimed at evaluating the effects, effectiveness and side effects of a given therapy. They also try, at the same time, to determine the practicability of a new therapy or the incidence of risk factors. These last aspects, however, will not be dealt with in the present context.

The evaluation of a therapy is based on comparisons. It should be made in such a way as to eliminate bias, keep the number of patients needed small, and the results of the trial apt to be generalized. Furthermore, the results should be self-explanatory, i.e. the results of other studies should not be needed to explain the present ones.

In practice two types of trials can be found: Those without a comparative therapy and those trials that have a control group. The so-called controlled clinical trials can be subdivided into those, where patients are assigned to trial groups at random and those, where assignment is not conducted at random. In trials without a control group, for instance, a so-called historical comparison will be carried out, i.e. the results will be compared to those of earlier data. Due to changes in the composition of patients, methods of diagnosis etc., this study design can lead to a bias. This means that differences observed may not be attributable to the different treatments but to other factors. The same applies to trials in which patients are not chosen at random for treatment. The best way to evaluate the effects, effectiveness and side affects of a therapy is the randomized controlled clinical trial.

The following is a discussion of some aspects to be taken into account apart from these general considerations, in planning, carrying out and evaluating a clinical trial.

Problems of planning

First of all it must be determined for which group of patients one wants to obtain information about the therapy to be tested. This is done, in most cases, by formulating so-called criteria of inclusion and exclusion. They determine, for example, which diagnoses, which degree of seriousness of a disease, which ages of the patients are to be included in the trial. Diseases that accompany the main disease, and thereby exclude patients from the trial, have to be defined.

Another important item is the definition of criteria for measuring the success of the therapy. These must be valid and reliable, i.e. they must measure the effects respectively the effectiveness and side effects of the therapy and not the effects of other factors. Also the definition of the criteria used must be reproducible. This is particularly important when several investigators are involved in a trial as this is often the case in multi-center trials. The following criteria are often applied in studies of cancer: Rate of remission, duration of remission, survival time and quality of life. The point, for example, must be clearly defined at which a patient has reached remission or at which he can be said to be relapsing. These definitions are binding for investigators participating in the trial.

In order to avoid any bias, the so-called confounding factors must be excluded. Confounding factors can be divided into those that are known and those that are unknown. In most cancer studies the ages of the patients and the stages of seriousness of the disease are confounding factors. Known confounding factors are eliminated by stratifying patients according to this factor. Groups of patients will be formed, for example, according to age and assigned to the treatments. This procedure guarantees an equal distribution of the confounding factor and thereby eliminates its harmful effects. Psychological factors, i.e. beliefs and prejudices of patients and investigators, form another class of confounding factors. To eliminate this source of danger, so-called simple – and double-blind trials are carried out. In the first case the kind of treatment administered is unknown to the patients, in the second case neither patient nor physician are aware of the therapy administered to the patient. This approach, however, is not always practicable. No blind-study, for example, is feasible in comparing irradiation and operation. The best protection against unknown confounding factors is randomization, i.e. the assignment of patients to treatments on a random basis. The same technique is applied with known confounding factors when additional stratification has rendered the study design so complicated that an orderly carrying-out of the trial is at risk.

The method of evaluation must be determined before the study begins. An answer must be given to the question whether statistical analysis is to follow the completion of the trial or whether interim analysis should be carried out. If interim analyses are decided upon, their time span must be fixed as well as the level of significance on which the statistical tests are to be carried out. As a rule of thumb a maximum of five interim analyses can be recommended.

Interim analyses are closely connected with terminating rules. Before the beginning of the study it must be determined which results of the interim analyses will lead to the termination of the trial. Moreover there must be criteria for the trial to be ended for an individual patient. It is only natural that not every contingency has been considered at the planning stage. Therefore the election of an advisory committee can be recommended for every major study.

Problems of realization

Out of the low incidence of certain diseases (e.g. gliomas) there arises the need for multicenter trials. Thus, as a rule, between twenty and thirty centers participate in cancer studies.

The number of data obtained per patient in a cancer study is usually very large. Thus, in a study of leukemia, which the author supervises, there will be 800 individual data for every patient. Also, due to the low incidence in the cancer field, a long duration of the trial must be envisaged. Accrural times of three years and follow-up phases of two years are common in cancer studies.

Out of this arises a number of organisational problems as well as problems of the quality of the data obtained. Psychological problems are also to be dealt with. The motivation of the physicians involved tends to dropt with the duration of the trial, a decrease in data quality is therefore to be expected. Statistics and data processing assist the head of the group. Thus the computer can print out reminders for overdue patient's sheets to be delivered. Moreover lists can be made reminding the centers to call in the patients at the right time. By programme checking mistakes made as wrong entries in the sheets can be discovered and corrections obtained. Patients not qualifying for participation can also be noted. Furthermore computer made graphs and charts showing the latest stage of the trial have proved useful in motivating the doctors who participate in the study.

Problems of evaluation

In evaluating cancer studies survival time is often at the center of interest. The success of a therapy is measured by the time passing until remission, by the duration of remission and the survival time. Very often the point of interest (e.g. recidive) is not reached by a number of patients by the time the study is evaluated. For these patients informations are not complete. In this case one speaks of censored observations. This type of data requires special methods of evaluation (e.g. life table methods). During evaluation one often discovers that in spite of careful planning confounding factors are unevenly distributed among the groups. In this case there are two possibilities: One is to stratify the data material and conduct the evaluation within the strata. The other, a so-called regression approach, takes the confounding factors into account numerically (e.g. logistic function, Cox model). More efficient, of course, is the elimination of confounding factors at the planning stage, but this, as already mentioned, is not always possible.

Special problems appear when the measured criteria are to be evaluated jointly. Since they are chronologically connected, their combination to a course of the disease and the examination of the effects of the therapy on that course suggest themselves. Problems of this nature require complicated methods of evaluation. The author is at present engaged in an effort to depict the course of various types of cancer by a mathematical model, more precisely by a stochiastic process. The influence of the therapy on the course of the disease can then be quantified by the changes of parameters of the mathematical model.

Summary

Due to the low incidence of the disease and the small differences of effects to be expected in cancer therapy, clinical trials in this field are generally conducted as multi-center studies. Often the influence of confounding factors in these studies is stronger than the effects of different therapies. These two facts lead to particular problems in the planning, realization and evaluation of trials. Statistics and data processing are providing methods for the adequate solution of these problems.

It goes without saying that the problems and solutions discussed in this paper represent only a limited selection of the problems dealt with in practice if a trial is to be conducted in the best possible way.

V Summary of the present state of chemotherapy of the supratentorial gliomas

Special and comparative pathology of the gliomas – experimental findings

If one considers the findings of special and comparative pathology and neuropathology, as well as experimental pathology a whole series of conclusions can be drawn about the special features of central nervous system tumours. Of absolutely basic significance however, particularly against the background of assessing the efficacy of any chemotherapy, is the classification of intrinsic brain tumours and the problems of grading. In neuropathology there are completely controversial opinions which allow one clearly to understand that the WHO classification published in 1979, just as might have been expected, represents a compromise between a large number of partly contradictory views and opinions. For the practical work of the neuropathologists and, indirectly also of the neurosurgeons, the retention of the old cytogenetic concept of tumour classification has not lost its significance; however, the slightest problems still exist here. The problem of grading of tumours and the consequences which arise from that as regards treatment and the assessment of its effectiveness, are really considerable. From one section of neuropathologists it has been suggested with much emphasis that because of the change in grading in the year 1979, it is only with the greatest reservations that actual historical control groups can now be used. A very special problem exists in that very frequently astrocytomas whose assessment of malignancy was based purely on the change in the scale of grading. This has meant that not a few astrocytomas which were earlier in Group II have now been placed in Group III (WHO). This inevitably leads to an apparent improvement in the survival times when they are compared with the period before 1972, which can then be wrongly interpreted, because of the use of historical control groups to assess the outcome of treatment.

Hence, one should accept the recommendation to use corresponding studies of chemotherapy only with contemporaneous control groups. Likewise it was regarded by all participants as most important that there should be a 'tumour reference centre' for neuropathological findings.

From the field of *comparative pathology* there were reports about spontaneous gliomas in animals, where, needless to say any clinical features or even surgical aspects are completely absent. Among most domestic animals brain tumours are certainly quite rare and it is only in the dog, and here predominantly in certain of the brachycephalic species, that one finds a relatively high incidence of gliomas. From a morphological aspect the various gliomas which occur in the dog are quite comparable with human tumours. Further morphological contributions were concerned with the use of immunological techniques, whose practical significance cannot yet be correctly assessed, as this specialised field is still in its developmental stages. Electron microscopic studies are concerned with the processes of cell death in gliomas, which apparently pursue a very typical course.

Another field whose future significance can still not be definitely estimated is that concerned with the *immune reactions* in gliomas and the significance of immunological mechanisms in the growth of these tumours. The observation also seems important that in corresponding investigations on the functional activity of the lymphocytes one can recognise a definite dependence on the stage to tumour growth. It would appear as if this difference in lymphocyte function is induced by the progressive growth of the tumour. Further investigations are dealing with the significance of the "natural killer (NK)-sensitivity".

These investigations took place on a human astrocytoma which had been kept in culture. They have shown that the cells are absolutely different in sensitivity in regard to the NK cells. The findings suggest that the resistant glioma cells are in a position to influence the protein biosynthesis in their surroundings. While no direct relationship to clinical problems is shown here, in the case of impulse cytophotometric investigation a relation of such a kind is quite possible. The well-differentiated gliomas show, as a rule, a pure diploid division of the DNA, but with more marked anaplasia pathological changes are also found in the DNA histograms, particularly in Grade IV tumours. An extension of these investigations is under way, with the possibility of making some pronouncements about the prognosis, even in human gliomas.

From the morphological point of view the occurrence of lymphocytic infiltrate has been observed in intrinsic brain tumours and it might be assumed that in the case of tumours the lymphocytes play a very active role, immunologically. It is shown that the extent of the lymphocytic infiltration even in tumours of similar classification, such as glioblastoma is very different. Even here firm statements relating to the prognosis or ultimately even in relation to the origin of the infiltrate, are still not possible.

Another paper reported on the *biochemical background* of the actions of neurooncogenic and also of chemotherapeutically effective agents. Finally there is a possible approach for the testing of the sensitivity of human tumours to chemotherapeutic agents, by the implantation of such gliomas. With the intracerebral implantation of a tumour cell suspension in mice there has been a success rate of about 50 per cent.

With this tumour model it should be possible to test the efficacy of cytostatics. Here also, further work is necessary in order to establish the clinical relevance of the method.

General and special diagnostic procedures for intrinsic brain tumours

As a result of the introduction of computer tomography the *diagnosis* of intrinsic brain tumours has for some years shown a striking improvement in precision and significance. Apart from information about the size and site of the tumour, opinions on the exact nature of the tumour are possible with a relatively greater chance of success. Their accuracy is estimated between 56 and 70%. By measuring the density of the tumour in Hounsfield units, further supplementary information is available. It is not possible at present to assess definitely what will be the significance in the future of supplementary procedures such as Positron Emission Tomography (PET). Other combined investigations appear to be quite interesting including the additional information provided by regional cerebral blood flow (rCBF), oxygen utilisation and also a report on regional glucose metabolism using the 18-fluorodesoxyglucose technique. From these investigations it is certain that much more information can be expected in the future, especially in relation to the peculiarities of glioma metabolism, about which at present few factors are known. Details are well-known about some of the older investigations by means of the estimation of regional cerebral circulation, such as the fall in regional circulation in the zone of oedema and its reversibility after treatment for the oedema. There were also reports on the influence of craniotomy on the above-mentioned factors.

The methods of *measuring the intracranial pressure* remain in the forefront of surgical care, among which measurement of the intraventricular pressure still yields the best results technically. However, in the case of tumours there are many instances where it cannot be used at all or only with considerable disadvantages, so that here one finds the main indications for epidural pressure measurements.

The indications are, in general, applied as follows. In the presence of obstructive hydrocephalus perhaps associated with tumours at the exit of the third ventricle, the aqueduct or even in the posterior fossa, intraventricular pressure measurements should still be attempted, at the same time considering the possibilities available for the relief of pressure. However if the ventricular system is small or is compressed and displaced, epidural pressure measurement should definitely be preferred. This should only be necessary pre-operatively in severe cases. Postoperatively the course of the pressure yields very useful information and allows one to recognise a rise of intracranial pressure perhaps the result of a severe brain swelling or a secondary haemorrhage, often before the appearance of any abnormal neurological signs. In comparison with the diagnostic procedures already mentioned, the EEG and acoustic and sensory evoked potentials give no useful additional information relating to the possible localisation of a supratentorial glioma. These features are also not influenced by radiotherapy or chemotherapy, but however, Misonidazol which is used as a *radiosensitizer* produces a reduction in the nerve conduction velocity as evidence of a subclinical neuropathy. Of rather more importance in the differential diagnosis is a not uncommon parasitosis of the central nervous system, namely *cysticercosis*. This appears only sporadically in Europe, however in India, Africa and Latin America a considerable morbidity can sometimes be identified. The clinical pictures produced by it can mimic exactly the symptoms of a tumour; however with the introduction of modern diagnostic methods they should present no problem in diagnosis for the expert.

It is generally accepted that the substances CEA (carcino-embryonic antigen) and TPA (tissue polypeptide antigen) act as tissue markers and the evidence for this has been reviewed. They were found in almost a half of the intrinsic brain tumours which were investigated, although actually in lower concentrations. The significance of these findings has been critically considered and so far they do not appear to be of any significance for clinical use.

A further contribution which links up to the possibilities of chemotherapy is concerned with the *in vitro* sensitivity of tumours cells to cytostatics. In this context a raised *in vitro* sensitivity against the particular cytostatic agent in relation to the survival time of the patient from whom the tumour cell cultures originated, also allows a definite conclusion on the *in vivo* sensitivity of the tumour. With further improvement this method could possibly be suitable as a screening test for the use of chemotherapy and for deciding the relevant protocols for treatment.

Fundamentals of operative treatment and radiotherapy

Although the central theme was chemotherapy, a consideration of *operative treatment* and also of *radiotherapy* proved to be necessary as both procedures play a decisive part in the results of the combined forms of treatment and are of significance for the newer aspects of oncology. Thus, the extent and the nature of the *changes produced* in the tumour and the brain tissue *by treatment* are of the greatest significance for the clinician, just as much as for the neuropathologist. While the detailed histological appearance of the actual late radiation damage is quite well-known, it has been shown on the other hand that the radiation-induced delayed necrosis in the tumour and in the surroundings can, as a result of tumour destruction and scar formation mimic a tumour recurrence both clinically and in the CT scan. It appears that the combination of radiotherapy and chemotherapy produces damage to the blood-brain barrier, as corresponding types of reaction such as "disseminated necrotising leuco-encephalopathy" and radiation necrosis, develop apparently more frequently under these conditions.

Among the long-term survivors late complications are found, such as progressive injury to the parenchyma, brain stem atrophy, diffuse gliosis and a communicating internal hydrocephalus, all clinical pictures which for their part also lead to a severe, often progressive damage to the patient. The nature and content of these therapy-induced changes are of the greatest importance for the clinician and particularly for the neurosurgeon.

Meanwhile the refinements of *surgical technique* through the microsurgical procedures has its own significance for glioma surgery. We are aware that for a long time the use of the operating microscope, with the appropriate armamentarium as well as the appropriate technique, in considering the existing tissue structures, can allow operations in regions which previously were fundamentally avoided by the operator.

This applies to the rostral basal ganglia and also to lesions in the vicinity of important centres in the dominant hemisphere.

The variation of the means of access through the sulci in the case of extensive space-occupying lesion and also through the gyri with preservation of the sulci and hence of a significant part of the vascular supply, allows the removal of tumours with, on the whole, definitely reduced risk of severe neurological deficits. It goes without saying that these techniques move away from the concept of "radical extirpation"; we are of course aware that conditions are completely different in the case of gliomas, as compared with carcinomas elsewhere in the body. Basically, in any case, the use of the microsurgical technique can substantially reduce both the extent and the severity of the deficits produced by operation.

The *total strategy* emerges from the report of a large neurosurgical clinic and it can be adapted in a similar manner to the procedures in all neurosurgical centres. Superficially situated tumours after whose total extirpation no serious additional neurological disturbances are to be expected will always be operated on. In the case of deeply situated lesions or those which involve functionally important regions, apart from a sophisticated neuroradiological diagnosis, a stereotaxic biopsy should be attempted before any open operation. Accordingly the entire strategy of treatment can be planned, including the possibilities of a total resection, a partial resection and the supplementary use of interstitial Curie-therapy.

Painstaking attention to preserving the vascular supply is of the greatest significance for the extent of the postoperative neurological disturbances. The fact that the treatment of peritumoral brain oedema is included in the planning of treatment, is summarised once again, against the background of the experimental and neuroradiological findings which have been known for a long time.

One paper was concerned with the problem of *repeat operations in the case of verified recurrences of gliomas,* a situation which unfortunately occurs very frequently. In agreement also with our own experiences the possibility of an operation on the tumour recurrence should be very carefully considered and, if at all possible, a positive decision made. The survival time of these patients can be quite markedly prolonged by one, occasionally even more repeat operations, in the course of which, it goes without saying that the details of the histological findings, the site, the rate of growth and the direction of spread, as well as the general condition of the patient must be taken into account.

The use of the *Ommaya reservoir* to give constant access to the ventricular system or even to other cavities after resection of a tumour, is also interesting from the point of view of intrathecal cytostatic agents. In considering a whole series of factors the complication rate of this procedure has now dropped to under 10%.

An important consideration from the surgical point of view is the fact, known for a long time, that the *operative mortality* defined by the authors reporting here as death within 30 days of the operation, which is 10% in patients under 60 years old, rises sharply to 23% in glioma patients over 60. Such figures with comparable results may well be reported from the majority of neurosurgical clinics. If one considers the present day results of glioma operations using microsurgical procedures it can be demonstrated that the postoperative mortality has very clearly fallen in recent years compared with earlier times but the global survival time has not really been influenced by the improvements in operative technique or by other methods such as intensive care and the methods of neuroanaesthesia.

One solitary paper is dedicated to an otherwise very neglected aspect of tumour treatment, namely neurophysiological investigations, with really interesting results. Thus, it is surprising that at the time of making the diagnosis 95% of all patients are already showing disturbances in the field of intellectual function. A third of the patients who were investigated after operation showed an increase in the involvement of their mental activities. On the other hand in 52.5% of the patients the operative intervention led to a definite improvement in the subjective findings so that there was a definite reduction particularly in the realm of "anxiety", "depression" and "dreaminess". Radiation therapy led to fluctuations in the intellectual efficiency, which because of increased irritability has an adverse effect on the intellectual capabilities. On the other hand, in the group of patients investigated here, (40 patients with gliomas) no organic effects on the brain could be identified as a result of the chemotherapy.

In view of the, in any case, very limited life expectation of glioblastoma patients and the fact verified in many investigations that *postoperative radiation therapy* definitely prolongs the time of survival, it seemed important to consider whether the stay in hospital during the treatment could be shortened. In this way it is suggested that the total tumour dose be limited to 35 Gy and the individual doses be made relatively high (single fractions of 3.5 Gy daily). The results show that the short term radiation with high single fractions with a total target dose limited to 35 Gy, is able to prolong the survival time.

All the papers on the results of radiotherapy show that this form of treatment has a secure place in the therapy of gliomas. That the results from different groups of workers are not identical, is not surprising.

The possibilities of *interstitial Curie-therapy* are explained in detail in one special contribution and its indications and uses are described. Interstitial Curie-therapy should be considered in all cases in which only a partial resection of the tumour was possible and a limited, circumscribed remnant of tumour remains, but it is, however, the only form of treatment in deep seated, but not too large tumours. It is no small advantage of this treatment that the strain of operation and the risks of implantation of the radioactive source are fortunately quite low.

Chemotherapy (fundamental principles, experiences, results, alternative methods)

The principles of chemotherapy in general were described in a series of papers, and particularly its use in intracranial tumours. In the chemotherapy of gliomas the problems of the blood-brain barrier and the lipoid solubility of the substances plays quite a decisive role. All the contributions to this part of the days proceedings strongly emphasized that a *statistically based plan of treatment* was an indispensible requirement, so that as a rule simultaneous control groups in randomised studies are absolutely necessary. On account of the relatively low morbidity, one cannot avoid here undertaking multicentric studies, a circumstance which compels particularly exact and painstaking drafting of the plan of study and the protocols of treatment.

At present the main agents in the chemotherapy of gliomas are the nitroso-urea derivatives (CCNU, BCNU, ACNU etc.) and in addition the use of a radiosensitizer (Misonidazole). Apart from therapy with only one of the nitroso-ureas mentioned studies have also been undertaken with *schemes of combined treatment,* which certainly in dealing with malignant tumours in other sites have definitely shown themselves superior to treatment with a single agent. The results of these various studies leave a general impression which cannot be said to be very hopeful. The EORTC study has already shown that no striking results can be achieved as regards the time of survival and this has been confirmed in a second large study from Scandinavia. Misonidazole has no effect on the survival time, although postoperative radiation clearly has a positive effect. The additional use of CCNU is unable to improve significantly the survival times. The possibility of poly-chemotherapy has been analysed is detail in other studies from Austria. Without wishing to go into endless details, it may be said that in general the results in patients with glioblastomas are bad, but in the case of anaplastic gliomas Grade III a clear improvement in the survival time is seen. The control group consisted of patients who had received only steroid, but no radiotherapy or chemotherapy. Radiation treatment alone and chemotherapy alone significantly lengthened the time of survival and the use of these two measures in addition to operative treatment showed relatively the best results. For instance, although dealing with a smaller number of patients, the value of BCNU on its own after operative treatment and radiotherapy has also been confirmed in further studies, while here a combination with VM 26, to be sure in a study not yet completed, has yielded no certain better results.

Among the newer nitroso-urea derivatives ACNU is particularly interesting. A study of astrocytomas and glioblastomas is reported here, which has been continued for about 3½ years. It is shown here that in a group of glioblastomas radiotherapy after the operation has a definitely positive effect on the survival time, that this effect cannot be improved by monotherapy with ACNU, although at ten percent the number of long-term survivors reaches a fairly high level. Despite this an ACNU effect on the factor "survival time" cannot be verified in the group of glioblastomas. In the case of the malignant astrocytomas who have, after operative treatment, still only life expectations (one year) of just 15% and do not reach the second year, radiation leads to a really significant improvement in the survival quotient with survival times of up to eight years. The 50% survival quota is about two years. An additional monotherapy with ACNU has a statistically very significant effect, with a prolongation of the life expectation to the 50% level of 3½ years. The side-effects of ACNU are, compared with other nitroso-urea derivatives altogether more favourable, in their spectrum and also in their intensity. A further report from the group working in Mainz, who reported on the investigations with ACNU, analysed the long-term surviving glioblastoma patients, the possible therapeutic approach, which can be deduced from these observations against the background of the special features of an oncological out-patient treatment. The great significance of the psychological problems and the avoidance of further admission to hospital by using O.P. oncological care were particularly stressed. Practical experience shows that ambulant oncological treatment in patients with gliomas is eminently possible and finally because of the limited life expectation many of these patients absolutely prefer admission to hospital.

The question, as to whether *pre-operative chemotherapy* and *radiotherapy* is suitable and promising was investigated on a relatively small group of patients and accepted with some reservations. Such a procedure is not however recommended as standard treatment for the majority of patients.

Among the procedures hitherto not adequately investigated, two authors reported on hyperthermia and one of these papers deals specifically with radiohyperthermia for human gliomas. The results here are not impressive. A further very detailed paper describes the possible significance of hyperthermia and hyperglycaemia in the treatment of peripheral malignant tumours, such as carcinomas and sarcomas. This report is also concerned with essentially theoretical considerations and illustrated with examples of a few cases. In conclusion what seemed to us of particular importance is a factual and rational explanation of the structure of a treatment protocol and the carrying out of studies of that kind. Assessed on the explanations of this paper it appears that a not insignificant part of the studies presented are scarcely adequate from a strictly statistical point of view.

The closing discussion between the participants from the various disciplines taking part, proved that further development involved not only the testing of the efficacy of possible new synthetic cytostatics, but a more extensive standardisation of neuropathological nomenclature, the development of methods for *in vitro* testing of tumour tissue sensitivity against particular drugs, apart entirely from the extraordinarily sketchy knowledge of the basic research, where in the coming years neuro-oncology will surely achieve some further progress. If one can for once deliberately ignore the particular details of the individual studies, there is no doubt that the use of cytostatics is able manifestly to improve the life expectancy of the patients with malignant astrocytomas.

In the individual papers the extent of this improvement is described very differently, however it can be noted in the majority of the investigations. The results can certainly not be described as pioneering! The advantages of chemotherapy using several agents as against using a single preparation, which have been absolutely substantiated with other tumours, have certainly not been confirmed so far, in the treatment of malignant gliomas. On balance the result of the very intensive concluding discussion signified for all participants, in spite of all the sceptical feelings, the urgent demand to pursue further the use of chemotherapy as a treatment for gliomas, to analyse it critically and to incorporate in the studies any newly appearing, possibly promising substances. There is at present a certain prospect of success even with the present measures, although hopes still remain essentially modest. Nevertheless, the most unfavourable results appear to be, as always, with the glioblastomas. For all the participants it was quite clear that the results of the studies will be confirmed all the sooner, the greater the number of centres taking part and hence the number of cases included in the studies. For this reason further investigations must be undertaken in the context of national and international multicentre studies.

List of contributors

Ahyai, A., Dr. med., Klinik und Poliklinik für Neurochirurgie, Robert-Koch-Straße 40, D-3400 Göttingen

Aleth, G., Dr. med., Ludwig-Boltzmann-Institut für klinische Neurobiologie, Krankenhaus Wien-Lainz, Wolkersbergenstraße 1, A-1130 Wien

Al-Hami, S., Neurochirurgische Univ.-Klinik, Langenbeckstraße 1, D-6500 Mainz

Ali-Osman, F., Dr. med., Brain Tumor Research Center, Univ. California, San Francisco, Ca 94143, USA

Altmannsberger, M., Dr. med., Allgemeinpathologie der Universität, Robert-Koch-Straße 40, D-3400 Göttingen

Ardenne, M. von, Prof. Dr. h. c. mult, Zeppelinstraße 7, DDR-8051 Dresden

Bamberg, M., Dr. med., Strahlenklinik des Univ.-Klinikums der GHS Essen, Hufelandstraße 55, D-4300 Essen 1

Beaney, R. P., Dr. med., MRC Cyclotron Unit, Hammersmith Hospital, Ducane Road, London W 12 OHS (GB)

Ben Hassel, M., Dr. med., Clinique Neuro-chirurgicale, CHU Pont de Chaillon, F-35000 Rennes

Beuningen, D. van, Priv. Doz. Dr. med., Institut für Strahlenbiologie und Strahlenphysik, Univ.-Klinikum der GHS Essen, Hufelandstraße 55, D-4300 Essen 1

Bilzer, Th., Dr. med., Abt. Allgemeine Pathologie, Inst. f. Tierpathologie, Ludwig-Maximilians-Univ., Veterinärstr. 13, D-8000 München 22

Blech, M., Dr. med., Klinik und Poliklinik für Neurochirurgie, Robert-Koch-Str. 40, D-3400 Göttingen

Bloom, H. J. G., Prof. Dr. med., Royal Marsden Hospital, Dapartment of Radiotherapy and Oncology, Fulham Road, London SW3 6JJ (GB)

Blümel, G., Prof. Dr. med., Institut für experimentelle Chirurgie der TU München, Ismaninger Straße 22, D-8000 München 80

Böker, D.-K., Dr. med., Neurochirurgische Univ.-Klinik, Sigmund-Freud-Straße 25, D-5300 Bonn 1

Bogdahn, U., Dr. med., Brain Tumor Research Center, Univ. California, San Francisco, Ca 94143, USA

Bohl, J., Dr. med., Patholog. Institut der Universität, Abteilung für Neuropathologie, Langenbeckstraße 1, D-6500 Mainz

Brandt, M., Prof. Dr. med., Chirurgische Univ.-Klinik, Lehrstuhl für Neurochirurgie, Jungeblodtplatz 1, D-4400 Münster

Brenner, R., Prof. Dr. med., Neurochirurgische Abteilung, Krankenhaus Rudolfsstiftung, Juchgasse 25, A-1030 Wien

Brock, M., Prof. Dr. med., Neurochirurgische Klinik und Poliklinik, Klinikum Steglitz der FU Berlin, Hindenburgdamm 30, D-1000 Berlin 45

Brooks, D. J., Dr. med., MRC Cyclotron Unit, Hammersmith Hospital, Ducane Road, London W12 OHS (GB)

Bruggmoser, G., Dr. med., Zentrum Radiologie, Abt. Röntgen- und Strahlentherapie, Klinikum der Albert-Ludwigs-Universität, Hugstetter Straße 55, D-7800 Freiburg i. Br.

Budach, V., Dr. med., Strahlenklinik des Univ.-Klinikums der GHS Essen, Hufelandstraße 55, D-4300 Essen 1

Chatel, M., Dr. med., Clinique Neuro-chirurgicale, CHU Pont de Chaillon, F-35000 Rennes

Darcel, F., Dr. med., Clinique Neuro-chirurgicale, CHU-Pont de Chaillon, F-35000 Rennes

Dawson, K. B., Dr. med., University of Cambridge, Department of Anatomy, Downing Street, Cambridge CB2 3DY (GB)

Eggert, H. R., Dr. med., Neurochirurgische Univ.-Klinik, Abt. allgemeine Neurochirurgie, Klinikum der Albert-Ludwigs-Universität, Hugstetter Straße 55, D-7800 Freiburg i. Br.

Ernst, H., Dr. med., Neurochirurgische Klinik und Poliklinik, Klinikum Steglitz der FU Berlin, Hindenburgdamm 30, D-1000 Berlin 45
Falk, W., Dr. med., Strahlenklinik und nuklear-medizinische Abteilung des Stadtkrankenhauses, Postfach 28, D-6050 Offenbach
Fankhauser, R., Prof. Dr. med., Univ. Bern, Institut für Vergleichende Neurologie, Bremgartenstraße 109a, CH-3001 Bern
Ferbert, A., Dr. med., Abteilung Neurologie der RWTH, Goethestraße 27–29, D-5100 Aachen
Flament, H., Dr. med., Ludwig-Boltzmann-Institut für klinische Neurobiologie, Krankenhaus Wien-Lainz, Wolkersbergenstraße 1, A-1130 Wien
Gebhard, L., Dr. med., Inst. für Neuropathologie, Univ.-Klinikum, GHS, Hufelandstraße 55, D-4300 Essen 1
Gilsbach, J., Dr. med., Neurochirurgische Univ.-Klinik, Klinikum der Albert-Ludwigs-Universität, Hugstetter Straße 55, D-7800 Freiburg i. Br.
Glees, J. P., Dr. med., F.Q.C.R. Consultant, The Royal Marsden Hospital, Dept. of Radiotherapy and Oncology, London & Surrey, Fulham Road, London SW3 6JJ (GB)
Glees, P., Prof. Dr. med., Dept. of Anatomy, University of Cambridge, Downing St., Cambridge CB2 3DY (GB)
Goebel, H. H., Prof. Dr. med., Abt. f. Neuropathologie des Patholog. Inst. d. Johannes-Gutenberg-Universität, Langenbeckstraße 1, D-6500 Mainz
Grisold, W., Dr. med., Ludwig-Boltzmann-Institut für klinische Neurobiologie, Krankenhaus Wien-Lainz, Wolkersbergenstraße 1, A-1130 Wien
Gullotta, F., Prof. Dr. med., Lehrstuhl für Neuropathologie der Universität, Domagkstraße 17, D-4400 Münster
Gutjahr, P., Prof. Dr. med., Univ.-Kinderklinik, Johannes-Gutenberg-Universität, Langenbeckstraße 1, D-6500 Mainz
Halama, J., Prof. Dr. med., Strahlenklinik und nuklear-medizinische Abteilung des Stadtkrankenhauses, Postf. 28, 6050 Offenbach a. M.
Halves, E., PD Dr. med., Neurologische Univ.-Klinik und Poliklinik, Kopfklinikum, Josef-Schneider-Straße 11, D-8700 Würzburg
Harders, A., Dr. med., Neurochirurgische Univ.-Klinik, Klinikum der Albert-Ludwigs-Universität, Hugstetter Straße 55, D-7800 Freiburg i. Br.
Hassler, W., Dr. med., Neurochirurg. Univ.-Klinik, Klinikum der Albert-Ludwigs-Universität, Hugstetter Straße 55, D-7800 Freiburg i. Br.
Hatlevoll, R., Dr. med., The Norwegian Radium Hospital, Montebello, Oslo – 3, Norwegen
Heiss, W. D., Prof. Dr. med., Neurologische Klinik, Krankenhaus Merheim, Ostmerheimerstraße 200, D-5000 Köln 91
Herbst, M., Dr. med., Strahlentherapeutische Klinik und Poliklinik der Univ. Erlangen-Nürnberg, Krankenhausstraße 12, D-8520 Erlangen
Herter, T., Dr. med., Chirurgische Univ.-Klinik, Lehrstuhl für Neurochirurgie, Jungeblodtplatz 1, D-4400 Münster
Hildebrand, J., Dr. med., Hôpital Erasme, Neurology, Cliniques Universitaires de Bruxelles, Route de Lennik 808, B-1070 Bruxelles
Hinkelbein, W., Dr. med., Zentrum Radiologie, Abt. Röntgen- und Strahlentherapie, Klinikum der Albert-Ludwigs-Universität, Hugstetter Straße 55, D-7800 Freiburg i. Br.
Holzgraefe, M., Dr. med., Neurolog. Abt. d. Univ. Göttingen, Robert-Koch-Straße 40, D-3400 Göttingen
Hürter, T., Dr. med., Krankenhaus Maria Hilf, Viersenerstraße 450, D-4050 Mönchengladbach
Hüwel, N., Dr. med., Neurochirurgische Universitäts-Klinik, Langenbeckstraße 1, D-6500 Mainz
Ilsen, H. W., Dr. med., Neurologische Klinik, Krankenhaus Merheim, Ostmerheimerstraße 200, D-500 Köln 91
Jaksche, H., Dr. med., Neurochirurgische Univ.-Klinik, D-6650 Homburg/Saar
Jellinger, K., Prof. Dr. med., Ludwig-Boltzmann-Institut für klinische Neurobiologie, Krankenhaus Wien-Lainz, Wolkersbergenstraße 1, A-1130 Wien
Jörg, J., Prof. Dr. med., Neurologische Universitäts-Klinik der GHS Essen, Hufelandstraße 55, D-4300 Essen 1

Kärcher, K. H., Prof. Dr. med., Allgemeines Krankenhaus der Stadt Wien, Universitätsklinik für Strahlentherapie und Strahlenbiologie, Alser Straße 4, A-1090 Wien
Kappos, L., Dr. med., Neurologische Universitäts-Klinik, Josef-Schneider-Straße 11, D-8700 Würzburg
Kargl, W., Dr. med., Neurologische Universitäts-Klinik, Josef-Schneider-Straße 11, D-8700 Würzburg
Kass, W., Dr. med. Universitätsklinikum der Gesamthochschule, Neurologische Klinik und Poliklinik, Hufelandstraße 55, D-4300 Essen
Keim, H., Dr. med., Strahlen- und Physikalisch-Therapeutische Abteilung des Städtischen Krankenhauses, D-8950 Kaufbeuren
Keiper, E., Dipl.-Psych., Neurologische Univ.-Klinik, Josef-Schneider-Straße 11, D-8700 Würzburg
Kessel, G., Dr. med., Neurochirurgische Universitäts-Klinik, Langenbeckstraße 1, D-6500 Mainz
Kirsch, J., Dr. med., Neurochirurgische Univ.-Klinik, Sigmund-Freud-Straße 25, D-5300 Bonn
Kleihues, P., Prof. Dr. med., Pathologisches Institut der Universität, Abteilung f. Neupathologie, Albertstraße 19, 7800 Freiburg.
Klug, W., Dr. med., Universitätsklinikum der Gesamthochschule, Institut für Med. Strahlenphysik und Strahlenbiologie, Hufelandstraße 55, D-4300 Essen
Kogelnik, H. D., Dr. med., Allgemein. Krankenhaus der Stadt Wien, Universitätsklinik für Strahlentherapie und Strahlenbiologie, Alser Straße 4, A-1090 Wien
Krauseneck, P., Prof. Dr. med., Neurologische Univ.-Klinik, Josef-Schneider-Straße 11, D-8700 Würzburg
Kühnert, A., Dipl.-Informatikerin, Institut für medizinische Statistik und Dokumentation, Johannes-Gutenberg-Universität, Langenbeckstraße 1, D-6500 Mainz
Lederer, T., Dr. med., Institut für Experimentelle Chirurgie, Techn. Universität, Ismaninger Straße 22, D-8000 München 80
Leenders, K. L., Dr. med., MRC Cyclotron Unit, Hammersmith Hospital, Ducane Road, London W12 OHS (GB)
Luginbühl, H., Prof. Dr. med., Universität, Institut für Tierpathologie, Länggass-Straße 122, CH-3012 Bern
Mahlmann, E., Dr. med., Neurochirurgische Univ.-Klinik, Langenbeckstraße 1, D-6500 Mainz
Mauersberger, W., Priv.-Doz. Dr. med., Neurochirurgische Univ.-Klinik, Sigmund-Freud-Straße 25, D-5300 Bonn 1
Mennel, H. D., Prof. Dr. med., Pathologisches Institut der Universität, Abteilung f. Neuropathologie, Robert-Koch-Straße 5, D-3550 Marburg
Mertens, H. G., Prof. Dr. med., Neurologische Univ.-Klinik, Josef-Schneider-Straße 11, D-8700 Würzburg
Müller, H., Dr. med., Neurochirurgische Klinik und Poliklinik, Klinikum Steglitz der FU, Hindenburgdamm 30, D-1000 Berlin 45
Mundinger, F., Prof. Dr. med., Abteilung für Stereotaxie und Neuronuklearmedizin, Neurochirurg. Univ.-Klinik, Hugstetter Straße 55, D-7800 Freiburg i. Br.
Nahser, H. C., Dr. med., Neurochirurgische Klinik, Univ.-Klinikum der GHS, Hufelandstraße 55, D-4300 Essen 1
Neiss, A., Prof. Dr., Gesellschaft für angewandte Mathematik und Informatik, Arabellastraße 5, D-8000 München 81
Oehr, P., Dr. med., Institut f. Nuklearmedizin der Universitäts-Klinik Bonn, Sigmund-Freud-Straße 25, D-5300 Bonn 1
Pecker, J., Prof. Dr. med., CHU Pont de Chaillon, F-35000 Rennes
Pegg, A. E., Dr. med., Patholog. Institut der Universität, Ludwig-Aschoff-Haus, Abt. Neuropathologie, Albertstraße 19, D-7800 Freiburg
Poploth, A., Dr. med., Neurolog. Klinik, Universitätsklinikum der GHS Essen, Hufelandstraße 55, D-4300 Essen
Polar Salinas, E., Dr. med., Clinica Delgado, Av. Angamos 490, Miraflores, Lima (Peru)
Potthoff, P. C., Prof. Dr. med., Neurochirurg. Abt. d. Univ. Ulm im Bezirkskrankenhaus, Reisenburger Straße 2, D-8870 Günzburg
Radebold, K., Dr. med., Neurochirurgische Univ.-Klinik, Joseph-Stelzmann-Straße 9, D-5000 Köln 41
Rama, B., Dr. med., Klinik und Poliklinik für Neurochirurgie, Universität Göttingen, Robert-Koch-Straße 40, D-3400 Göttingen

Rebmann, A., Dr. med., Universitätsklinikum der Gesamthochschule, Institut für Med. Strahlenphysik und Strahlenbiologie, Hufelandstraße 55, D-4300 Essen
Richard, K. E., Prof. Dr. med., Neurochirurgische Universitäts-Klinik, D-5000 Köln 41
Richter, E., Dr. med., Neurologische Universitäts-Klinik, Josef-Schneider-Straße 11, D-8700 Würzburg
Roggendorf, W., Dr. med., Neurochirurgische Klinik und Poliklinik, Klinikum Steglitz der FU, Hindenburgdamm 30, D-1000 Berlin 45
Rosenblum, M. L., Dr. med., Brain Tumor Research Center, Univ. California, San Francisco, Ca 94143, USA
Rupniak, H. T. R., Dr. med., Brain Tumor Research Center, Univ. California, San Francisco, Ca 94143, USA
Scarabin, J. M., Dr. med., CHU Pont de Chaillon, F-35000 Rennes
Schandelmaier, C., Dr. med., Neurochirurg. Univ.-Klinik, Hugstetter Straße 55, D-7800 Freiburg
Scheef, W., Dr. med., Robert-Janker-Klinik, Baumschulallee 12, 5300 Bonn 1
Schlechtingen, J., Dr. med., Robert-Janker-Klinik, Baumschulallee 12, D-5300 Bonn 1
Schlie, M., Dr. med., Patholog. Inst. der Universität Mainz, Abteilung f. Neuropathologie, Langenbeckstraße 1, D-6500 Mainz
Schmidt, M., Dr. med., Neurologische Universitäts-Klinik, Josef-Schneider-Straße 11, D-8700 Würzburg
Schwarz, M., Dr. med., Neurochirurgische Universitäts-Klinik, Langenbeckstraße 1, D-6500 Mainz
Seeger, W., Prof. Dr. med., Neurochirurgische Universitäts-Klinik, Klinikum der Albert-Ludwigs-Univ., Hugstetter Straße 55, D-7800 Freiburg i. Br.
Seybold, D., Dr. med., Neurologische Universitäts-Klinik, Josef-Schneider-Straße 11, D-8700 Würzburg
Spaar, F. W., Prof. Dr. med., Neuropathologische Abt., Robert-Koch-Straße 40, D-3400 Göttingen
Spoerri, O., Prof. Dr. med., Klinik und Poliklinik für Neurochirurgie, Robert-Koch-Straße 40, D-3400 Göttingen
Sprich, M., Dr. med., Neurochirurg. Univ.-Klinik, Hugstetter Straße 55, D-7800 Freiburg
Stadler, B., Dr. med., Allg. Krankenhaus der Stadt Wien, Univ.-Klinik für Strahlentherapie und Strahlenbiologie, Alser Straße 4, A-1090 Wien
Stavrou D., Prof. Dr. med., Institut f. Therpathologie der Universität München, Veterinärstraße 13, D-8000 München 22
Stochdorph, O., Prof. Dr. med., Institut f. Neuropathologie, Thalkirchner Straße 36, D-8000 München 2
Streffer, C., Prof. Dr. med., Institut f. Strahlenbiologie und Strahlenphysik, Univ.-Klinikum der GHS, Hufelandstraße 55, D-4300 Essen 1
Szepesi, T., Dr. med., Allgemeines Krankenhaus der Stadt Wien, Universitätsklinik für Strahlentherapie und Strahlenbiologie, Asler Straße 4, A-1090 Wien
Thomas, D. G. T., MECP FRCSE, Senior lecturer, Dept. of Neurological Surgery, The National Hospital, Queen Square, London, WC1E 3BG (GB)
Trappe, A., Dr. med., Institut f. experimentelle Chirurgie der Technischen Universität München, Ismaninger Straße 22, D-8000 München 80
Vandevelde, M., Doz. Dr. med., Universität Bern, Institut für vergleichende Neurologie, Bremgartenstraße 109a, CH-3001 Bern
Volc, D., Dr. med., Ludwig-Boltzmann-Institut für klinische Neurobiologie, Krankenhaus Wien-Lainz, Wolkersbergenstraße 1, A-1130 Wien
Voth, D., Prof. Dr. med., Neurochirurgische Universitäts-Klinik, Langenbeckstraße 1, D-6500 Mainz
Wannenmacher, M., Prof. Dr. Dr. med., Zentrum Radiologie, Abt. Röntgen- und Strahlentherapie, Klinikum der Albert-Ludwigs-Universität, Hugstetter Straße 55, D-7800 Freiburg i. Br.
Weigel, K., Dr. med., Abt. für Stereotaxie und Neuronuklearmedizin, Neurochirurg. Univ.-Klinik, Hugstetter Straße 55, D-7800 Freiburg i. Br.
Weiss, R., Dr. med., Ludwig-Boltzmann-Institut für klinische Neurobiologie, Krankenhaus Wienz-Lainz, Wolkersbergenstraße 1, A-1130 Wien
Wessely, P., Dr. med., Allg. Krankenhaus der Stadt Wien, Univ.-Klinik für Strahlentherapie und Strahlenbiologie, Alser Straße 4, A-1090 Wien
Wiestler, O., Dr. med., Pathologisches Institut der Universität, Abteilung f. Neuropathologie, Albertstraße 19, D-7800 Freiburg

Wilhelm, H., Dr. med., Neurologische Univ.-Klinik der GHS Essen, Hufelandstraße 55, D-4300 Essen 1
Wöber, G., Dr. med., Neurochirurgische Abteilung, Krankenhaus Rudolfsstiftung, Juchgasse 25, A-1030 Wien
Zänker, K. S., Dr. Dr. med., Institut für experimentelle Chirurgie, der Technischen Universität München, Ismaninger Straße 22, D-8000 München 80
Zeile, G., Prof. Dr. med., Abteilung der I. Medizinischen Universitäts-Klinik und Poliklinik, Johannes-Gutenberg-Universtiät Mainz, Langenbeckstraße 1, D-6500 Mainz

Author's index

Subject index

Bei Fragen zur Produktsicherheit wenden Sie sich bitte an:
If you have any questions regarding product safety,
please contact:

Walter de Gruyter GmbH
Genthiner Straße 13
10785 Berlin
productsafety@degruyterbrill.com